# Paediatric
# pocket comp

To my parents, brother and sisters

# Paediatric pocket companion

**Michael D. Harari,** MB, BS, FRACP
Consultant Paediatrician, Department of Paediatrics,
Hadassah University Hospital, Mount Scopus, Jerusalem
Formerly: Clinical Lecturer, University of Cambridge,
Department of Paediatrics, Addenbrooke's Hospital, Cambridge

**Butterworth–Heinemann**
London Boston Singapore Sydney Toronto Wellington

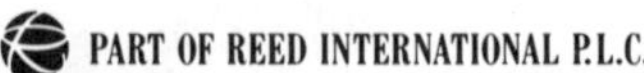

PART OF REED INTERNATIONAL P.L.C.



First published 1991



**British Library Cataloguing in Publication Data**

Harari, Michael D.
Paediatric pocket companion.
1. Paediatrics
I. Title
618.92

ISBN 0-7506-1001-8

**Library of Congress Cataloging-in-Publication Data**

Harari, Michael D.
Paediatric pocket companion/Michael D. Harari.
p. cm.
Includes bibliographical references.
Includes index.
ISBN 0-7506-1001-8
1. Pediatrics–Handbooks, manuals, etc. I. Title.
[DNLM: 1. Pediatrics–handbooks. WS 39 H254p]
RJ48.H346 1991
618.92–dc20
DNLM/DLC 90 16030
for Library of Congress CIP

Composition by Genesis Typesetting, Laser Quay, Rochester, Kent
Printed and bound in Great Britain by Courier International Ltd, Tiptree, Essex

# Foreword

Few Senior House Officers in paediatrics will have had previous postgraduate experience of looking after sick children – yet it is their advice and help which is initially sought when a child is taken to hospital.

This pocket book was written by Dr Harari when he was working as a Senior Registrar/lecturer at Addenbrooke's Hospital in the late eighties. Dr Harari received his paediatric education in the world-famous Children's Hospital at Melbourne and subsequently worked in Papua New Guinea where he found himself responsible for the care of very ill children in primitive conditions without the back-up that a hospital provides in what is called the 'developed world'. He decided to write this book when he realized how dependent British Senior House Officers are on their Registrars for elementary advice on what to do in the anxious period between the arrival of a new patient and the arrival of the Consultant responsible for their care. This is a critical time during which mistakes of omission or commission can be very serious and there is little opportunity for consulting standard text books.

A Senior House Officer will find in this book nearly everything that he or she needs to know in order to deal sensibly with the many and various conditions that lead to a child's being referred to hospital, both what to do and how to do it. It will be of help to General Practitioners, Registrars and to non-paediatricians who may find themselves responsible for the management of paediatric cases. There is room for a House Officer to insert new material or instructions from his or her Registrar and/or Consultant, based on their own experience. Not every Consultant will find him/herself in agreement with everything in the text but the information given is practical, precise and backed up by the relevant references. If its advice is taken, a Senior House Officer will live up to the adage primum non nocere.

John A. Davis
Cambridge, 1990

# Preface

This book originally was conceived as a handbook for Senior House Officers (SHOs) in Paediatrics, at Addenbrooke's Hospital, Cambridge. It was felt that SHOs quite reasonably ask clinical questions that require answers based not just on theory available in textbooks, but that need further moulding to fit clinical situations. The book was written to offer just such a perspective, aimed at the level of what a registrar or SHO would like to know from a senior registrar or consultant clinician about given clinical paediatric problems. It is my hope that doctors working in paediatric departments will find some of that information here, and that medical students who require a clinical orientation to their ward attachments will find the approach of this book to be of some use.

Some issues are given more weight than others. This is not always due to their relative importance or frequency in paediatrics, but may be a reflection of the difficulty in managing the problem, however uncommon, new information that is not yet found in larger textbooks, or occasionally my own familiarity with the topic. The converse applies to issues given scant attention, which also may have been sacrificed in the interests of keeping down the size and price of the book. The book does not attempt to cover any aspect of specialized neonatology except some of the illnesses that are likely to appear after the child has already been discharged from hospital. There are several impressive small books on neonatal care already available in the UK. For the purposes of this book, the word 'neonate' loosely refers to a child under one month of age; 'infant' means a child from one month to one year; 'toddler' from one year to age three or four.

The English language obliges us to use masculine or feminine pronouns in the third person singular when describing people. I felt that consistently using the masculine form was preferable to constructing cumbersome sentences. I apologize to those whom this offends.

Oliver Cromwell, while addressing the Scottish Lords, said: 'I beseech you in the bowels of Christ. Think it possible that you may be mistaken.' I urge all readers to apply that to me when they read the book, and to themselves when they practise its teaching and advice.

M.D.H.

## Note concerning references

Most chapters contain a section on 'Further reading' which offers references aimed at justifying the particular therapeutic philosophy advocated in the chapter, as well as a representation of some divergent views. There are also some references found in the body of the text to support small items of dogma. If a reference justifies a small piece of dogma and in addition contributes to a better overall understanding of the topic, I have placed the author's name and year of publication in the body of the text with the reference itself appearing under the 'Further reading' section. If a topic has no references offered, it is likely that most of the information can be found in standard textbooks.

# Acknowledgements

I wish to acknowledge a debt of gratitude to my teachers and peers at the Royal Children's Hospital, Melbourne, where I underwent all my years of paediatric training, and to the people of the Papua New Guinea highlands and Goroka Base Hospital where as a paediatrician I gained more than I gave. Both places taught me much about what was important in caring for children, and their influence permeates the whole book. Both convinced me of the need for and the possibility of training good general consultant paediatricians in this modern age of expanding knowledge and subspecialization, regardless of the sophistication of the society.

I owe thanks to numerous people in Cambridge, Jerusalem and Melbourne for helping me prepare this book; Helen Hatfield for ongoing encouragement, friendship, secretarial help, and keeping me organized, and Heather Cheesley and Paula Sewell who, with Mrs Hatfield, typed the first draft. Kimberley Walker did all original drawings; Janet Rennie made major contributions to the chapters on neonatal jaundice, cystic fibrosis and cyanotic heart disease, as did Nick Bishop to the article on TPN. Many colleagues at Addenbrooke's read parts of the book and made constructive suggestions. The book owes much to the encouragement of Julia Pearce, along with that of several other dear friends in Cambridge. Simon Rose was a source of consistent inspiration; Arnold Shmerling, Stanley Korman and Lionel Lubitz reviewed much of the final draft. The book's flaws are mine; they have been diminished by the help of all these people.

Professor John Davis has now retired. The book was his idea, and was nourished by his input. It is a very modest addition to his legacy at Addenbrooke's Hospital.

# Contents

Chapter 1

# Emergencies

## 1.1 Cardiopulmonary resuscitation (CPR)

*All emergency information is provided in Table 1.1.*

### GOLDEN RULES

1. Cardiac arrest predominantly occurs secondary to hypoxia or hypovolaemia. Primary myocardial disease is rare.
2. Always address airways and breathing before commencing external cardiac massage (ECM).
3. If cardiac output is not responding to CPR, reconsider the adequacy of airway and breathing support.

### PROCEDURE – THE ABC OF RESUSCITATION

#### A – Airway

Clear it with suction or finger sweep. Pull jaw forwards – infants should be in the 'sniffing position' with a small pillow under the occiput, i.e. neck flexed, head slightly extended. N.B. Extreme hyperextension of the neck will obstruct the airway.

#### B – Breathing

Mouth to mouth (mouth to mouth and nose in infants) expired air resuscitation (EAR) is effective even from inexperienced practitioners. Bag and mask ventilation is not always effective because of the difficulty in securing a seal. Endotracheal intubation is best, but precious minutes may be squandered by an inexperienced person when EAR may be perfectly adequate.

Give $O_2$. If using mouth to mouth EAR the resuscitator can put an oxygen catheter in his own or the patient's mouth to increase inspired $O_2$ concentration in the recipient.

Endotracheal tube (ETT) size – formula for the size in mm is (Age/4) + 4. Use uncuffed tube. Insert tube to the distance specified in Table 1.1.

**Table 1.1 Cardiopulmonary resuscitation (From Shann, F. A. and Duncan, A. (1987) *Drug Doses in Paediatric Intensive Care*, Royal Children's Hospital, Melbourne, with permission)**

| *Age* (yr) | *Birth* | | 1 | 2 | | 3 | | 4 | 5 | 6 | 7 | 8 | 9 | 10 | 11 | | 12 | 13 | yr |
|---|---|---|---|---|---|---|---|---|---|---|---|---|---|---|---|---|---|---|---|
| *Weight* (kg) | 3 | 5 | 10 | | | | | 15 | | 20 | | 25 | | 30 | | 35 | | 40 | kg |
| *Sodium bicarbonate* 8.4%<br>2 ml/kg stat | 6 | 10 | 20 | | 25 | | | 30 | | 40 | | 50 | | 60 | | 70 | | 80 | ml |
| *Sodium bicarbonate* 8.4%<br>1 ml/kg/10 min arrest time | 3 | 5 | 10 | | | | | 15 | | 20 | | 25 | | 30 | | 35 | | 40 | ml |
| *Adrenaline* 1:10 000<br>0.1 ml/kg, repeat if no response | 1 | | 1 | | | | | 1.5 | | 2 | | 2.5 | | 3 | | 3.5 | | 4 | ml |
| *Calcium chloride* 10%<br>0.2 ml/kg (max. 10 ml) | 1 | 1 | 2 | | | | | 3 | | 4 | | 5 | | 6 | | 7 | | 8 | ml |
| *Calcium gluconate* 10%<br>0.5 ml/kg (max. 20 ml) | 2 | 3 | 5 | | | | 7 | | | 10 | | | | 15 | | | | 20 | ml |

| | | | | | | | | | | | | | | |
|---|---|---|---|---|---|---|---|---|---|---|---|---|---|---|
| *Lignocaine* 1% 0.1 ml/kg (1 mg/kg), then 20–40 µg/kg/min | 0.5 | | 1 | | | | 1.5 | 2 | 2.5 | 3 | 3.5 | | 4 | ml |
| *Volume expansion*. Initially 10 ml/kg, repeat ×2–3 if required | 30 | 50 | 100 | | 125 | | 150 | 200 | 250 | 300 | 350 | | 400 | ml |
| *Endotracheal tube* Internal diameter (mm) | 3.0 | 3.5 | 4.0 | 4.5 | | | 5.0 | 5.5 | 6.0 | 6.5 | | 7.0 | | mm |
| *Endotracheal tube (oral)* Length at lip (cm) | 8.5 | | 11 | 12 | | 13 | 14 | 15 | 16 | 17 | | 18 | | cm |
| *Endotracheal tube (nasal)* Length at nose (cm) | 10.5 | | 14 | 15 | | 16 | 17 | 19 | 20 | 21 | | 22 | | cm |
| *Cardioversion*. Atrial arrhythmia 1 J/kg | 3 | 5 | 10 | | | | 15 | 20 | 25 | 30 | 35 | | 40 | J |
| *Cardioversion*. Ventricular arrthymias 5 J/kg | 15 | | 50 | | | | 75 | 100 | 125 | 150 | 175 | | 200 | J |

Watch the motion of chest wall to assess adequacy of ventilation. In prolonged resuscitation insert a nasogastric tube (NGT) to prevent gastric distension which will splint the diaphragm.

## C – Circulation

External cardiac massage ideally requires that the child be on a hard surface.

1. Infant. Encircle the chest with two hands, the fingers meeting at the back. Use the thumbs to compress the heart at a level two-thirds of the way down the sternum. Sternal depression should be 2–3 cm.
2. Infants and toddlers. Place two or three fingers two-thirds of the way down the sternum.
3. Children > 4 years of age. Use the 'heel' of the hand on the lower one-third of the sternum and compress it about 4 cm. The heart should be massaged or squeezed rather than punched. Compression should be regular, uninterrupted and smooth, and should occupy 50% of the cardiac compression cycle. Heart massage to breath ratio should be at 5:1; however, *there should not be a pause in the ECM* each time a breath is given. Recommended rates of ECM and ventilation are shown in Table 1.2.

**Table 1.2 Ventilation–compression ratios and rates in one- and two-person cardiopulmonary resuscitation (From Tibballs, J. (1988) *Aust. Paediatr. J.*, 24, 230, with permission)**

| | *Teenager* | *Child/infant* | *Newborn* |
|---|---|---|---|
| *Two-person resuscitation* | | | |
| Breaths/min | 12 | 20 | 24–30 |
| Compressions/min (ratio 1:5) | 60 | 100 | 120–150 |
| *One-person resuscitation* | | | |
| Breaths/min | 8 | 12 | 16 |
| Compressions/min | 60 | 90 | 120 |

## D – Drugs (see Table 1.3)

### *1 Route*

**1.1 Endotracheal tube** Adrenaline, atropine, lignocaine can be given in conventional doses via the endotracheal tube (the UK Resuscitation Council (1987) recommends using twice the usual dose of adrenaline: *Lancet* (1987) **i**, 1098. Dilute with a volume of normal (0.9%) saline according to body size (newborn 1 ml, infant 3 ml, preschool and school children 5–10 ml). Inject into ETT and disperse with bag ventilation.

**Table 1.3 Algorithm for management of asystole–bradycardia, ventricular fibrillation and electromechanical dissociation (From Tibballs, J. (1988) *Aust. Paediatr. J.*, 24, 230, with permission)**

| *Asystole–bradycardia* | *Ventricular fibrillation* | *Electromechanical dissociation* |
|---|---|---|
| Basic CPR | Basic CPR | Basic CPR |
| ↓ | ↓ | ↓ |
| Intubate, ventilate with $O_2$, IV access | Defibrillate 2–5 J/kg | Intubate, ventilate with $O_2$, IV access |
| ↓ | ↓ | ↓ |
| Adrenaline 0.01 mg/kg IV or ETT | Intubate, ventilate with $O_2$, IV access | Adrenaline 0.01 mg/kg IV or ETT |
| ↓ | ↓ | ↓ |
| Sodium bicarbonate 1 mmol/kg IV | Sodium bicarbonate 1 mmol/kg IV | Sodium bicarbonate 1 mmol/kg IV |
| ↓ | ↓ | ↓ |
| Atropine 20 μg/kg IV or ETT | Defibrillate | Consider repeating adrenaline, bicarbonate (according to blood gases). Exclude hypovolaemia, pneumothorax, pericardial tamponade |
| ↓ | ↓ | |
| Consider repeating adrenaline, sodium bicarbonate (according to blood gases), pacing | Lignocaine 1 mg/kg IV or ETT | |
| | ↓ | |
| | Defibrillate | |
| | ↓ | |
| | Consider repeated sodium bicarbonate, adrenaline, bretylium, lignocaine | |

**1.2 Intravenous** Insert a peripheral IV line as soon as possible. During emergencies, the external jugular vein is the obvious choice for cannulation. A central line is often of use, although insertion by the occasional resuscitationist is not recommended. The internal jugular approach is the safest (see Section 4.5).

**1.3 Intraosseous** See Section 4.6.

**1.4 Intracardiac** Insert a narrow gauge needle vertically through the fourth or fifth interspace immediately to the left of the sternum to avoid lung puncture. Cease massage and ventilation during needling. Blood should be aspirated before injection.

### *2 Asystole*

**2.1 Adrenaline** 0.1 ml/kg of a 1:10 000 solution, i.e. a normal 1:1000 ampoule diluted by a factor of 10 in normal saline (0.01 mg/kg).

**2.2 Sodium bicarbonate** 1 ml of 8.4% = 1 mEq. Initial dose 2 mEq/kg, then 0.5–1 mEq/kg for every 10 min of ongoing arrest. Side effects – hypernatraemia, hyperosmolarity, $CO_2$ retention unless adequate ventilation is established.

**2.3 Atropine** Uses: bradycardia, bradyarrhythmias, 2° and 3° heart-block, asystole. Dose: 0.02 mg/kg. Repeat as necessary.

**2.4 Volume expansion** Useful in most arrests as a treatment of unrecognized hypovolaemia or in anticipation of capillary leak after the arrest. Use 10 ml/kg of normal (0.9%) saline or colloid (Haemaccel, human albumin solution).

### *3 Ventricular tachyarrhythmia/antiarrhythmics*

**3.1 Lignocaine 1%** Used after DC shock. Bolus 0.1 ml/kg (= 1 mg/kg). Repeat ×1 if unsuccessful. Then commence infusion at 20–55 μg/kg/min.

**3.2 Bretylium tosylate** Useful as a second-line antiarrhythmic, after DC shock and lignocaine. Dose: 5–10 mg/kg IV bolus for ventricular fibrillation. Onset of action: up to 15 min. Then try repeating the DC shock, as bretylium may aid conversion. If arrhythmia persists, repeat loading dose every 15 min to a total max. of 30 mg/kg. If responds, dose may be repeated after 2 h and again every 6–8 h IV or IM. Alternatively, commence an infusion at 5–15 μg/kg/min.

**3.3 Bicarbonate** As above.

## E – Electric cardioversion

Used for ventricular fibrillation/tachycardia (VF or VT).

### *1 Size of paddle*

4.5 cm in infants, 8 cm in children, 14 cm in adults.

### *2 Placement of paddles*

**2.1 Anterior – posterior** One paddle over the precordium, the other behind the heart (between the scapulae).

**2.2 Anterior chest wall** One paddle to the right of the sternum, below the clavicle, the other just below and to the left of the left nipple.

### *3 Dose*

For VF or VT, start with a 2–4 J/kg shock (some advocate 5 J/kg). In VT, use synchronized mode, in VF use non-synchronized mode. Atrial arrhythmias respond to 1 J/kg shock. If an arrhythmia is unresponsive to DC shock, consider the possibility of poor contact (insufficient gel) or malposition of paddles.

### Ongoing management

1. Assess all methods of resuscitation continually by observing chest movement, colour, pulses, pupils (i.e. brain perfusion).
2. Check electrolytes, urea, arterial gases, Hb, as soon as possible after commencing resuscitation.
3. Insert NGT and aspirate gastric contents.
4. Obtain a good history from parents/staff about antecedent events, e.g. drug ingestion, accidental or non-accidental injury.

### Note

The American Heart Association (1986) no longer recommends calcium in the treatment of asystole (*J. Am. Med. Ass.* (1986) **255**, 2841–3044). Its use should be restricted to the treatment of hypocalcaemia, hyperkalaemia, and calcium channel blocker toxicity. It may be of use in electromechanical dissociation after exclusion of remediable causes such as hypovolaemia, pneumothorax, haemo/pneumopericardium. Dose: Ca gluconate 10%, 0.5 ml/kg (max. 20 ml); Ca chloride 10%, 0.2 ml/kg (max. 10 ml). *Caution – calcium potentiates digitalis-induced dysrhythmias.*

## Further reading

Tibballs J. (1988) Practical aspects of advanced paediatric cardiopulmonary resuscitation. *Aust. Paediatr. J.*, **24**, 228–234

# 1.2 Emergency management of complete laryngeal obstruction

This contingency will predominantly occur in the context of croup or epiglottitis. The management of an inhaled or ingested foreign body is considered in Chapter 7. In general, one should attempt the procedure with which one is most familiar. For those inexperienced in resuscitation, the following protocol is advised.

*If an experienced paediatric anaesthetist is present.* They will usually use orotracheal intubation, often followed by nasotracheal intubation.

*If they are on their way.* Give '100% oxygen' with bag and mask ventilation.

*If an anaesthetist is unavailable.* Make a single attempt at orotracheal intubation using an ETT (one-half size smaller than usual, i.e. Age/4 + 4 – ½) with an introducer. If not immediately successful, perform a cricothyroid puncture with a 12 G needle, or cricothyroidotomy (Figure 1.1).

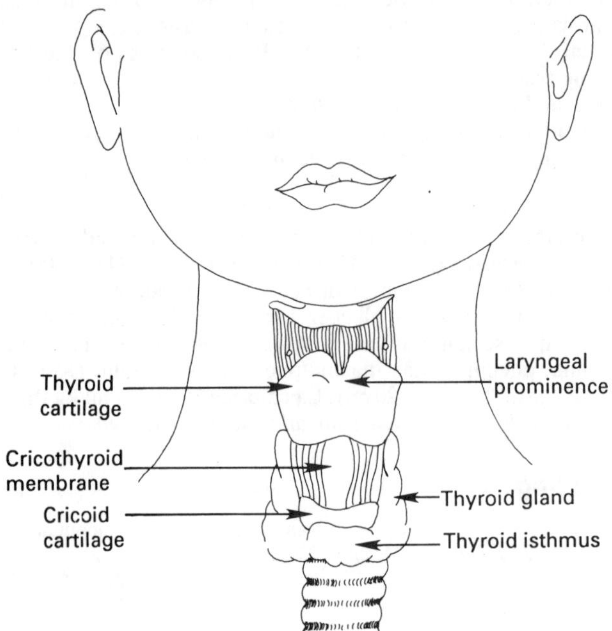


**Figure 1.1** Cricothyroid membrane in relation to laryngeal prominence

## 1.3 Cricothyroidotomy and puncture

In complete upper airway obstruction it is not always possible to intubate the child via the endotracheal route. Cricothyroidotomy or puncture can be done by an inexperienced person and it is safer and quicker than tracheostomy

### CRICOTHYROID PUNCTURE

#### 1 Equipment

Large-bore IV cannula or needle.
Bag and $O_2$ source.

Portex connector – taken from a size 3 mm ETT.
Rolled-up towel or pillow.

**2 Method**

Place towel under shoulders to extend neck.
Keep head scrupulously in midline.
Place left thumb and middle finger on larynx.
Palpate cricothyroid membrane with index finger – see Figure 1.1.
Insert needle or IV cannula through membrane and withdraw stylet.
Connect Portex connector to cannula or needle.
Connect bag and $O_2$ to connector and use rapid ventilation with high-flow $O_2$.

### CRICOTHYROIDOTOMY

**1 Equipment**

Rolled-up towel/pillow.
Curved artery forceps.
Scalpel blade and handle.
Suction equipment.
Small endotracheal tube: 2.5 mm for <5 yr; 3.0 mm for >5 yr.
Anaesthetic bag with compatible fitting for ETT.
$O_2$ source with tubing compatible with bag.

**2 Method**

*The thyroid isthmus is a very vascular structure* – great care must be taken when stabbing the cricothyroid membrane with the scalpel. Place rolled-up towel under shoulders to keep neck extended. Keep head scrupulously in midline. Hold larynx with thumb and middle finger. Palpate cricothyroid membrane with index finger – see Figure 1.1. Make 2–3 cm vertical incision through the skin (it makes it easier to remain in the midline than if a horizontal incision is used). Stab cricothyroid membrane with scalpel blade, sharp side up. Dilate the opening with artery forceps. Insert ETT through the gap between the open blades of the forceps. Connect to the bag and $O_2$.

## 1.4 Burns: major and minor

### 1.4.1 Severe burns

Rapid appraisal by a plastic surgeon, rapid insertion of a short large-bore IV catheter and early skin cover are important in preventing shock and infection, and minimizing cosmetic and functional damage.

## EVALUATION OF THE PATIENT

*1 Remove all clothing*

*2 Weigh the child*

*3 Check vital signs*

*4 Assess the burn*

**4.1 Surface area (SA)** (see Figure 1.2) Degree of shock corresponds to the SA burnt. The younger the child, the greater the likelihood of shock. Burns >10% of body SA require admission and insertion of IV line, if necessary through burnt tissue. For extensive burns, early placement of a central venous catheter (CVC) is helpful.

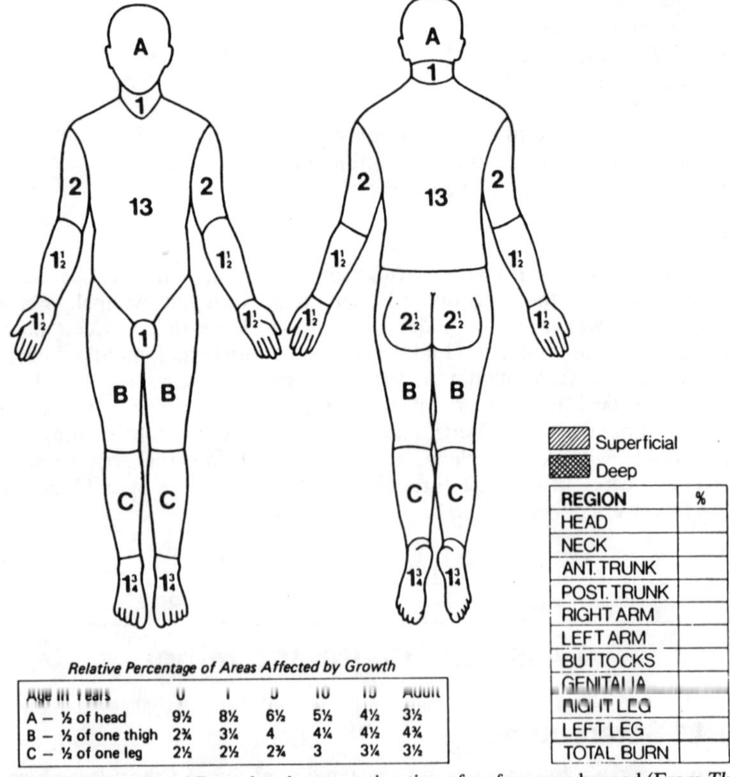


*Relative Percentage of Areas Affected by Growth*

| Age in Years | 0 | 1 | 5 | 10 | 15 | Adult |
|---|---|---|---|---|---|---|
| A – ½ of head | 9½ | 8½ | 6½ | 5½ | 4½ | 3½ |
| B – ½ of one thigh | 2¾ | 3¼ | 4 | 4¼ | 4½ | 4¾ |
| C – ½ of one leg | 2½ | 2½ | 2¾ | 3 | 3¼ | 3½ |

| REGION | % |
|---|---|
| HEAD | |
| NECK | |
| ANT. TRUNK | |
| POST. TRUNK | |
| RIGHT ARM | |
| LEFT ARM | |
| BUTTOCKS | |
| GENITALIA | |
| RIGHT LEG | |
| LEFT LEG | |
| TOTAL BURN | |

**Figure 1.2** Lund and Browder charts – estimation of surface area burned (From *The Paediatric Handbook* (1989) Royal Children's Hospital, Melbourne, with permission)

**4.2 Depth** Partial thickness: painful, erythematous, moist, blisters. Full thickness: painless, dry, whitish or charred.

**4.3 Circumferential burns** Check distal blood flow.

**4.4 Respiratory burns** Explosions or heat injury in a confined space. Preliminary evidence of a respiratory burn includes oropharyngeal burns, stridor, tachypnoea, cyanosis.

## MANAGEMENT

### *1 Insert large-bore IV or CVC*

Send blood for cross-match, FBC, U+E. If unable to secure venous access, intraosseus fluid may be given (see Section 4.6).

### *2 Fluids and electrolytes*

Burns >10% of body SA require IV fluids. A CVC with pressure transducer may be required in anticipation of impending major fluid shift.

**2.1 Fluid volume needed**

1. Expected losses: 3 ml/kg/% body SA involved for the first day.
2. Maintenance fluids: 100 ml/kg/day 1st 10 kg<br>50 ml/kg/day 2nd 10 kg<br>25 ml/kg/day thereafter
3. Rate of infusion:<br>First 8 h after the burn – one-half expected losses + one-third maintenance.<br>Second 8 h – one-quarter expected losses + one-third maintenance.<br>Third 8 h – one-quarter expected losses + one-third maintenance.<br>Second 24 h – one-half previous day's expected losses + maintenance.<br>Third 24 h – normal maintenance.

These are only suggested guidelines. After the initial resuscitation, one should tailor IV fluids to urine output (increase input if urine output <1 ml/kg/h) or central venous pressure (CVP).

**2.2 Type of fluid** Half of the replacement fluid should be human albumin solution. The rest should be normal saline. Hartmann's solution or 0.45% NaCl + 2.5% dextrose. It is uncommon to need blood transfusion within the first 18 h.

**2.3 Electrolytes** Urine $K^+$ losses may be enormous because of the large adrenal response to the stress. However, massive cell lysis and the possibility of compromised renal function should make one cautious about giving $K^+$ routinely in IV fluids.

### *3 Urine output*

Probably the best indicator of intravascular volume apart from CVP. Aim for urine output of >1 ml/kg/h.

**3.1 Insert indwelling urinary catheter** Do not give diuretics. With rare exceptions, poor urine output means that the child is hypovolaemic and requires more volume replacement.

### 4 Analgesia

Morphine 0.1 mg/kg IV (*do not give it IM*). Repeat as necessary or commence infusion at 10–50 µg/kg/h (i.e. 0.5 mg/kg in 50 ml 5% dextrose at 1–5 ml/h). Give bolus doses (0.1 mg/kg if not on infusion, otherwise 0.05 mg/kg) to cover any distressing procedures, or use ketamine (see Section 4.4).

### 5 Tetanus toxoid

0.5 ml IM if no booster given in the past 5 years. Otherwise see Chapter 6.

### 6 Topical care

Apply silver sulphadiazine over entire burn area. Rare side effects are sulphonamide sensitivity (rash) and leucopenia (reversible). Wounds may be nursed open (face, genitalia, chest) or closed.

### 7 Surgery

Fasciotomies are performed on circumferential burns if there is possible circulatory occlusion. Early debridement and escharotomies are commonly done. The main goal of treatment is that the burned area should be covered with skin as soon as possible.

### 8 Respiratory management

Facial burns may require early intubation or insertion of tracheostomy in anticipation of worsening facial oedema. Rapid sequence intubation is used for emergency situations (see Section 1.6). For progressive stridor, an inhalational anaesthetic should be used with an ENT surgeon standing by should tracheostomy be necessary (see Section 7.7). Inhalational burns will usually only affect the upper airway (steam affects lower as well and is a notable exception); however, severe chemical injury to the lungs can occur when the toxic products of combustion are inhaled. If a child requires an inspired $O_2$ concentration of >50%, then elective intubation and positive end expiratory pressure should be considered. Prophylactic antibiotics should not be given for chemical pneumonitis.

The possibility of carbon monoxide or cyanide poisoning should be considered if the fire occurred in a confined space. If so, measure carboxyhaemoglobin and thiocyanate levels and give 100% $O_2$ via face mask (see Section 5.2).

### 9 Antibiotics

Generally they should not be used prophylactically, but the choice must remain that of the plastic surgeon responsible for the child. If used, penicillin is the drug of choice.

*10 Nutrition*

Gastric dilatation and vomiting may occur. Most children will tolerate small volumes of liquids within 8 h of the burn. Aim to have full enteral nutrition by 2–3 days. Tube feeding with high-caloric feeds may be necessary; however, if it is initially not well tolerated, use TPN.

### 1.4.2 Superficial burns

Superficial burns of less than 10% of the body can be managed with outpatient treatment unless they are on the face, neck, hands, feet or perineum. Infants under 12 months often need admission.

MANAGEMENT

*1 Debride*

Cleansing of wound

*2 Non-stick dressing*

Several layers of Jelonet or tulle gras (for clean wound, otherwise use Bactigras) followed by an absorbent dressing (e.g. gauze).

*3 Immobilize*

*4 Follow-up*

Leave the Jelonet dressing untouched for 7–10 days. The outer absorbent dressing may be changed sooner. Burns treated in outpatients usually heal within 3 weeks, but if the unhealed area is >3 cm diameter, refer the child to a surgeon for skin grafting.

Pain, fever and very offensive dressings suggest infection. The dressings may need more frequent changing and antibiotics should be considered.

### Further reading

Solomon, J. R. (1986) Burns. In *Clinical Paediatric Surgery* (eds Jones, P. G. and Woodward, A.) Blackwell Scientific Publications, Melbourne

## 1.5 Anaphylaxis

The rapid onset of at least one of:

1. Angio-oedema – laryngeal, pharyngeal, glossal oedema. Can cause severe upper airway obstruction.
2. Bronchospasm.
3. Hypotension – also tachycardia.

Urticaria is a frequent accompaniment.

## IMMEDIATE TREATMENT

### *1 Adrenaline*

1:10 000 (i.e. 1:1000 ampoule diluted 10-fold) 0.1 ml/kg IV – repeat p.r.n. If IV access cannot be secured, give 0.01 ml/kg of undiluted 1:1000 adrenaline subcutaneously.

### *2 Colloid*

Use 10 ml/kg of human albumin solution or Haemaccel (if no colloid available, use normal saline) for hypotension. May be repeated.

### *3 Treat bronchospasm*

**3.1 Salbutamol** Nebulize with $O_2$.

**3.2 Aminophylline** 5 mg/kg IV over 10 min, then 1 mg/kg/h infusion.

**3.3 IV adrenaline infusion** at 0.2–1.0 μg/kg/min. Put 0.6 mg/kg adrenaline in 50 ml of 5% dextrose. 1 ml/h = 0.2 μg/kg/min.

### *4 Upper airway obstruction*

**4.1 Mask** $O_2$.

**4.2 Nebulized adrenaline** with $O_2$:

Racemic adrenaline 2.25%, 0.5 ml/kg/dose made up to 2 ml, *or*
Adrenaline 1:1000 (0.1%), 0.25–0.5 ml/kg/dose – max. 5 ml.
Rarely, endotracheal intubation is needed.

### *5 Hydrocortisone 10 mg/kg IV*

Later onset of action.

### *6 Antihistamines*

Of little value acutely. Most useful for urticaria.

## AETIOLOGY

It is a life-threatening allergic reaction caused by immunoglobulin E (IgE) triggered release of vasoactive amines from mast cells, and activated complement.

The most common causes in children are: allergy extracts – used in desensitization or skin testing; foods; insect stings; antibiotics and other drugs.

# 1.6 Emergency endotracheal intubation

Those inexperienced in endotracheal intubation should realize that good oxygenation and ventilation can usually be achieved with bag and mask ventilation until help arrives. If ventilation is nevertheless inadequate or if the child cannot protect his airway because of decreased conscious state, endotracheal intubation may be necessary.

## INDICATIONS

An anaesthetist is unavailable *and* the child has respiratory or cardiorespiratory failure or is unable to protect his airway.

## METHOD

Always assume that the child has a full stomach – use cricoid pressure. It is best to use no anaesthetic at all if the child is unconscious (e.g. under conditions of CPR or severe head injury). If the child is still conscious, use rapid sequence intubation ('crash induction').

## METHOD OF RAPID SEQUENCE INTUBATION

### *1 Prepare all equipment*

(a) Yankaeur suction catheter – check that the suction works.
(b) $O_2$ – check amount left in cylinders.
(c) Bag and mask – check the fittings.
(d) Laryngoscope – check the light and battery. Have a spare available.
(e) Suitable ETT – size = Age/4 + 4. Have ETT half a size bigger and smaller as well. An introducer should be inserted into the ETT.
(f) Magill's forceps.
(g) Suxamethonium 1 mg/kg – drawn up.
(h) Atropine 0.02 mg/kg – drawn up in syringe with suxamethonium.
(i) Pancuronium 0.1 mg/kg.
(j) Nasogastric tube (NGT).
(k) ?Fentanyl 10 μg/kg.
(l) Linen tie.
(m) Check anticipated distance of ETT insertion (see Table 1.1).

### *2 Method*

Pass the NGT if child is conscious and alert. Aspirate stomach.
Preoxygenate with 100% $O_2$ – use 'anaesthetic' bag and mask. Continue for 10 min, circumstances permitting.
Cricoid pressure – maintain until ETT and NGT are in position.

Rapid IV injection of suxamethonium, atropine (± fentanyl or thiopentone first, but these may drop BP and, for an inexperienced doctor, may complicate a tense situation). After a period of twitching, full relaxation is achieved which allows ready intubation.
Insert orotracheal tube to the predicted distance (see Table 3.1).
Look at the chest movement, auscultate both lungs, and assess colour to verify correct insertion of ETT.
Secure ETT with linen tie and tape.
At the first sign of movment in the child, administer pancuronium.
In the event of head injury or encephalopathy, a neurological assessment should first be carried out.

### *Contraindications to suxamethonium (succinylcholine)*

Burns, major trauma with severe muscle injury, denervated muscle, spinal cord transection all may cause severe hyperkalaemia after suxamethonium administration. If it nevertheless must be given, pretreatment with a small dose of non-depolarizing blocker (e.g. pancuronium 0.02 mg/kg) may prevent this phenomenon.

Chapter 2

# Drugs

## 2.1 Drug doses

- *Verify all uncommonly used drugs from other sources before use.*

In this collection of drug doses and schedules, the notation 6 h or /6 h means six hourly or every six hours.

**Acetazolamide**. 3–7.5 mg/kg/8 h oral for glaucoma, epilepsy or mountain sickness prophylaxis. Max. 1.0 g/day.
**Acetylcysteine**. 200 mg/ml. Meconium ileus equivalent: 2.5 ml/6–8 h oral. Dilute with soft drink. Paracetamol poisoning (?use oral methionine instead): 150 mg/kg IV over 15 min, then 50 mg/kg over 5 h, then 100 mg/kg over 16 h (see Table 5.3, Section 5.5). For cystic fibrosis, 2 ml 20% soln by inhalation.
**ACTH**. Infantile spasms: 150 u/m$^2$ IM daily. In infants this is usually 40 u IM. Adjust dose to response. Decrease over 4 weeks. Synacthen test: tetracosactin (long acting) 250 μg × 1 for short test, or 0.5 mg IM/12 h × 4 days for long test.
**Acyclovir.** Herpes simplex: 5 mg/kg/8 h IV over 1 h. Oral 100 mg/4–6 h in <2 yr, 200 mg/4–6 h if >2 yr. Encephalitis: 10 mg/kg/8 h IV over 1 h. Herpes zoster: 10 mg/kg *or* 500 mg/m$^2$/8 h IV over 1 h × 7 days. Zoster prophylaxis in immunosuppressed children: 0–5 yr 200 mg/6 h oral for 21 days. 6–10 yr 400 mg/6 h, >10 yr 800 mg/6 h.
**Adrenaline**. Cardiac arrest + anaphylaxis: 0.1 ml/kg of 1:10 000 (= 10 μg/kg) IV or via ETT. Repeat p.r.n. Croup: 0.25 ml/kg/dose of 1:1000 (max. 5 ml) by inhalation *or* racemic adrenaline 2.25% 0.05 ml/kg/dose by inhalation.
**Albumin**. See Human Albumin Solution.
**Alcuronium**. 5 mg/ml 0.25 mg/kg IV over 1 min, then 0.05 mg dose. Incompatible with bicarbonate, thiopentone.
**Allopurinol**. 3–4 mg/kg/8 h oral (10 mg/kg/day). Adult dose 600 mg/day. N.B. Lower dose of 6-mercaptopurine (MP) by 25% if used concurrently.
**Aluminium hydroxide**. Gel: 400 mg in 10 ml. For phosphate binding. 0.1 ml/kg/8 h. Maintain serum phosphate below 1.8 mmol/litre.

**Amikacin**. 7.5 mg/kg/12 h (daily in first week of life preterm). Max. 500 mg/dose. Incompat. heparin.
**Aminocaproic acid (EACA)**. Prophylaxis: 70–100 mg/kg/6 h. Treatment: 100 mg/kg, then 30 mg/kg/h oral or IV until bleeding stops, then as for prophylaxis.
**Aminophylline**. Asthma: 5–6 mg/kg IV over 20 min. Then 1 mg/kg/h as infusion (max. 50 mg/h) or 5 mg/kg/6 h (max. 250 mg) over 15 min. Omit loading dose if patient has already received oral theophylline. In severe asthma administer $O_2$ concurrently. Theophylline level 55–110 µmol/litre (× 0.18 = µg/ml). 1 mg aminophylline = 0.8 mg theophylline.
**Amiodarone**. 5 mg/kg IV over 1 h, then 5–15 µg/kg/min. Oral 4 mg/kg/8 h for 1 week, then /12 h for 1 week, then daily. Level 0.5–2.5 µg/ml. N.B. Very long half-life. Reduce dose of digoxin and warfarin. Monitor thyroid, liver, lung and eye function.
**Amitriptyline**. Tab. 10, 25 mg. Enuresis: 25–50 mg nocte. Cease after 1 month if ineffective.
**Amoxycillin**. Syr. 125 mg or 250 mg/5 ml; cap. 250, 500 mg. 10–20 mg/kg/8 h IV, IM, oral. Severe infection: 50 mg/kg/6 h. Max. 4 g/day.
**Amphotericin B**. Mouth infection: <1 yr, 100 mg suspension/6 h, retained in mouth; >1 yr, 10 mg lozenge sucked slowly. Gut: oral 100–200 mg 6 h after meals. Systemic infection: test dose 1 mg in 20 ml 5% dextrose over 1 h. Then 0.25 mg/kg/day, infuse over 6 h. Increase gradually to max. 1 mg/kg day. Protect from light.
**Ampicillin**. Normally 15–25 mg/kg/6 h IV, IM, oral. Severe infection: 50 mg/kg/4 h (/12 h, 1st week of life; /6 h for age 2–4 weeks). Max. 10 g/day.
**Ascorbic acid**. Scurvy: 100 mg/8–12 h × 10 days oral. Urine acidification (see Section 5.1): 25 mg/kg/6 h.
**Aspirin**. Avoid using as an antipyretic/analgesic. The exceptions are – anti-inflammatory: 20–30 mg/kg/6 h × 3 days, then 30 mg/kg/12 h. Salicylate level: 1.0–2.0 mmol/litre (× 13.8 = mg/100 ml). Antiplatelet: 3–5 mg/kg/day.
**Atenolol**. IV 0.05 mg/kg/5 min till response (max. 0.2 mg/kg). Oral 1–2 mg/kg/12–24 h.
**Atracurium**. 0.5 mg/kg, then 5–10 µg/kg/min infusion.
**Atropine**. Premedication: 0.02 mg/kg IV or IM (max. 0.6 mg). Also used with suxamethonium for depolarizing neuromuscular blockade and with neostigmine for reversal of non-depolarizing blockade.
**Atrovent**. See Ipratroprium.
**Augmentin**. See Clavulanic acid.
**Azlocillin**. 25–50 mg/kg/8 h.
**Aztreonam**. 30 mg/kg/dose 12 h (neonates), 8 h (1–4 weeks), 6 h (>1 month) IV.

**Baclofen**. 5 mg/day. Inc. by 5 mg every 3 days. <5 yr max. 30 mg/day, 6–8 yr max. 40 mg/day, >8 yr max. 60 mg/day.
**Beclomethasone**. Neb. soln 50 µg/ml 1–2 ml/6–12 h. Metered aerosol:

50 μg or 250 μg/puff. 100–500 μg/6–12 h. Rotacap (if <8 years): 100, 200 μg/cap., 100–500 μg/6–12 h.
**Bendrofluazide**. 2.5, 5 mg. <12 months: 1.25 mg, 1–4 yr: 2.5 mg, >4 yr: 2.5–5 mg daily. Give $K^+$ supplements.
**Benorylate**. In juvenile chronic arthritis (JCA). Tab. 750 mg. Susp. 2 g/5 ml, 50–100 mg/kg/12 h. Take with or after meals. N.B. Adjust dose to salicylate level – see Aspirin.
**Benztropine**. 0.02 mg/kg IM, IV. Repeat 15 minutely p.r.n.
**Benzyl penicillin**. See Penicillin G.
**Bicarbonate**. Neonates: mmol deficit = B. excess × Wt/2 IV. Older: B. excess × Wt/3. *Give half the calculated amount.*
**Blood transfusion**. Packed cells: Volume (ml) = (Desired Hb − Current Hb) × Wt (kg) × 3 *or* 10 ml/kg raises Hb 3 g%. Whole blood: Volume = (Desired Hb − Current Hb) × Wt × 6.
**Bretylium**. 5–10 mg/kg IV over 15 min, then 5–15 μg/kg/min infusion or repeat loading dose every 15 min till max. 30 mg/kg, then again after 2 h and again 6 hourly thereafter.

**Calcium**. Daily requirements 1 mmol/kg.
**Calcium chloride**. 10% (0.7 mmol/ml Ca) 0.2 ml/kg slow IV. Daily req. 2 ml/kg. Very corrosive if extravasates.
**Calcium gluconate**. 10% (0.22 mmol/ml Ca) 0.5 ml/kg slow IV. Daily req. 5 ml/kg. Inotropic infusion 0.1–0.4 ml/kg/h.
**Calcium resonium**. See Resonium.
**Captopril**. 0.3 mg/kg increasing slowly to 1.0 mg/kg/8 h oral.
**Carbamazepine**. 2 mg/kg/8 h increasing over 2 weeks to 10 mg/kg/8 h. Max. 1.2 g/day. Initially causes profound sedation. Level 20–50 μmol/litre (×0.24 = μg/ml), not a good indicator of anticonvulsant effect.
**Cefaclor** (Ceclor). 10–15 mg/kg/8 h oral. Max. 2 g/day.
**Cefamandole**. Severe infection: 40 mg/kg/6 h IV. Usually 25 mg/kg/8 h IV.
**Cefazolin** (Kefzol). 10–35 mg/kg/8 h IV. Max. 6 g/day.
**Cefotaxime**. 30–50 mg/kg/6 h IV (1st week of life 50 mg/kg/8 h).
**Ceftazidime**. 30–50 mg/kg/6–8 h IV, IM.
**Ceftriaxone**. Severe infection 100 mg/kg once daily IV or IM (inject with 1% lignocaine). Normally 60 mg/kg/24 h.
**Cefuroxime**. 35 mg/kg/8 h IV, IM. Max. 9 g/day.
**Cephalexin**. 10–15 mg/kg/6 h oral.
**Cephalothin**. 20 mg/kg/6 h IV, IM.
**Charcoal**. 0.5–1.0 g/kg oral or NGT. May repeat hourly with 0.25 g/kg.
**Chloral hydrate**. 50 mg/kg (max. 1.0 g) oral for sedation or premedication.
**Chloramphenicol**. 40 mg/kg stat, then 25 mg/kg/6 h (9+ weeks) or 8 h (5–9 weeks). IV, IM, oral. Max. 4 g/day. Avoid using in neonates. Level 20–30 mg/litre peak, <15 mg/litre trough. Interacts with phenytoin, phenobarbitone, rifampicin. See Section 8.3.
**Chloroquine base**. Treatment: 10 mg/kg/day × 3 days *or* 4 mg/kg/8 h IM. Change to oral as soon as possible. Prophylaxis: 5 mg/kg/dose oral once a week. Chloroquine phosphate 250 mg = 150 mg base. Chloroquine

sulphate 200 mg = 150 mg base. Syr. 50 mg base/5 ml. Inj. 200 mg base/5 ml.
**Chlorothiazide**. 10 mg/kg/12–24 h oral (adult 0.5–2 g/day).
**Chlorpheniramine**. Oral: 0.1 mg/kg/8 h (adult 8–10 mg/day). Subcutaneous (SC) or IV: 0.25 mg/kg (max. 10 mg) × 1.
**Chlorpromazine**. 0.5–1.0 mg/kg slow IV, IM, oral, for sedation, antipyretic, antinausea. Max. 2 mg/kg/24 h. For extrapyramidal side effects (S/E) give benztropine.
**Cimetidine**. 5–10 mg/kg/6 h IV, oral. Admin. IV soln over 30 min. Max. 200 mg/dose. Binds microsomal cytochrome $P_{450}$, and may potentiate phenytoin, theophylline, warfarin.
**Ciprofloxacin**. 5–10 mg/kg/12 h IV, oral.
**Clavulanic acid** – with amoxycillin or ticarcillin. Use normal antibiotic dose.
**Clonazepam**. Status epilepticus: neonates 0.25 mg; children 0.5 mg; adults 1 mg (25–40 μg/kg/dose) IV. Oral 0.01 mg/kg/8 h. Avoid long-term use.
**Clonidine**. 5 μg/kg IV over 5 min. Oral 1–4 μg/kg/8 h. Migraine: 0.5 μg/kg/12 h oral.
**Cloxacillin**. 25–50 mg/kg/6 h oral, IV.
**Codeine phosphate**. Analgesic: 0.5 mg/kg/4 h oral. Antitussive: 0.25 mg/kg/6 h.
**Cortisone acetate**. 0.2 mg/kg/6 h or 20–25 mg/m$^2$/day (physiological).
**Cotrimoxazole** – doses are given as trimethoprim : sulphamethoxazone. Amp. 16:80 mg/ml. Mixt. 8:40/ml. Tab. 80:400 mg or 160:800 (forte). Dose: 4:20 mg/kg/12 h oral, IV over 1 h. Pneumocystis: 5–10:25–50 mg/kg/6 h oral, IV.
**Cromoglycate** – see Sodium cromoglycate.
**Cyproheptadine**. 0.1 mg/kg/8 h oral. Usual dose: 2–6 yr, 2 mg/8 h; >6 yr, 4 mg/8 h. Uses: migraine prophylaxis, antipruritic, appetite stimulant.

**DDAVP (desmopressin)**. 5–10 μg/12–24 h (0.05–0.10 ml) intranasal for diabetes insipidus. For mild–mod. FVIII deficiency or von Willebrand's disease, use 0.03 μg/kg IV over 1 h/12–24 h.
**Desferrioxamine**. Iron poisoning: 10–15 mg/kg/h IV (max. 80 mg/kg/24 h), or 40 mg/kg/6 h IM. Thalassaemia: 500 mg per unit of blood. 1–3 g/5 ml SC overnight, 5–6 nights/wk.
**Dexamethasone**. 0.1 mg/kg IV, IM stat, then 0.05 mg/kg/6 h IV, oral.
**Dextrose**. Neonates require 8–12 mg/kg/min. Hyperkalaemia – see Section 5.7.
**Diazepam** – procedures, premedication, convulsions: 0.2 mg/kg IV, oral, rectal, *not IM*. Repeat as necessary. Suppos. and rectal soln 5 mg, 10 mg. N.B. Respiratory depression, especially with barbiturates and other sedatives.
**Dicyclomine**. 0.5 mg/kg/dose 15 min before meals. Up to ×4/day (max. 15 mg/kg/dose). Apnoea has been reported in children <6 months.
**Digoxin**. 5 μg/kg/12 h oral. Elix. 50 μg/ml, tab. 125, 250 μg, inj. 500 μg/2 ml. Level 0.4–2.0 ng/ml (×1.28 = nmol/litre). Rapid digitaliz-

ation (rarely indicated) is with loading dose 15 μg/kg followed by 5 μg/kg after 6 h oral or slow IV.

**Dihydrocodeine**. Not recommended <7 years. 0.5 mg/kg/6–8 h p.r.n. oral, IM.

**Dimercaprol** (BAL). Heavy metal poisoning: 3 mg/kg/3 h IM for 2 days, then 6 h for 2 days, then 12 h for 6 days.

**Diphenhydramine**. 1.25 mg/kg/6 h oral, IV, IM. For antihistamine, anaphylaxis or sedation.

**Dobutamine**. As per Dopamine (see below).

**Docusate sodium** (dioctyl sodium sulphosuccinate). Syr. 12.5 mg/5 ml. Tab. 100 mg, 4 weeks–12 months: 12.5 mg t.d.s. 1–4 yr: 12.5–25 mg t.d.s. >4 yr: 25–50 mg t.d.s.

**Dopamine**. Inotropic dose: 5–15 μg/kg/min. Renal dose: 2 μg/kg/min. If one puts 15 mg/kg in 50 ml 5% dextrose, then 1 ml/h = 5 μg/kg/min.

**Edrophonium** (Tensilon). Draw up 100 μg/kg. Give one-fifth of it IV. If tolerated, give the rest. For myaesthenia gravis test.

**Enalapril**. 0.2–1.0 mg/kg daily. Start with lower dose first. Adult usual maintenance dose 10–20 mg daily, max. 40 mg.

**Erythromycin**. 8–15 mg/kg/6 h oral or slow IV.

**Ethambutol**. 10–15 mg/kg/day oral.

**Ethosuximide**. Start at 2.5 mg/kg/8 h oral. Increase gradually once a week to a max. of 15 mg/kg/8 h. Therapeutic range (not very helpful) 40–100 μg/litre.

**Factor VIII concentrate** – normally 20 u/kg, major bleeds (psoas haematoma) 30 u/kg, head injury 50 u/kg.

**Fansidar** (pyrimethamine 25 mg, sulphadoxine 500 mg). Treatment: <4 yr, one-half tab. × 1; 4–8 yr, 1 tab.; 9–14 yr, 2 tabs. Prophylaxis: <4 yr, one-quarter tab. weekly; 4–8 yr, one-half tab.; 9–14 yr, three-quarters tab.

**Fentanyl**. 2–5 μg/kg/dose (N.B. Respiratory suppression). Infusion: loading dose 5 μg/kg, then 2–4 μg/kg/h if not ventilated or 5–10 μg/kg/h if ventilated.

**Ferrous gluconate and sulphate**. 12% of gluconate is elemental iron (300 mg tab. has 35 mg Fe). 30% of sulphate is elemental iron (200 mg tab. has 60 mg Fe). Treatment of iron deficiency: 6 mg/kg/day elemental iron for 3 months (give vitamin C as well). Physiological requirement 1 mg/kg/day.

**Flecainide**. Supraventricular tachycardia (SVT) 2 mg/kg IV over 10–15 min (max. 150 mg), then infuse at 1.5 mg/kg/h for 1 h, then 0.25 mg/kg/h. Oral dose: in adults 100–200 mg/12 h; in children, manufacturer uncertain. Start at 2 mg/kg/12 h. Increase gradually over 2 weeks to max. 4 mg/kg/12 h.

**Flucloxacillin**. 25–50 mg/kg/6 h IV, IM, oral (12 h 1st week of life, 8 h 2–4 weeks).

**Flucytosine (5-FC)**. 50 mg/kg/8 h oral, IV over 30 min. Peak level 25–50 μg/ml. Decrease dose in renal disease.
**Fludrocortisone**. 5 μg/kg daily oral (max. 0.2 mg). Tab. 0.1 mg.
**Folic acid**. Treatment 0.2 mg/kg/day. Adult 10 mg/day.
**Folinic acid**. Methotrexate rescue: 5–15 mg/6 h IV, IM, oral for 2 days.
**Fresh frozen plasma**. 10–20 ml/kg. In DIC, contains all clotting factors.
**Frusemide**. 1 mg/kg/6–12 h IV, IM, oral. In prerenal renal failure, after adequate volume replacement try 5 mg/kg IV × 1.
**Fusidic acid**. Syr. 250 mg = sodium fusidate 175 mg. Injection diethanol amine fusidate 580 mg = 500 mg sodium salt. All doses as sodium salt. 6.5–8 mg/kg/8 h IV over 6 h or oral 10–12.5 mg/kg/8 h. Level 40–400 μmol/litre (× 0.52 = μg/ml).

**(Infant) Gaviscon**. Infant: one-half to 1 sachet with feeds p.r.n. (<2 months, not more than one-half sachet per feed). Child: 1 sachet after food. Contains $Na^+$ 4 mmol/sachet. Liquid: 5 ml after feed.
**Gentamicin**. 2.5 mg/kg/8 h (2.5 mg/kg/12 h in first week of life), IV, IM, max. 80 mg/dose. Level: trough <2 mg/litre, peak 5–10 mg/litre. Decrease dose in renal disease. Intraventricular: 1 mg.
**Glucagon**. 20 μg/kg/day. Max. 1 mg/day.
**Glyceryl trinitrate**. 1.5 μg/kg/min. Titrate dose against response.
**Griseofulvin**. Microsize preparation 10–15 mg/kg/day (max. 1 g/day), ultramicrosize preparation 5–10 mg/kg/day (max. 670 mg/day), oral with meals in one or two divided doses. Usual course is 6–12 weeks. For tinea of scalp, nails, skin after histological confirmation.

**Haloperidol**. 25 μg/kg IV, IM for severe agitation, then give smaller doses 2 hourly, gradually increasing to 25 μg/kg/12 h IV, IM. Oral dose 0.5 mg/dose once daily, increase by 0.25 mg/day every week till symptoms controlled (max. 7 mg/day). N.B. extrapyramidal S/E.
**Heparin**. 1 mg = 100 u. 150 u/kg start, then 15–25 u/kg/h. Adjust infusion according to kaolin partial thromboplastin time (KPTT) 2–3 × control.
**Human Albumin Solution (HAS)**. 10–20 ml/kg IV.
**Hydralazine**. 0.2–0.4 mg/kg IV, IM stat, then 0.1–0.2 mg/kg/4–6 h. Oral: 0.2 mg/kg/12 h, gradual increase to max. 2.0 mg/kg. Associated with drug-induced lupus.
**Hydrochlorothiazide**. 1–1.5 mg/kg/12–24 h oral.
**Hydrocortisone**. 3–5 mg/kg/4–6 h IV, IM (painful), or infusion 1 mg/kg/h.
**Hydroxycobalamin** – see Vitamin $B_{12}$.
**Hydroxyzine** (Atarax). 0.5 mg/kg/6 h. Max. 400 mg/day.
**Hyoscine hydrobromide**. Premedication: 0.01 mg/kg. See Papaveretum.

**Imipenem–cilastatin**. Serious infection: 25 mg/kg/6 h over 30 min (neonate 12 h). Normally 10–15 mg/kg/6 h.
**Imipramine**. Enuresis: 25–50 mg nocte. >10 yr may try 75 mg nocte.
**Immunoglobulin**. Hypogammaglobulinaemia: 6% soln, 6.5 ml/kg IV over 4 h monthly or 0.6 ml/kg IM of 16% soln every 3 weeks. Hepatitis A

prevention 0.1 ml/kg IM. Measles and varicella (see Chapter 6), Kawasaki syndrome (see Section 11.11), ITP (see Subsection 9.8.1).
**Indomethacin**. For juvenile chronic arthritis 1.0–3.0 mg/kg/day in 2–3 divided doses (max. 200 mg/day).
**Infusions**. 1 mg/kg of anything diluted in 50 ml at 1 ml/h = 0.33 μg/kg/min.
**Insulin**. 0.1 u/kg IV or SC. Hyperkalaemia: give it with 1 g/kg IV dextrose bolus (2 ml/kg 50% dextrose).
**Ipecacuanha**. 6–12 months 10 ml × 1 only. 1–2 yr 15 ml, 2–3 yr 20 ml, 3–4 yr 25 ml, >4 yr 30 ml. Repeat ×1 after 30 min if no emesis.
**Ipratropium bromide**. 0.4–1.0 ml of 0.025% soln diluted to 2 ml or mixed with $\beta_2$ agonist via nebulizer 4–6 h. Metered aerosol 2–4 puffs 6–8 h (36 μg per puff).
**Iron**. See Ferrous gluconate and sulphate.
**Isoniazid (INAH)**. 10–15 mg/kg/day. Pyridoxine concurrently if using the higher dose.
**Isoprenaline**. 0.1–1.0 μg/kg/min. Put 0.3 mg/kg in 50 ml 5% dextrose at 1 ml/h = 0.1 μg/kg/min.

**Ketamine**. 1–2 mg/kg/IV, or 4–6 mg/kg IM. Give atropine 0.01 mg/kg IV/IM with induction. As procedure is about to end, give diazepam 0.1 mg/kg. Anaesthesia: infusion 10–20 μg/kg/min. Analgesia: 4 μg/kg/min.
**Ketoconazole**. 5 mg/kg/12–24 h oral.

**Labetolol**. Hypertensive emergency: 1–3 mg/kg/hourly IV infusion. 2 mg/kg/12 h oral. Can increase gradually to 20 mg/kg/12 h.
**Lactulose**. Laxative: 0.5 mg/kg/12–24 h. Liver failure: 1 mg/kg/6 h.
**Lignocaine**. 1% = 10 mg/ml. 1 mg/kg IV stat and then 20–55 μg/kg/min infusion. Max. dose for local anaesthetic: 4 mg/kg (6 mg/kg with adrenaline – not for digital block).
**Loperamide.** 0.08–0.24 mg/kg/day in 2–3 divided doses. Max. 15 mg/day.

**Magnesium**. Requirements: 0.2–0.4 mmol/kg/day. Hydroxide mixture contains $Mg^{2+}$ 13.5 mmol/10 ml, inj. Mg sulphate 50% has 4.1 mmol/2 ml.
**Magnesium sulphate 50%**. 1 ml = 50 mg elemental magnesium = 2.1 mmol. Deficiency 0.2 ml/kg/12–24 h IM or slow IV. Give 3–4 doses. Cathartic/laxative 1 ml/kg/8–12 h oral × 2 days. Acts within 1 h. Anticonvulsant 0.4 ml/kg IV.
**Magnesium trisilicate**. Antacid 0.3–0.5 ml/kg p.r.n. Contains 6 mmol $Na^+$/10 ml. Reduces absorption of oral iron.
**Maloprim** (pyrimethamine 12.5 mg, dapsone 100 mg). Malaria prophylaxis: <4 yr, one-quarter tab.; 4–8 yr, one-half tab.; 8–12 yr, three-quarters tab.; >12 yr, 1 tab. weekly.
**Mannitol**. 0.25–0.5 g/kg/dose IV. Beware repeated doses. Use only if serum osm. <325 mmol/litre.
**Mebendazole**. Antihelminthic: 100 mg/12 h × 3 days. For threadworms 100 mg once, repeat after 3 weeks.

**Metaraminol**. 0.01 mg/kg stat. Repeat p.r.n. For tetraology of Fallot turns and as temporary treatment of acute vasodilatation hypotension. Contraindicated in hypovolaemia.
**Methyl phenidate**. For hyperactive and inattentive children, 20 mg/m$^2$/day. Start with half-dose and progressively increase over 4–6 weeks.
**Methyl prednisolone**. Asthma 1–2 mg/kg/4 h IV.
**Methylene blue**. For methaemoglobinaemia induced by nitrites, aniline dyes, chlorates, nitrobenzene, sulphurs, quinones, etc. 1–2 mg/kg IV as 1% solution over 5 min. Repeat 1–3 h if needed. Max. total dose 7 mg/kg.
**Metoclopramide**. 0.1 mg/kg/6 h IV, oral. Avoid anti-emetics in children (except in oncology) because dystonic reactions are common. Treatment of dystonic reaction is benztropine or diphenhydramine.
**Metronidazole**. *Giardia*: 5–7.5 mg/kg/8 h oral, suppos. For 7–10 days *or* 40 mg/kg once daily × 3 days. Anaerobic infection: 7.5 mg/kg/6 h IV (max. 4 g/day) or 5–10 mg/kg/8 h oral (max. 2 g/day). Symptomatic intestinal or invasive amoebiasis 10–15 mg/kg/8 h. oral (max. 2.25 g/day) × 5–10 days. *Trichomonas vaginalis*: >13 yr, 2 g oral × 1. Partner must also be treated. N. B. Antabuse reaction with alcohol.
**Mexiletine**. 5 mg/kg IV over 15 min, then 5–20 µg/kg/min. Oral: 5 mg/kg/8 h.
**Mezlocillin**. 50 mg/kg/4 h or 75 mg/kg/6 h IV.
**Miconazole**. Antifungal: 10–15 mg/kg/8 h. IV over 30 min. Oral = one-half IV dose. Topical: apply 2% cream at each nappy change.
**Microlette**. Micro-enema. 5 ml PR as necessary.
**Midazolam**. 0.1–0.2 mg/kg IV repeat p.r.n. S/E hypotension (treat with 10–20 ml/kg of normal saline) and hypoventilation. Some advocate higher doses (*Lancet* (1988) **ii**, 565).
**Morphine**. 0.1–0.2 mg/kg/2–4 h IV, IM. Infusion 10–50 µg/kg/h. There is no dose limit for those receiving palliative treatment.

**Nalidixic acid**. 12.5 mg/kg/6 h oral. Take with meals. Caution in renal, liver failure. Not for infants <3 months. UTI prophylaxis: 12.5 mg/kg nocte. S/E photosensitivity. Do not use if creatinine clearance is <10 ml/min/1.73 m$^2$.
**Naloxone**. 0.1 mg/kg IV, IM, SC (max. 2 mg) or intratracheal. Repeat as necessary or commence infusion 5–10 µg/kg/h IV because half-life is shorter than that of the opiates. Amp. 400 µg/ml and neonatal 40 µg/2 ml.
**Naproxen**. 5–7.5 mg/kg/12 h oral. Max. 1.0 g/day.
**Neomycin**. 12.5–25 mg/kg/6 h oral.
**Neostigmine**. 0.05 mg/kg IV. For reversal of neuromuscular blockade or myaesthenia gravis test, add atropine 0.02 mg/kg.
**Netilmicin**. 2.5 mg/kg/8 h IV (max. 100 mg/dose).
**Nifedipine**. Hypertension: 0.1–0.2 mg/kg/8 h initially. Increase to 0.3–0.5 mg/kg/8 h orally.
**Nitrazepam**. 0.25 mg/kg/12 h, max. 5 mg. Hypnotic or anticonvulsant.
**Nitrofurantoin**. 1.25–2 mg/kg/6 h. Prophylaxis: 2.5 mg/kg dose nocte. Adult dose: 100 mg. Take with meals. Contraindicated in renal disease.

**Nitroglycerine**. See Glyceryl trinitrate.
**Nitroprusside**. 0.5–5 μg/kg/min IV. Protect from light. Measure thiocyanate levels if used at >5 μg/kg/min.
**Noradrenaline**. 0.1–0.5 μg/kg/min.
**Nystatin**. Susp. 100 000 u/ml. Pastilles 100 000 u. Tab. 500 000 u. Ointment 100 000 u/g. Oral thrush: 1 ml on tongue after each feed (oncology children 5 ml/4 h). Intestinal: 1–5 ml with meals. >5 yr: use 500 000 u/6 h. Napkin thrush: topical nystatin with each nappy change.

**Omnopon**. See Papaveretum.
**Oxybutynin**. 5 mg/8 h oral, for neurogenic bladder.

**Pancuronium**. 0.1 mg/kg IV p.r.n.
**Papaveretum**. 0.4 mg/kg IM or 0.2. mg/kg IV slowly. Half-life of 3 h. Papaveretum/hyoscine preparation (20 mg/0.4 mg/ml) is available for premedication, 0.2 ml/kg IM.
**Paracetamol**. 10–15 mg/kg/4–6 h oral, suppos.
**Paraldehyde**. 1 ml = 1 g. Rectal: 0.25 ml/kg mixed with equal volume of arachis or olive oil, or normal saline (max. 10 g/dose). Repeat after 10 min p.r.n. NGT: 0.25 ml/kg diluted in water or saline. IM: 0.15 ml/kg deep injection. Repeat p.r.n. IV: 100 mg/kg over 20 min, then 20 mg/kg/h infusion, made up in normal saline as a 5% solution, delivered via non-PVC tubing (0.4 ml/kg/h).
**(D)-Penicillamine**. For lead, gold, mercury poisoning, 10 mg/kg/12 h. Give pyridoxine 10 mg concurrently.
**Penicillins**:
**Benzathine penicillin** (Bicillin). 1.2 million units. Good for monthly IM prophylaxis against group A streptococci in rheumatic fever. Not currently marketed in the UK.
**Penicillin G** (benzyl penicillin, crystalline penicillin). Serious infection 60 mg (100 000 u)/kg/4 h. Otherwise 30 mg/kg/4–6 h. Intraventricular 0.1 mg/kg. 1 million units = 600 mg.
**Penicillin V** (phenoxymethyl penicillin). 7–15 mg/kg/6 h oral. Prophylaxis: 12.5 mg/kg/12 h.
**Procaine penicillin**. 1000 u = 1 mg. 25–50 mg/kg/day IM.
**Pentamidine**. Pneumocystis: 4 mg/kg/day IM. × 10–14 days.
**Pethidine**. 1 mg/kg/dose IV, IM. Repeat 2–3 hourly.
**Phenobarbitone**. Status 15–20 mg/kg IV over 10 min (20–30 mg/kg in neonates) or IM. After 12 h continue with maintenance dose of 4–5 mg/kg/24 h oral (adolescents 3–4 mg/kg/day). Max. 200 mg/day. Level 80–120 μmol/litre (× 0.23 = mg/litre).
**Phenoxybenzamine**. In pheochromocytoma: oral 0.1 mg/kg/12 h. Slow IV 0.5–1 mg/kg single dose.
**Phentolamine**. In pheochromocytoma: 20–50 μg/kg/min.
**Phenytoin**. In status epilepticus, 15–20 mg/kg IV over 30 min. Max. 1 g/dose. Then 2–4 mg/kg/12 h oral. Level 40–80 μmol/litre (× 0.25 = mg/litre).

**Pholcodeine**. Linctus 0.2–0.4 mg/kg/6–12 h. Max. dose 10 ml.
**Physostigmine**. See Tricyclic antidepressants (Section 5.10). Anticholinesterase.
**Phytomenadione**. See Vitamin K.
**Piperacillin**. 50 mg/kg/6 h IV over 30 min. Max. 24 g/day.
**Pizotifen**. Usually 0.5 mg mane, 1.0 mg nocte. For treatment of migraine.
**Platelets**. 4–6 u/m$^2$ or 0.2 u/kg over 15 min.
**Potassium**. 1 g KCl = 13.4 mmol. Requirements 2–4 mmol/kg/day. Max. infusion rate 0.4 mmol/kg/h. 'Slow K' tablet = 8 mmol $K^+$; 'Sando K' effervescent = 12 mmol; 'Kay-Cee-L' syrup = 1 mmol/ml. Hyperkalaemia – see Section 5.7.
**Prazosin**. 0.01 mg/kg test dose oral (N.B. First dose hypotensive effect), then 0.05–0.1 mg/kg/6–12 h.
**Prednisolone**. 1–2 mg/kg/day. Nephrotic syndrome 60 mg/m$^2$/day, single morning dose, max. 28 days. If relapsing frequently, can try 40 mg/m$^2$ on alternate days.
**Primaquine**. To eradicate *Vivax* malaria: 0.15 mg/kg/12 h × 14 days. Exclude G-6-PD deficiency first.
**Primidone**. Start with 125 mg/day. Increase over several weeks to 4–8 mg/kg/8 h. Monitor serum primidone or phenobarbitone. Adult dose: 750–1500 mg/day.
**Probenicid**. 10 mg/kg/6 h oral. Max. 2 g/day. As an adjunct to penicillin therapy or rarely as a uricosuric.
**Prochlorperazine**. Anti-emetic, anti-vertigo. 0.05 mg/kg/8 h IV, IM or 0.1 mg/kg/8–12 h oral. Avoid in children (unless on cancer chemotherapy) because of dystonic S/E which will require benztropine or procyclidine.
**Procyclidine**. 0.1–0.2 mg IM, IV slowly for dystonic reactions. Repeat after 20 min.
**Proguanil**. Malaria prophylaxis daily: 25 mg < 12 months, 50 mg 1–4 yr, 75 mg 5–8 yr, 100 mg 8–12 yr, 200 mg > 12 yr.
**Promethazine**. Antihistamine: 0.5 mg/kg/8–12 h IV, IM or oral (adult 20–25 mg). Sedation 0.75–1.0 mg/kg single dose. Elixir 5 mg/5 ml, tab. 10, 25 mg.
**Propranolol**. 0.02–0.1 mg/kg (max. 3 mg/dose) slow IV. Oral dose 0.5 mg/kg/6–12 h initially. Increase as necessary to max. 18 mg/kg/day.
**Protamine sulphate**. 1 mg for each 100 u heparin, slow IV. Repeat p.r.n.
**Prothrombinex** (Factors II, IX, X). 1 ml/kg IV.
**Pyrantel**. 11 mg/kg/dose × 1 for pinworm or roundworm. For hookworm, same dose daily for 3 days.
**Pyrazinamide**. 10–15 mg/kg/12 h oral daily.
**Pyridoxine**. Fitting neonate 50 mg/kg IV, preferably under EEG control.

**Quinine**. Resistant falciparum malaria: 20 mg/kg IM or IV over 4 h, then 7.5 mg/kg/8 h IM or IV over 1 h. When awake, give 10 mg/kg/8 h oral for 5 days. Finish course with one dose of fansidar.

**Ranitidine**. 1 mg/kg/8 h IV over 5 min. Oral 3 mg/kg/12 h. Does not have androgenic effects or major drug interactions.
**Resonium**. 1 g/kg/4 h via NGT (give magnesium sulphate or lactulose) or PR.
**Rifampicin**. TB: 15 mg/kg (max. 600 mg) daily oral on empty stomach. *Haemophilus influenzae* and meningococcus prophylaxis: 10 mg/kg/12 h (adult 600 mg/day; child under 1 month 5 mg/kg/12 h) for 2 days (meningococcus) or 4 days (*H. influenzae*). Long-term use: monitor SGOT. Administer 1 h before or 2 h after meals. Stains urine and soft-contact lenses orange.

**Salbutamol**. Oral: 0.1–0.15 mg/kg/6 h. Metered aerosol: 1–2 puffs 4–6 h (100 μg/puff). Resp. soln: 5 mg/ml. Nebules: 2.5 mg/2.5 ml. 2.5 mg/4 h all ages. N.B. Nebulize with $O_2$ for sicker children. Rotacap (available as 200 or 400 μg): 200–400 μg/6 h. IV infusion: 5 μg/kg/min.
**Senna**. Tab. 7.5 mg, syr. 7.5 mg = 5 ml. 3.75–7.5 mg nocte <5 yr, 7.5–15 mg 5–10 yr, 15–30 mg >10 yr.
**Sodium**. 30% NaCl = 4.5 mmol Na/ml. Normal saline = 0.15 mmol/ml. 1 g NaCl = 17 mmol Na. Requirements: 2.5–4 mmol/kg/day.
**Sodium cromoglycate** (INTAL). Spincap 20 mg, nebules 20 mg/2 ml. 20–40 mg/8 h.
**Sodium nitroprusside**. See Nitroprusside.
**Sodium valproate**. See Valproate.
**Spironolactone**. 1.0–1.25 mg/kg/12 h oral.
**Stemetil**. See Prochlorperazine.
**Streptomycin**. 20 mg/kg/day IM (adult dose 1 g).
**Sucralfate**. Tab. 1 g, one-quarter tab./6 h <2 yr, one-half tab./6 h 3–12 yr, 1 tab./6 h >12 yr. Doses may be doubled and tried 12 hourly. Tablets may be dispersed in water. Avoid combined use with antacids or $H_2$ antagonists. Reduces absorption of phenytoin.
**Sulphasalazine**. 10–25 mg/kg/6 h, then taper to 10 mg/kg/6 h. Max. 4 g/day.
**Suxamethonium**. 1 mg/kg/dose IV.

**Tensilon**. See Edrophonium.
**Terbutaline**. Oral: 0.75 μg/kg/6–8 h. Tab. 5 mg, syr. 1.5 mg/5 ml. Metered aerosol: 250 μg/puff, 1–2 puffs/4–6 h. Nebulizer: 10 mg/ml 5–10 mg p.r.n. Subcut.: 10 μg/kg, max. 300 μg. Amp.: 500 μg.
**Tetracosactrin** (Synacthen). See ACTH.
**Tetracycline, oxytetracycline**. Not advised in <8 yr because of enamel hypoplasia and permanent discoloration of teeth. 3.5–7 mg/kg/8 h IV or 10 mg/kg/6 h oral given 1 h before or 2 hr after meals. Acne in adolescents: 250 mg/8 h orally. Reports of benign intracranial hypertension with long-term use in acne sufferers.
**Theophylline**. Asthma: 5 mg/kg/6 h oral. Slow-release preparations 8–10 mg/kg/12 h. Level 55–110 μmol/litre (10–20 μg/ml).
**Thiopentone**. 4–5 mg IV (N.B. Hypotension is common. Treat with normal saline 10–20 ml/kg stat). Then 1–3 mg/kg/h infusion (the higher

dose may be needed initially until the fat stores are saturated), level 150–200 μmol/litre (× 0.24 = μg/ml).
**Thyroxine**. Infants 25 μg/day oral. Older children 4–5 μg/kg/day (adults 100–200 μg/day).
**Ticarcillin**. 50–75 mg/kg/6 h IV. Reconst. 1 g + 1.5 ml = 1 g/2 ml.
**Tinidazole**. 50 mg/kg single dose. Repeat × 1 in 24–48 h. For *Giardia*.
**Tobramycin**. 2.5 mg/kg/8 h IV (max. 100 mg) (<2-week-olds give 18–24 h). Level 5–10 mg/litre peak, <2 mg/litre trough.
**Tolmetin**. 5–10 mg/kg/8 h oral (max. 2.0 g/day).
**Tranexamic acid**. 15 mg/kg/12 h slow IV. 30 mg/kg/8 h oral. Reduce dose in renal failure.
**Trimeprazine** (Vallergan). Sedative: 3 mg/kg/dose × 1 oral, 1 mg/kg/dose IM. Antihist.: 0.25 mg/kg/6 h oral.
**Trimethoprim**. 4–5 mg/kg/12 h oral (adult 200 mg/dose). 3 mg/kg/12 h slow IV. For moderate or severe renal impairment, increase dosing interval to 18 hourly or 24 hourly, respectively. Prophylaxis: 2.5–5 mg/kg nocte. Pneumocystis – see Cotrimoxazole.

**Vallergan**. See Trimeprazine.
**Valproate**. Initially 5 mg/kg/12 h oral. Increase weekly by 5–10 mg/kg/day until fits are well controlled or until 30 mg/kg/12 h (occasionally may go to 40 mg/kg/12 h). Drug level 0.3–0.7 mmol/litre (× 144 = μg/ml). The correct dose is that which controls the fits. Drug levels correlate poorly with seizure control.
**Vancomycin**. 10–15 mg/kg/8 h IV over 30–60 min. Peak level 25–40 mg/litre. Trough 5–10 mg/litre. Intraventricular 5 mg/dose/48 h.
**Vasopressin**. 0.3 u/kg run in over 30 min for GI bleed. Repeat in 1–2 h if bleeding continues. Aqueous: 2–10 u/8 h IM, SC. Oily: 2.5–5 u IM every 2–4 days p.r.n.
**Verapamil**. SVT: 0.1–0.2 mg/kg IV over 10 min (max. 10 mg/dose). Repeat in 30 min if needed. Contraindicated with beta-blockers. May cause sudden hypotension and asystole. Oral 1–2 mg/kg/8 h.
**Vitamin $B_{12}$** (hydroxycobalamin). 20 μg/kg/dose IM. Treatment: daily for 1 week, then weekly. Prophylaxis: monthly. Oral dose 70–100 μg/dose.
**Vitamin C** (ascorbic acid). Scurvy: 100 mg/day for 10 days. Urine acidification 10 mg/kg/6 h. Normal daily requirement 35–50 mg.
**Vitamin D**. Calcitriol (1,25-dihydroxy $D_3$) for vitamin D resistance, chronic renal failure, hypoparathyroidism 0.025 mg/day starting dose. In nutritional rickets, malabsorption or liver disease: ergocalciferol ($D_2$) 10 000 u (250 μg) daily for a month. Then manage as per ‘prevention’. Prevention of nutritional rickets: calcium + vitamin D compound tab. containing 500 u $D_2$. Take 1 daily. No other low-dose preparation is available in the UK. All patients on vitamin D should have Ca measured regularly. Normal daily requirements 400 u.
**Vitamin K** (phytomenadione). 0.2–0.3 mg/kg IM, SC (if unavoidable, can be given by slow IV). Max. 10 mg. For vitamin K deficiency, 2.5–20 mg/day oral.

**Warfarin**. 200 μg/kg/day (prothrombin time ratio 2:1). Antidote: vitamin K 0.2 mg/kg IM or slow IV. N.B. Increased anticoagulation with aspirin, barbiturates, sulphurs, chloral hydrate, etc.

## Further reading


*Alder Hey Book of Children's Doses* (1982) Alder Hey Children's Hospital, Liverpool

Benitz, W. E. and Tatro, D. S. (1981) *The Pediatric Drug Handbook*, Year Book Medical Publishers, Chicago

*British National Formulary* (1988) British Medical Association, London

Gilman, A. G., Goodman, L. S., Rall, T. W. and Murad, F. (eds.) (1985) *Goodman and Gilman's The Pharmacological Basis of Therapeutics*, Macmillan, London

Insley, J. (1986) *A Paediatric Vade-Mecum,* Lloyd-Luke, London

*Paediatric Pharmacopoeia* (1985) Royal Children's Hospital, Melbourne

Shann, F. A. and Duncan, A. (1987) *Drug Doses in Paediatric Intensive Care,* Royal Children's Hospital, Melbourne

Yip, C. L. W. and Tay, S. H. J. (1989) *A Practical Manual on Acute Paediatrics,* PG Publishing, Singapore


# 2.2 Relative activity of adrenal corticosteroids

| | *Glucocorticoid activity* | *Mineralocorticoid activity* | *Biological half-life** |
|---|---|---|---|
| Cortisone acetate | 1 | 1 | S |
| Hydrocortisone | 1.25 | 1.25 | S |
| Prednisolone | 5 | 1 | I |
| Prednisone | 5 | 1 | I |
| Betamethasone | 50 | – | L |
| Dexamethasone | 40 | – | L |
| Fludrocortisone | 10 | 500 | S |

* S (short) = 8–12 h; I (intermediate) = 12–36 h; L (long) = 36–72 h.

## 2.3 Maternal drugs and breast feeding

| *Probably safe* | *Drugs to avoid* | *Absolute contraindication* |
|---|---|---|
| Paracetamol | Anthroquinones (laxatives) | Antineoplastic drugs |
| Alpha-methyldopa | Atropine | Bromocryptine |
| Ampicillin | Bromides | Carbimazole |
| Antihistamines* | Calciferol | Chloramphenicol |
| Aspirin | Danthron | Diethylstilboestrol |
| Chlorpromazine* | Ethanol | Ergots (migraine doses) |
| Codeine* | Metronidazole | Gold salts |
| Digoxin | Narcotics | Immunosuppressants |
| Frusemide | Oral contraceptives (progesterone-only pill is allowable) | Iodides |
| Haloperidol* | Oestrogens | Phenindione |
| Hydralazine | Primidone | Radioisotopes |
| Indomethacin | Reserpine | Cimetidine |
| Methadone* | Marijuana† | Thiouracil† |
| Phenobarbitone* | | |
| Phenytoin | | |
| Prednisolone | | |
| Theopyhylline | | |
| Warfarin | | |
| Carbamazepine | | |
| Beta-blockers (metoprolol†) | | |
| Thiazides | | |
| Antimicrobials (all transfer into breast milk in limited amounts): | | |
| cephalosporins | | |
| ampicillin | | |
| isoniazid | | |
| nalidixic acid‡ | | |
| nitrofurantoin‡ | | |
| rifampicin | | |
| cotrimoxazole‡ | | |
| tetracycline | | |

* Causes mild sedation.
† Concentrates in breast milk.
‡ Causes haemolysis in G-6-PD deficiency.

## Further reading


Behrman, R. E. and Vaughan, V. C. (1987) *Nelson: Textbook of Pediatrics,* WB Saunders, Philadelphia, p. 364.

Committee on Drugs, American Academy of Pediatrics (1983) The transfer of drugs and other chemicals into human breast milk. *Pediatr.* **2**, 375–383.

# 2.4 Prescribing for children

Special care is needed when prescribing for neonates (first 30 days of life) because the distribution, metabolism and excretion of a drug may be vastly different from that of infants. Virtually all children need to have the adult dose of a medicine adjusted until they are post-pubertal or reach (an arbitrary) 50 kg.

## DETERMINING A DOSE

### *1 Paediatric pharmacopoeia* – the safest way

If none is available the dose may be calculated from the adult dose using age, body weight, surface area or a combination of those parameters.

### *2 Body weight* – The average adult weighs 70 kg

A paediatric dose in mg/kg can be obtained by dividing the adult dose by 70. This is unreliable because young children have a high metabolic rate and there is no good reason why dose should be in direct proportion to body weight. Obese children would receive higher doses than necessary. Important drugs should probably be calculated according to height, age or surface area.

### *3 Surface area (SA)*

An adult male has a body SA of approximately 1.8 $m^2$.

$$\text{Approximate dose} = \frac{\text{SA } (m^2)}{1.8} \times \text{Adult dose}$$

A body surface area normogram is given in Chapter 3 (Figure 3.2).

### *4 Percentage method*

For drugs which have a wide margin between therapeutic and toxic dose, it is reasonable to use the following table:

| *Age* | *Ideal weight* (kg) | *Height* (cm) | *Surface area* ($m^2$) | *Per cent adult dose* |
|---|---|---|---|---|
| Term baby | 3.4 | 50 | 0.23 | 12.5 |
| 3 mo | 5.6 | 59 | 0.32 | 18 |
| 6 mo | 7.7 | 67 | 0.40 | 22 |
| 1 yr | 10 | 76 | 0.47 | 25 |
| 3 yr | 14 | 94 | 0.62 | 33 |
| 5 yr | 18 | 108 | 0.73 | 40 |
| 7 yr | 23 | 120 | 0.88 | 50 |
| 10 yr | 30 | 132 | 1.10 | 60 |
| 12 yr | 38 | 148 | 1.25 | 75 |
| 14 yr | 50 | 166 | 1.50 | 80 |

Adapted from *British National Formulary* (1988) British Medical Association, London, and from Shann, E. A. and Duncan, A. (1987) *Drug Doses in Paediatric Intensive Care*, Royal Children's Hospital, Melbourne.

# 2.5 The child with a history of penicillin allergy

Many children requiring antibiotics give a history of adverse reactions to prior treatment with penicillins. The exact nature of the reaction should be ascertained. In many cases the child can safely be given an oral penicillin challenge, although occasionally the first dose should be administered in a hospital, or else an alternative antibiotic sought such as erythromycin. There is a high cross-reactivity between penicillins and cephalosporins. None of the tests listed below, apart from an oral challenge, is of much use in assessing the child with suspected allergy.

## TESTS FOR POSSIBLE PENICILLIN ALLERGY

### *1 Skin prick test*

Use benzyl penicillin (0.06 g/ml) and phenoxymethyl penicillin (0.05 g/ml) on the forearm. Use saline and histamine (1 mg/ml) as controls. A weal larger than 3 mm is considered positive.

### *2 Intradermal testing*

See Chandra, R. G., *et al.* (1980) *Arch. Dis. Child.*, **55**, 857–860.

### *3 Radioallergosorbent test (RAST)*

This is of use in anticipating IgE-mediated reactions which are rare. False-negative results may be obtained because only major determinants are tested or because specific IgE titres will wane over several months. False-positive results occur when IgE levels are high.

### *4 Oral challenge*

This is probably the only way of identifying true penicillin allergy. A heredity of atopic disease does not increase the chance of adverse reaction to subsequent challenge. A child who was aged less than 4 years at the time of the initial reaction is much less likely than one over 4 years to react to oral challenge. The nature of the initial reaction, as described below, should determine one's attitude to subsequent oral challenge.

## TYPES OF REACTION

### *1 Acute anaphylaxis* – a type 1 hypersensitivity reaction

It is rare and is an absolute contraindication to challenge with penicillins and cephalosporins. Carbapenems (imipenem) and monobactams (aztreonam) also have a beta-lactam ring and should be avoided, although anaphylaxis is much less likely.

### *2 Exanthem without pruritus*

Not a contraindication to oral challenge which may even be given at home.

### *3 Urticaria, pruritus, swollen joints, facial oedema*

11–42% of these children will show some clinical reaction to oral challenge, although the risks of anaphylaxis are negligible. Nevertheless, if there is a convenient alternative antibiotic it should be used, otherwise the first oral challenge dose should be given in a doctor's surgery or hospital, with some adrenaline at hand.

### *4 Diarrhoea*

Most likely to be due to the illness for which the antibiotic was prescribed or antibiotic-induced diarrhoea (*Clostridium difficile* is the major culprit). This is not a contraindication to oral challenge.

## PARENTERAL PENICILLIN

Almost all deaths from anaphylaxis have resulted from parenteral administration of the drug. A child with a history of previous exanthematous reaction to penicillin can be given parenteral penicillin in a hospital setting. Those who have had more severe reactions to penicillin should not have parenteral beta-lactam drugs. If no suitable alternative can be found or penicillin is urgently needed, a small parenteral dose may be given (0.1 ml of 100 u/ml benzylpenicillin) which is increased in 15–20 steps at 20 min intervals to reach the normal dose (Ackroyd, J. F. (1989) *Lancet*, **i**, 335, and Holgate (1988)). After the course is completed the child should not necessarily be considered non-allergic.

## Further reading

Anon (1989) Penicillin allergy. *Lancet*, **i**, 420

Graff-Lennevig, V., Hedlin, G. and Linfors, A. (1988) Penicillin allergy – a rare condition? *Arch. Dis. Child.*, **63**, 1342–1346

Holgate, S. T. (1988) Penicillin allergy: how to diagnose and when to treat. *Br. Med. J.*, **296**, 1213–1214

Sher, T. H. (1983) Penicillin hypersensitivity – a review. *Pediatr. Clin. N. Am.*, **30**, 161–176

## 2.6 Drug-induced haemolysis in glucose-6-phosphate dehydrogenase (G-6-PD) deficiency

The following drugs and chemicals have been known to produce a haemolytic anaemia in subjects with G-6-PD deficiency:

**Antimalarials**
Primaquine
Pamaquine
Quinacrine
Quinine

**Sulphonamides**
Cotrimoxazole
Sulphapyridine
Sulphisoxazole
Salicylazosulphpyridine (Salazopyrin)
Diaminodiphenylsulphone (DDS)
Sulphoxone (Diasone)

**Analgesics and related compounds**
Acetylsalicylic acid
Acetophetidin (Phenacitin)
Para-aminosalicylic acid (PAS)
Acetanilide
Aminopyrine

**Nitrofurans**
Nitrofurantoin (Furadantin)
Nitrofurazone (Furacin)

**Miscellaneous**
Water-soluble vitamin K analogues
Chloramphenicol
Nalidixic acid (Negram)
Naphthalene
Aniline dyes
Methylene blue
Quinidine
Probenecid
Dimercaprol (BAL)

Fava (broad) beans may also produce haemolysis.

Chapter 3

# Normal data

*For normal haematological data, see Section 9.13.*
*For normal CSF findings, see Section 8.1.*

## 3.1 Endotracheal tube (ETT) size

Endotracheal tubes in children under about 7 years of age are uncuffed. There must be a small air leak around them, otherwise there is a risk of post-extubation tracheal stenosis. If the air leak is too large, it becomes impossible to ventilate the child adequately and a larger one must be inserted. If the tube is inserted too far, it may enter the right main bronchus and the unventilated left lung will then shunt unoxygenated blood and may collapse.

The specifications for correct endotracheal tube placement are found in Table 3.1.

**Table 3.1 Endotracheal tube specifications (From Shann, F. and Duncan, A. (1987) *Drug Doses in Paediatric Intensive Care*, Royal Children's Hospital, Melbourne, with permission)**

| *Age* | *Wt* (kg) | *Int. dia.* (mm) | *Ext. dia.* (mm) | *At lip* (cm) | *At nose* (cm) | *Suction catheter* (Fr.) |
|---|---|---|---|---|---|---|
| Newborn | <1 | 2.5 | 3.4 | 5.5 | 7 | 6 |
| Newborn | 1 | 3.0 | 4.2 | 6 | 7.5 | 7 |
| Newborn | 2 | 3.0 | 4.2 | 7 | 9 | 7 |
| Newborn | 3 | 3.0 | 4.2 | 8.5 | 10.5 | 7 |
| Newborn | 3.5 | 3.5 | 4.8 | 9 | 11 | 8 |
| 3 mo | 6 | 3.5 | 4.8 | 10 | 12 | 8 |
| 1 yr | 10 | 4.0 | 5.4 | 11 | 14 | 8 |
| 2 yr | 12 | 4.5 | 6.2 | 12 | 15 | 8 |
| 3 yr | 14 | 4.5 | 6.2 | 13 | 16 | 8 |
| 4 yr | 16 | 5.0 | 6.8 | 14 | 17 | 10 |
| 6 yr | 20 | 5.5 | 7.4 | 15 | 19 | 10 |
| 8 yr | 24 | 6.0 | 8.2 | 16 | 20 | 10 |
| 10 yr | 30 | 6.5 | 8.8 | 17 | 21 | 12 |
| 12 yr | 38 | 7.0 | 9.6 | 18 | 22 | 12 |
| 14 yr | 50 | 7.5 | 10.2 | 19 | 23 | 12 |
| Adult | 60 | 8.0 | 11.0 | 20 | 24 | 12 |
| Adult | 70 | 9.0 | 12.2 | 21 | 25 | 12 |

Int., internal; Ext., external; dia., diameter.

# 3.2 Blood gases and SI units

| *[$H^+$]* (mmol/litre) | *pH* | *[$H^+$]* (mmol/litre) | *pH* |
|---|---|---|---|
| 25 | 7.60 | 75 | 7.13 |
| 30 | 7.52 | 80 | 7.10 |
| 35 | 7.46 | 85 | 7.07 |
| 40 | 7.40 | 90 | 7.05 |
| 45 | 7.35 | 95 | 7.02 |
| 50 | 7.30 | 100 | 7.00 |
| 55 | 7.26 | 105 | 6.98 |
| 60 | 7.22 | 110 | 6.96 |
| 65 | 7.17 | 115 | 6.94 |
| 70 | 7.15 | 120 | 6.92 |

Approximate conversion: to convert hydrogen ion concentration to pH, subtract $H^+$ concentration from 80. The result can be inserted after the figure 7 and the decimal point.

For example, for $H^+$ concentration of 45 mmol/litre: $80 - 45 = 35$. Hence pH = 7.35.

This only works well when pH is close to the normal physiological range of 7.35–7.45.

| $Po_2$ and $Pco_2$ | | $Po_2$ and $Pco_2$ | |
|---|---|---|---|
| (mmHg) | (kPa) | (mmHg) | (kPa) |
| 7.5 | 1 | 75 | 10 |
| 15 | 2 | 82.5 | 11 |
| 22.5 | 3 | 90 | 12 |
| 30 | 4 | 97.5 | 13 |
| 37.5 | 5 | 105 | 14 |
| 45 | 6 | 112.5 | 15 |
| 52.5 | 7 | 120 | 16 |
| 60 | 8 | 127.5 | 17 |
| 67.5 | 9 | 135 | 18 |

Conversion factor: multiply kPa by 7.5 to convert to mmHg.

Normal values:

| | Arterial | Venous |
|---|---|---|
| pH: | | |
| newborn | 7.33–7.49 | |
| 1 day | 7.25–7.43 | |
| 2 days – adult | 7.35–7.45 | 7.31–7.42 |
| $Pco_2$: | | |
| <2 yr | 26–42 mmHg | |
| >2 yr | 33–46 | 40–50 |
| $Po_2$: | | |
| newborn | 65–75 mmHg | |
| older | 80–100 | 25–50 |
| Actual bicarbonate | 18–25 mmol/litre | |
| Base excess: | | |
| newborn | −10 to −2 | |
| older | −4 to +3 | |

# 3.3 Normal dentition

Dental age is a crude indicator of skeletal maturity or nutritional status. The loose association of eruption of teeth and age is demonstrated in the formula:

Approximate age in months (max. 24) = Number of teeth + 6

If no teeth have erupted by 12 months of age in a child with normal skeletal growth who is thriving, a dental opinion should be sought.

## PRIMARY OR DECIDUOUS TEETH ($n$=20)

| | *Central incisors* | *Lateral incisors* | *Cuspids* | *First molar* | *Second molar* |
|---|---|---|---|---|---|
| Age (months) of eruption | 6–8 | 7–9 | 16–18 | 12–14 | 20–26 |

## SECONDARY OR PERMANENT TEETH ($n$=32)

| | *Central incisors* | *Lateral incisors* | *Cuspids* | *First bicuspids* | *Second bicuspids* | *First molar* | *Second molar* | *Third molar* |
|---|---|---|---|---|---|---|---|---|
| Age (yr) | 6–8 | 7–9 | 9–12 | 10–12 | 10–12 | 6–7 | 11–13 | 17–21 |

# 3.4 Some biochemistry values

*N.B. There is marked variation in normal or therapeutic range between different laboratories and between different methods used for most assays. Consult your laboratory for their own reference values.*

**Alanine aminotransferase** (formerly SGPT). <1 yr <60 u/litre; >1 yr <40 u/litre. Comes from liver, skeletal muscle, heart and kidney.
**Albumin**. See Proteins
**Alkaline phosphatase**. 150–550 u/litre during infancy and childhood. Higher values during periods of rapid growth. Adult values are <150 u/litre. Comes from bone, liver, kidney and intestine. Isoenzymes can be measured.
**Ammonia**. <60 μmol/litre (<100 in newborn). Send heparinized blood to laboratory on ice.
**Amylase**. 20–120 u/litre. Comes from pancreas or salivary glands.
**Antistreptolysin-O titre (ASOT)**. >300 u suggests recent streptococcal infection.
**Aspartate aminotransferase (AST)** (formerly SGOT). <1 yr < 100 u/litre (normal range not well defined in infancy); 1–5 yr <50 u/litre; 5–15 yr <45 u/litre. Comes from cardiac and skeletal muscle, liver, kidney, red blood cells.

**Bicarbonate**. See Section 3.2.
**Bilirubin (total)**. 1 month old–adult <17 μmol/litre (<1 mg/dl). Higher values of mainly unconjugated bilirubin are seen in the neonatal period.

**Calcium**. Total calcium, newborn 1.8–3.0 mmol/litre (× 4 = mg/100 ml), >7 days, 2.15–2.75 mmol/litre. Lower in hypoalbuminaemia. Ionized calcium 1.0–1.35 mmol/litre. Decreased in alkalosis.
**Carbamazepine**. Therapeutic range 20–50 μmol/litre (× 0.24 = μg/ml).
**Carnitine**. Total 60–70 μmol/litre; free carnitine 40–50 μmol/litre.
**Carotene**. 1.0–4.6 μmol/litre (50–250 μg/100 ml).

**Chloramphenicol**. Peak therapeutic level taken 1 h after dose, 15–30 mg/litre.
**Chloride**. 96–106 mmol/litre.
**Cholesterol**. <1 yr < 5.0 mmol/litre; >1 yr 3.0–5.5 mmol/litre (× 38.5 = mg/dl). Values based on blood taken after 12 h fast.
**Complement**. C3, 80–160 mg/100 ml; C4, 0–6 months 7–26 mg/100 ml, >6 months 10–40 mg/100 ml. Both are acute phase reactants.
**Cortisol**. 0800 h 190–740 nmol/litre; 2000 h 30–300 nmol/litre. Random levels are virtually meaningless. Best measured after appropriate stimulation or suppression test.
**Creatine kinase**. <1 yr <390 u/litre; >1 yr 50–250 u/litre. Comes from skeletal, cardiac and smooth muscle, and brain. Increased levels after physical exercise or IM injections. Suspected carriers of Duchenne's muscular dystrophy should be tested on 3 separate occasions.
**Creatinine**. <5 yr <0.05 mmol/litre; 5–10 yr <0.08 mmol/litre; >10 yr <1.0 mmol/litre (× 11.3 = mg/dl). Levels relate to muscle mass.
**Creatinine clearance** – see Section 13.3

**Dehydroepiandrosterone sulphate (DHEA-S)**. <6 months <5 µmol/litre; 6 months–7 yr <0.5 µmol/litre; 8–9 yr <3 µmol/litre. Male: 10–12 yr <6, 13–19 yr 3–12. Female: 10–12 yr <8, 13–19 yr 1–12. Comes from adrenal glands.
**Digoxin**. Therapeutic range 0.5–2.0 ng/ml (×1.28 = mmol/litre). Take blood 8–24 hours after a dose.
**1,25-Dihydroxyvitamin D**. 40–150 pmol/litre.

**Free erythrocyte protoporphyrin**. <1.4 µmol/litre (<80 µg/100 ml) of RBC. Used for investigation of lead poisoning and porphyria. Increased in iron deficiency and chronic disease anaemia.

**Gamma-glutamyl transferase (GGT)**. <1 month <375 u/litre; 1–2 months < 250; 2–4 months < 135; 4–6 months < 75; 6 months–15 yr <50. Adult male <75; adult female <55. Comes from liver and pancreas.
**Gentamicin**. Peak level 5–10 mg/litre, 30 min after completion of infusion. Trough <2, taken just prior to a dose.
**Glucose**. 1–3 days 1.8–4.5 mmol/litre; 4 days–1 month 2.2–5.0 mmol/litre; >1 month 2.5–6.1 mmol/litre (×18 = mg/dl).
**Growth hormone**. Random values are of no use. Must perform stimulation test (sleep, exercise, insulin, arginine, L-dopa). Peak response level of >20 milliunits/litre excludes deficiency.

**Haemoglobin $A_{1c}$ (glycosylated Hb)**. Expressed as percentage of total haemoglobin. Normally 3.5–6.1%. Diabetic with reasonable control 9–10%.

**Immunoglobulins**. See Section 3.5.
**Insulin**. <145 pmol/litre or <20 microunits/litre. Fasting.

**Iron**. <1 yr 5–13 μmol/litre (30–70 μg/dl); >1 yr 9–27 μmol/litre (50–150 μg/dl)
**Iron binding capacity – total (TIBC)**. >1 yr 45–72 μmol/litre (250–400 μg/dl).

**Lactate**. 1–2 mmol/litre (venous) = 9–18 mg/dl. Arterial level is slightly lower. Level is higher in newborn (up to 3 mmol/litre), haemolysis, delayed separation of serum.
**Lactate dehydrogenase (LDH)**. Adults 80–250 u/litre.
**Lead**. 0–1.4 μmol/litre (0–30 μg/dl) in heparinized blood.

**Magnesium**. 0.70–1.0 mmol/litre (1.4–2.0 mEq/litre).

**Osmolality**. 270–295 mmol/kg of water.

**Paracetamol**. See Section 5.5
**Phenobarbitone**. Therapeutic range 80–120 μmol/litre (× 0.23 = mg/litre).
**Phenytoin**. Therapeutic range 40–80 μmol/litre (× 0.25 = mg/litre).
**Phosphate**. Birth 1.60–3.10 mmol/litre; 1 month–2 yr 1.3–2.4; >2 yr 1.1–1.8 (× 3.1 = mg/dl).
**Potassium**. Newborn 4.0–6.5 mmol/litre; 1 wk–3 months 4.0–6.2; 3 months–1 yr 3.7–5.6; >1 yr 3.7–5.2.
**Proteins**. Total protein: 0–6 months 45–75 g/litre; 6 months–2 yr 54–75 g/litre; >2 yr 55–80 g/litre. Albumin: 0–1 months 23–46 g/litre; 1 month–1 yr 30–48 g/litre; >1 yr 33–58 g/litre. Total globulins: 0–1 month 10–30 g/litre; 1 month–1 yr 13–28 g/litre; >1 yr 15–38 g/litre.

**Renin activity (plasma)**. <4 yr <10 ng/ml/h; 4–15 yr <6. Adult upright 0.9–4.5 ng/ml/h.

**Salicylate**. See Section 5.6.
**Serum glutamic oxaloacetic transaminase (SGOT)**. See Aspartate aminotransferase.
**Sodium**. Newborn 133–142 mmol/litre. Infant and older 135–145–mmol/litre.

**Theophylline**. Therapeutic range 55–110 μmol/litre (× 0.18 = mg/litre).
**Thiopentone**. Anaesthetic therapeutic range 150–200 μmol/litre.
**Thyroid function**:
**Thyroxine ($T_4$), total:**
days 2–3, 115–275 nmol/litre (= 9–22 μg/100 ml)
day 4–1 month, 100–245
1–4 months, 90–200
4–12 months, 70–165
>1 yr, 70–155

Thyroid-stimulating hormone (TSH):
1–3 days, <45 milliunits/litre
3–7 days, <25
>7 days, <5
Thyroxine-binding globulin (TBG):
Adult 10–30 mg/litre. Higher but ill-defined values in children.
Triiodothyronine ($T_3$):
Adults 1.4–3.5 nmol/litre (90–220 ng/100 ml). Values may be 10–15% higher in infants and early childhood.
Triiodothyronine resin uptake ($T_3RU$):
25–35%.
High $T_3RU$ suggests hyperthyroidism (or deficiency of TBG).
Low $T_3RU$ suggests hypothyroidism or high TBG (e.g. oestrogen therapy, pregnancy).

**Tobramycin**. Identical to gentamicin pharmacokinetics and range.

**Urea**. Newborn 2.9–10.0 mmol/litre (= 8–28 mg/100 ml as urea nitrogen); >1 month, <6.7 mmol/litre.

**Uric acid** (urate). 0.12–0.36 mmol/litre.

**Vancomycin**. Peak level 25–40 mg/litre through 5–10 mg/litre.

**Vitamins**:
Vitamin A, 1.0–3.0 µmol/litre.
Vitamin D, 25-hydroxy $D_3$ 20–80 nmol/litre (8–30 ng/ml); 1,25-dihydroxyvitamin D 40–140 pmol/litre.
Vitamin E, 7.0–12.0 µmol/litre (0.3–0.5 mg/100 ml).

**Zinc**. 10–22 µmol/litre (70–145 µg/100 ml).

## 3.5 Levels of immunoglobulins

The graphs in Figure 3.1 (p. 42) demonstrate the variations in immunoglobulin levels with age.

## 3.6 Growth charts

See Growth and Development Record charts (Figures 3.2–3.7, pp. 43–50).

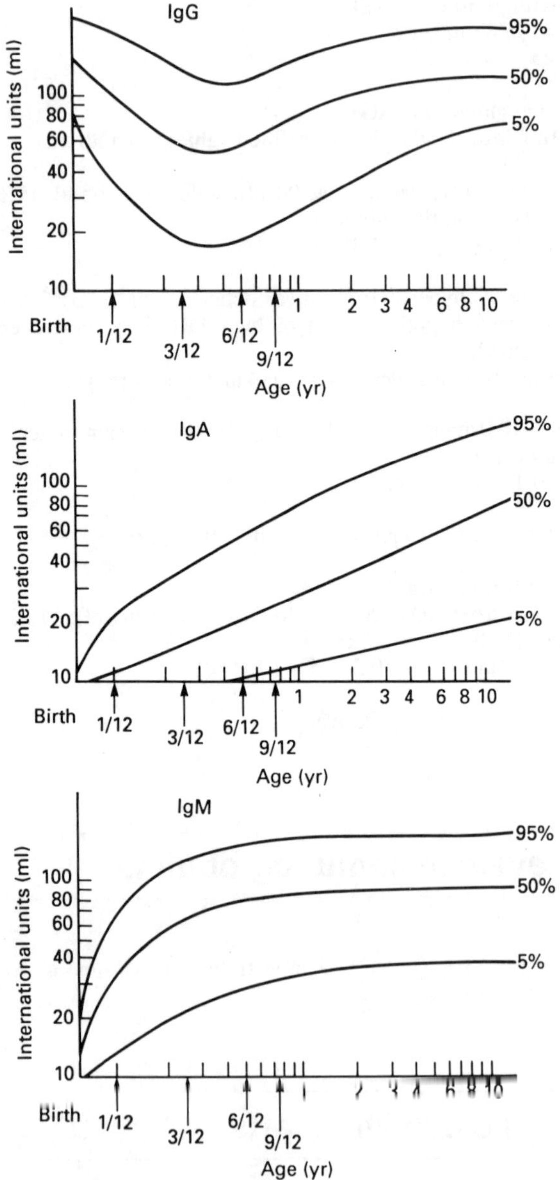


**Figure 3.1** Variations in serum immunoglobulin levels with age. The scales are logarithmic. 5th, 50th and 95th centiles are shown. Conversion factors of iu/ml to mg/100 ml are as follows: IgG 8.06 × iu/ml; IgA 1.42 × iu/ml; IgM 0.85 × iu/ml (From *The Paediatric Handbook* (1989) Royal Children's Hospital, Melbourne, with permission)

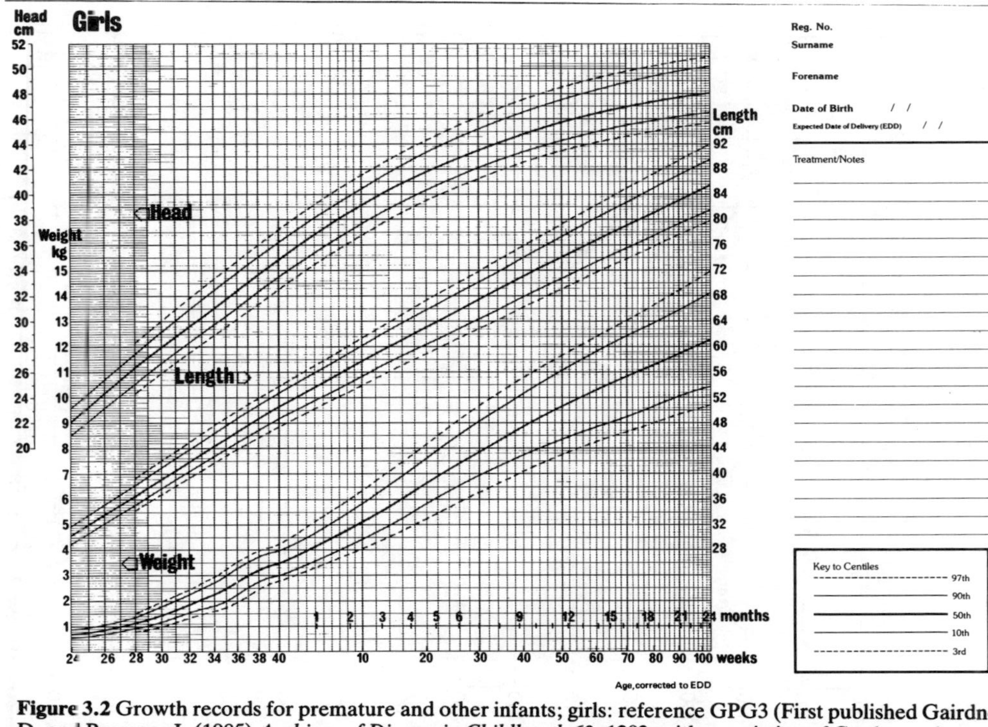


**Figure 3.2** Growth records for premature and other infants; girls: reference GPG3 (First published Gairdner, D. and Pearson, J. (1985) *Archives of Disease in Childhood,* **60**, 1202, with permission of Castlemead Publications, Ware)

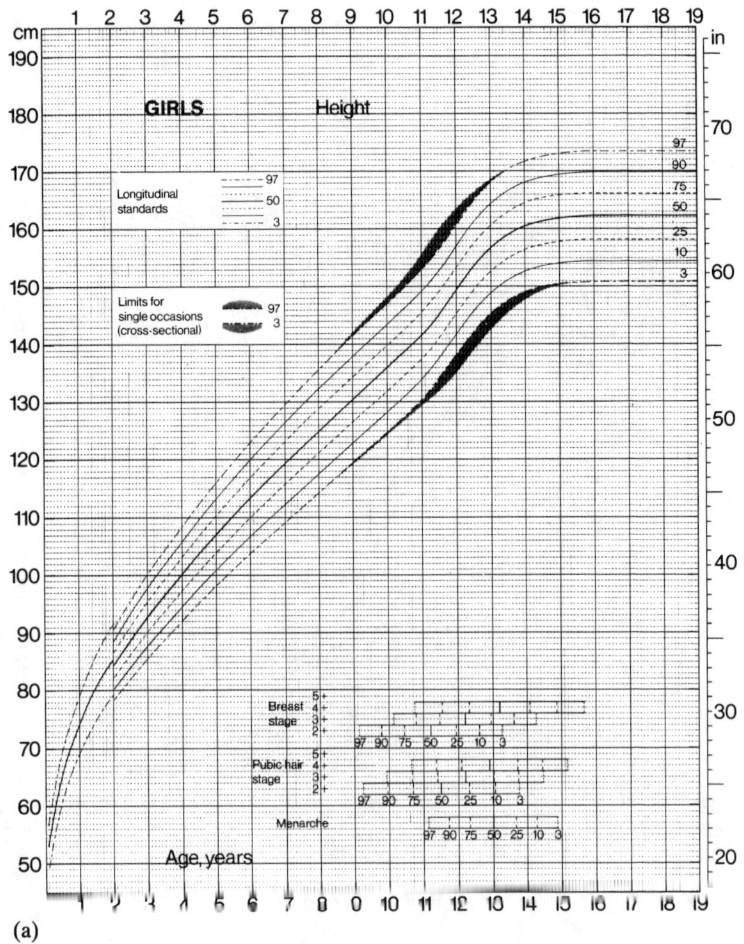


(a)

**Figure 3.3** Growth records for height (a) and weight (b) attained 0–19 years; girls: reference 12A (First published Tanner, J. M. and Whitehouse, R. H. (1975) *Archives of Disease in Childhood,* **51**, 170, with permission of Castlemead Publications, Ware)

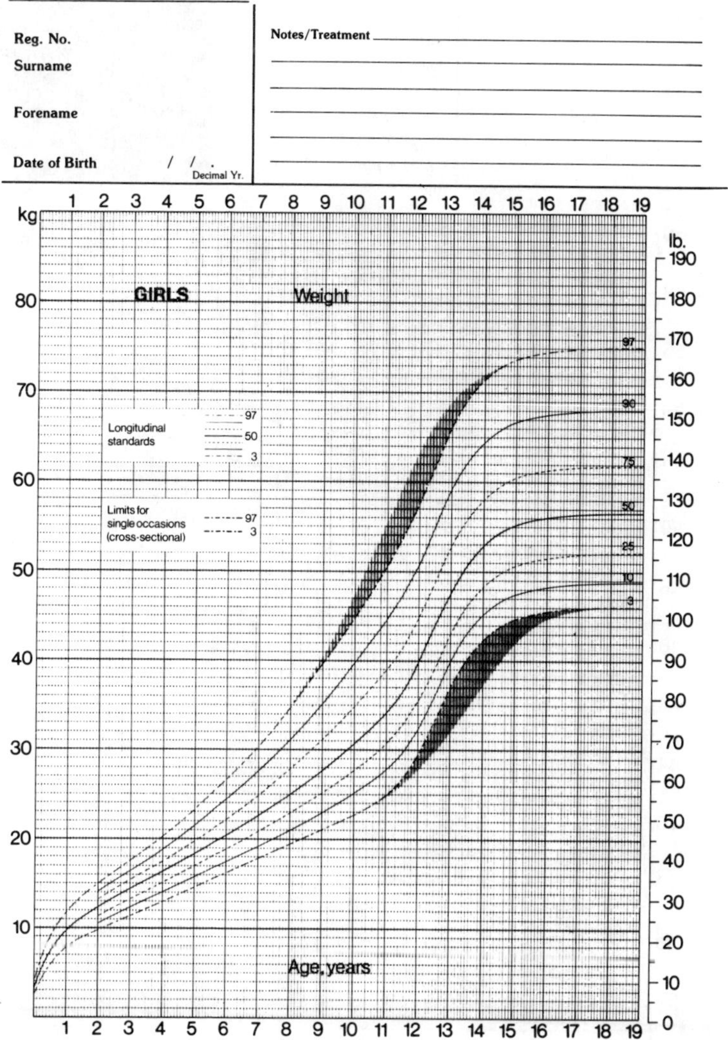
Reg. No.
Surname
Forename
Date of Birth / / .
Decimal Yr.
Notes/Treatment
GIRLS
Weight
Longitudinal standards
97
50
3
Limits for single occasions (cross-sectional)
97
3
Age, years
kg
lb.
97
90
75
50
25
10
3

(b)

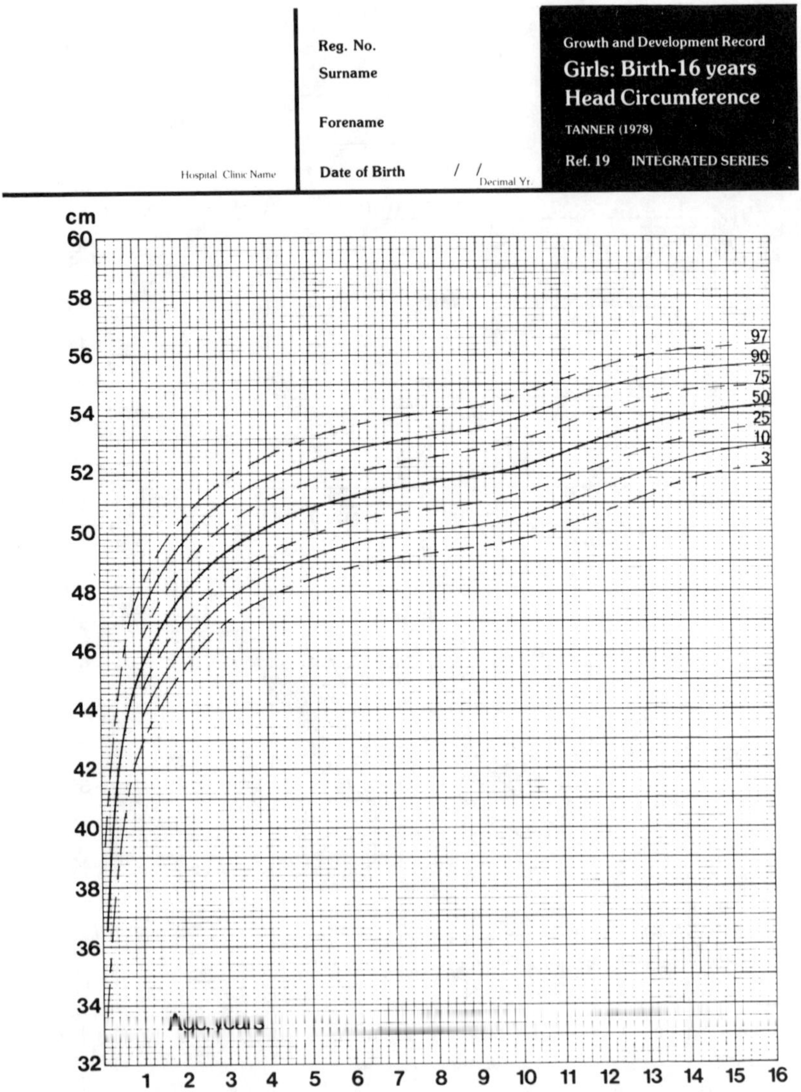

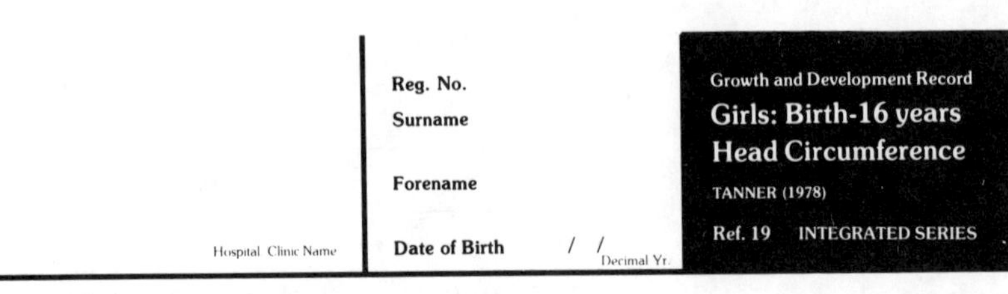


**Figure 3.4** Head circumference 0–16 years; girls: reference 19 (From Tanner, J. M. (1978) Physical growth and development. In *Textbook of Paediatrics* (eds Forfar, J. O. and Arneil, G. C.), with permission of Castlemead Publications, Ware)

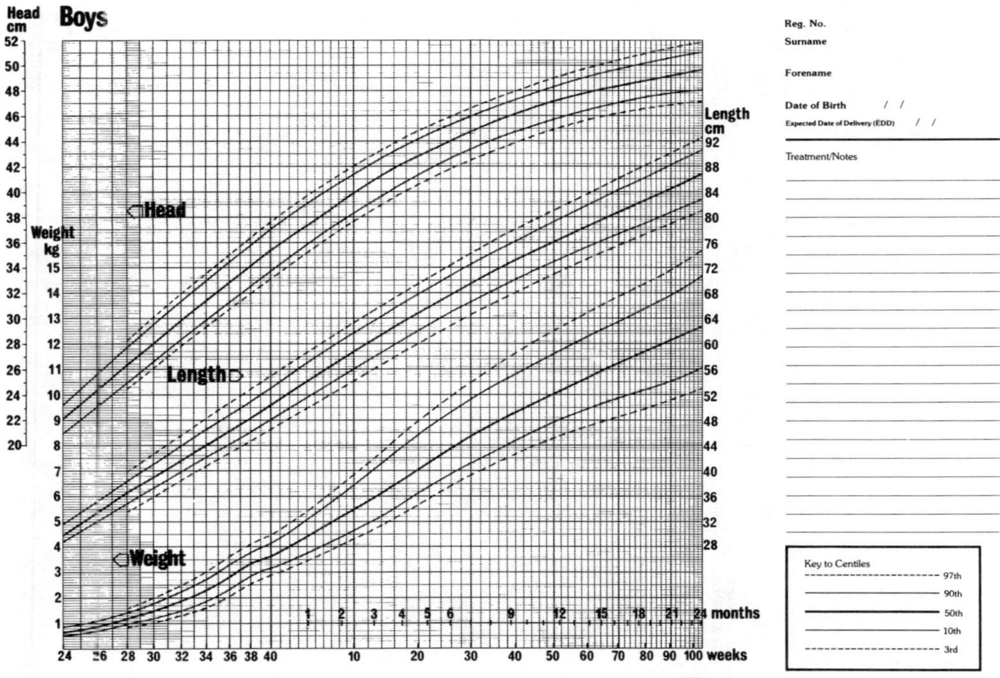


**Figure 3.5** Growth records for premature and other infants; boys: reference GPB3 (First published Gairdner, D. and Pearson, J. (1985) *Archives of Disease in Childhood*, **60**, 1202, with permission of Castlemead Publications, Ware)

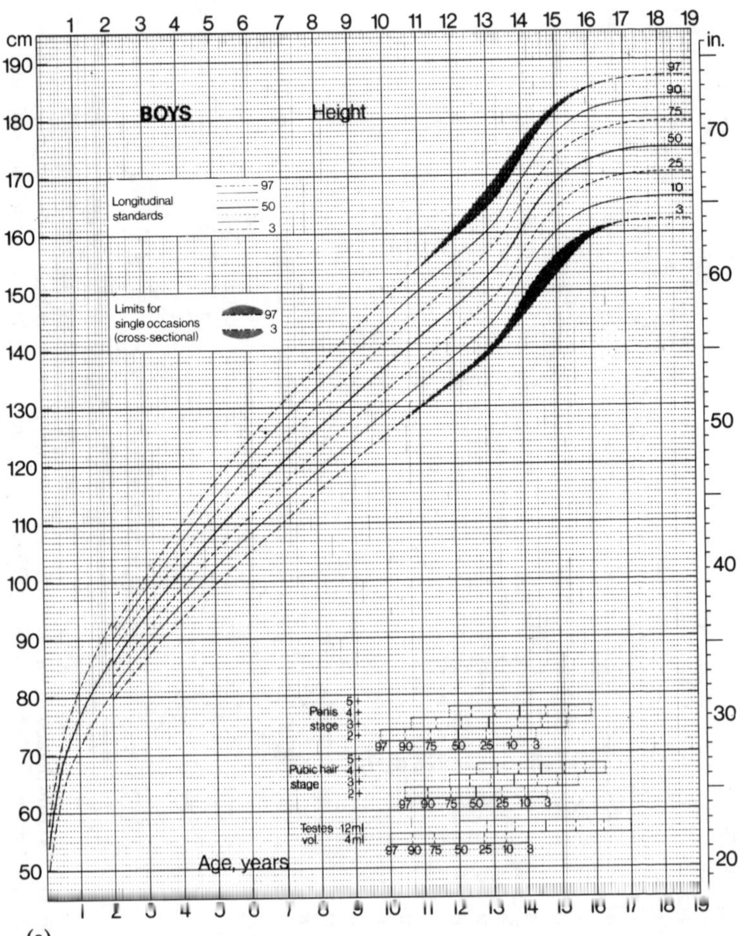


(a)

**Figure 3.6** Growth records for height (a) and weight (b) attained 0–19 years; boys: reference 11A (First published Tanner, J. M. and Whitehouse, R. H. (1975) *Archives of Disease in Childhood,* **51**, 170, with permission of Castlemead Publications, Ware)

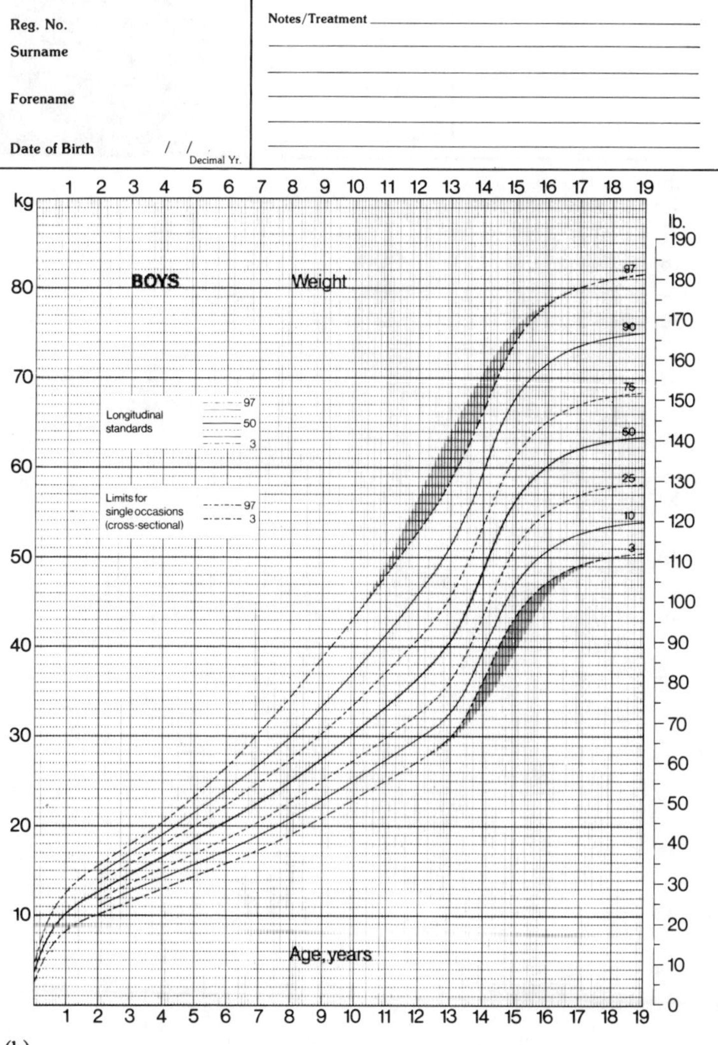
Reg. No.
Surname
Forename
Date of Birth
/ /
Decimal Yr.
Notes/Treatment
kg
lb.
BOYS
Weight
Longitudinal standards
97
50
3
Limits for single occasions (cross-sectional)
97
3
97
90
75
50
25
10
3
Age, years

(b)

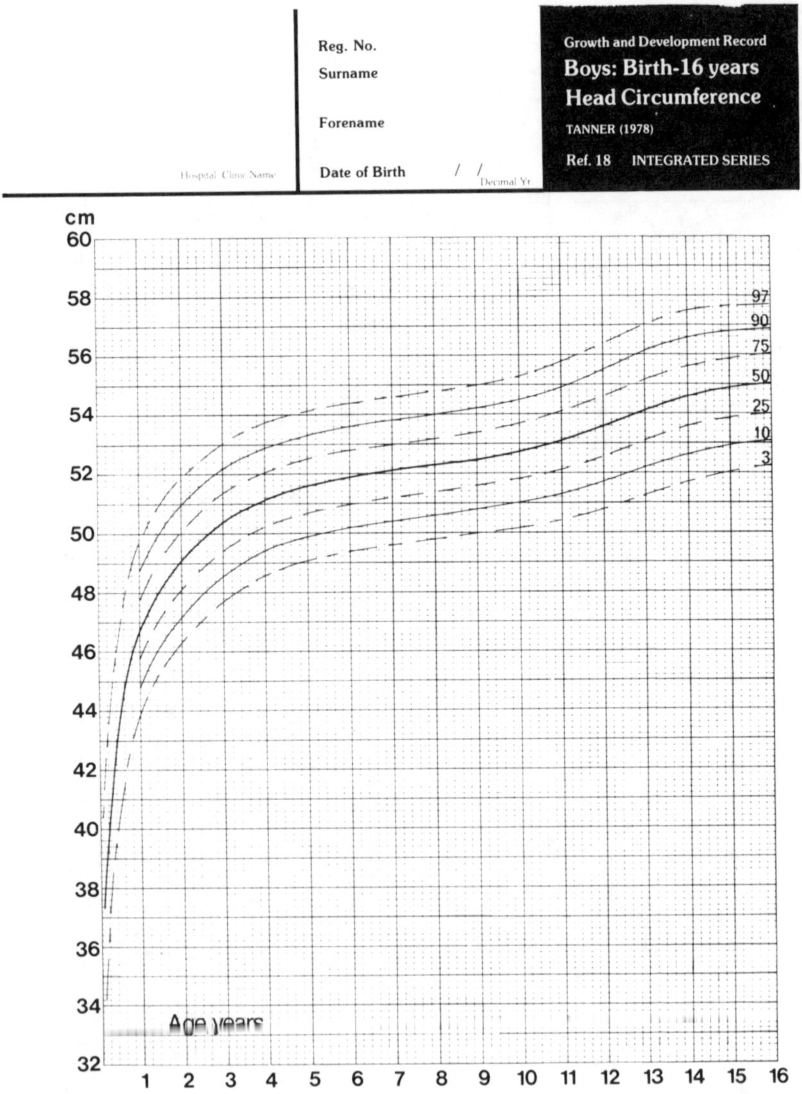

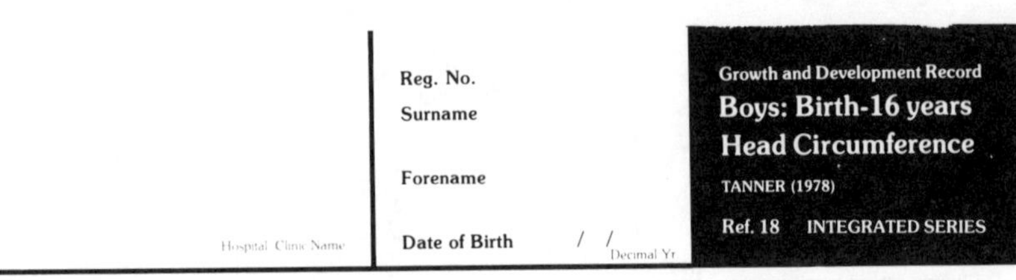


**Figure 3.7** Head circumference 0–16 years; boys: reference 18 (From Tanner, J. M. (1978) Physical growth and development. In *Textbook of Paediatrics* (eds Forfar, J. O. and Arneil, G. C.), with permission of Castlemead Publications, Ware)

## 3.7 Body surface area (SA)

The conventional way to assess SA is with a body surface area nomogram. SA is the point on the scale th̶at ̶ ̶rossed by a line joining height and weight (Figure 3.8, p. 54).

There are alternative ways ̶ which the approximate SA can be calculated:

$$1.\ \text{SA}\ (\text{m}^2) = \sqrt{\frac{\text{Height (cm)} \times \text{Weight (kg)}}{3600}}$$

(From Lam, T. K. and Leung, D. T. Y. (1988) *New Engl. J. Med.*, **318**, 1130)

$$2.\ \text{SA}\ (\text{m}^2) = \frac{[4 \times \text{Weight (kg)}] + 7}{\text{Weight (kg)} + 90}$$

## 3.8 Some developmental milestones

Table 3.2 may be used for very basic developmental assessment.

**Table 3.2 Screening of child development* (From the Denver Developmental Screening Test and the Royal Children's Hospital, Melbourne, Residents' Handbook, with permission)**

| *Age* | *Gross motor* | *Fine motor–adaptive* | *Language* | *Personal–social* |
|---|---|---|---|---|
| 1 M | Lifts head momentarily while prone (0–3 W) | Visual following to midline (0–5 W) | Alerts to sound | Watches face (0–4 W) |
| 2 M | Lifts head momentarily to erect position when sitting | Hands predominantly open | Vocalizes (0–7 W) | Smiles responsively (0–7 W) |
| 3 M | Lifts head to 90° while prone (0–10 W) | Visual following past midline (0–10 W) | Laughs (6–10 W) | |
| 4 M | Head steady when held erect (6–17 W) | Plays with hands together (6–15 W) | Goos and gurgles | Excited by approach of food |
| 5 M | No head lag when pulled to sitting (3–6 M)<br>Rolls over (2–5 M) | Grasps rattle (10–18 W)<br>Reaches for object with palmar grasp (3–5.5 M) | Squeals (6–18 W) | Smiles spontaneously (6W–5 M) |
| 6 M | Lifts head forward when pulled to sit (9–19 W) | Passes block hand to hand (4.5–7.5 M) | Turns to voice (3.5–8.5 M) | Friendly to all-comers |
| 8 M | Maintains sitting position without support (5–8 M) | Reaches well with either hand | Repetition of syllables, e.g. ba ba, Dada; waves bye bye | Feeds self biscuit; tries to get toy out of reach (5–9 M) |
| 10 M | Stands holding on (5–10 M) | Index finger approach | 'Mum', 'Dad' without meaning (6–10 M) | |

| | | | | |
|---|---|---|---|---|
| 12 M | Walks holding on to furniture (7.5–12.5 M) | Crude finger thumb grasp (7–11 M) | Imitates speech sounds (6–11 M) | Gives up toy |
| 15 M | Walks alone (11.5–15 M) | Neat pincer grasp of pellet (9–15 M) | 'Mum', 'Dad' with meaning | Indicates wants (10.5–14.5 M) |
| 1.5 Y | Walks well (11.5–18 M) | Tower of 2 blocks (12–20 M) | 3 words other than 'Mum', 'Dad' (12–20 M) | Drinks from cup (10–17 M) |
| 2 Y | Walks up steps without help (14–22 M) | Scribbles (12–24 M) | Points to one named body part (14–23 M) | Feeds self with spoon (12–24 M) |
| 2.5 Y | Throws ball (15–32 M) | Builds tower of 4 blocks (15–26 M) | Combines 2 words (14–27 M) | Helps in house – simple tasks (15–24 M) |
| 3 Y | Pedals tricycle (21 M–3 Y) | Imitates vertical line (18 M–3 Y) | Uses 4-word sentences | Puts on clothes (2–3 Y) |
| 4 Y | Balances on 1 foot (2.75–4.25 Y) | Copies square | Gives 1st and last name (2–4 Y) | Dresses with supervision (2.25–3.5 Y) |
| 5 Y | Hops on 1 foot (3–5 Y) | Draws man in 3 parts (3–5.5 Y) | Knows some colours (3–5 Y) | Dresses without supervision (2.5–5 Y)<br>Knows age |

* Figures in brackets indicate 25th–90th centiles; W = weeks, M = months, Y = years.

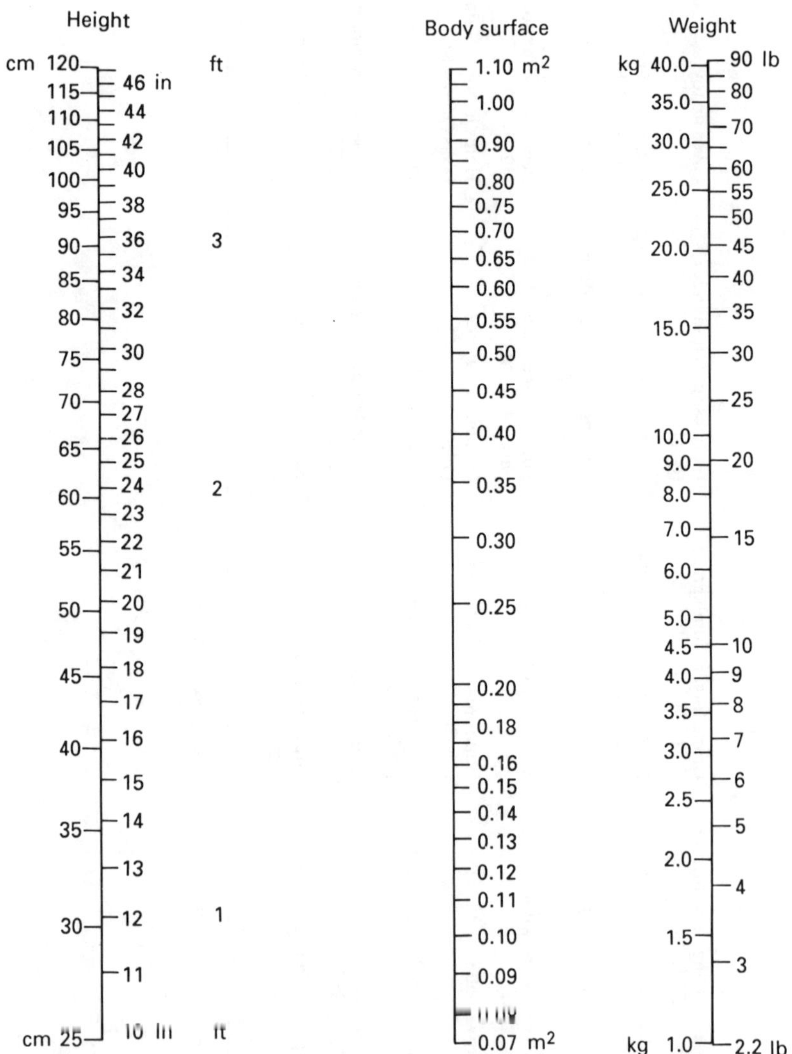


**Figure 3.8** Surface area nomogram. Body surface area may be calculated from the person's height and weight. Plot height and weight on the appropriate scale, and join them with a straight line. Surface area is the point at which this line intersects the central scale

Chapter 4

# Procedures

## 4.1 Measurement of blood pressure (BP)

The mercury sphygmomanometer is the most practical technique available. For young children, accurate recordings may only be possible with the Doppler ultrasound.

To cover the age range of 0–14 years one should have available a minimum of 3 cuffs; recommended bladder sizes are 4 × 13 cm, 8 × 18 cm and 12 × 35 cm (adult cuff). One should use the largest cuff width that covers the upper arm yet still allows the bell of the stethoscope to be placed over the brachial artery in the cubital fossa. The bladder should encircle the arm. If the cuff is too small, the blood pressure will be overstated. The child must be seated and at rest.

Measuring of systolic pressure is preferred because of its greater accuracy and consistency. The diastolic pressure is probably best identified from the Korotkoff phase IV (muffling) rather than phase V (disappearance).

Blood pressure centiles in children are given in Section 13.2. Children with increased height for age, and weight for age, tend to have higher BPs than their peers. Relating BP to height or weight may be more sensible than relating it to age.

### Further reading

De Swiet, M., Dillon, M. J., Littler, W. *et al.* (1989) Measurement of blood pressure in children. *Br. Med. J.*, **299**, 497

Dillon, M. J. (1988) Blood pressure. *Arch. Dis. Child.*, **63**, 347–349

## 4.2 Suprapubic aspiration (SPA) of urine

This technique is the best and most consistent way of collecting uncontaminated urine in suspected UTI. (N.B. Always have a sterile urine collection bottle open and ready during this procedure.) The child will often void spontaneously while the skin and equipment are being prepared, and thus a clean catch specimen may be obtained. The technique may be used on children <2 yr of age.

### EQUIPMENT

1. 23 G disposable needle fitted to a 2 ml syringe.
2. 70% alcohol skin preparation.

### METHOD

1. Have the child lying with his head on your right (for a right-handed practitioner).
2. Immobilize the child – an experienced assistant is invaluable.
3. Prepare the lower abdomen with alcohol.
4. Locate the symphysis pubis with your pronated left hand. The genitalia should be visible between your 2nd and 3rd fingers such that an imaginary straight line can be drawn to the umbilicus. This helps you remain in the midline.
5. With your right hand, insert needle into the skin crease 1–2 cm above the symphysis. The bladder is often a full needle length below the skin (only 1–2 cm in neonates).

- *Pay scrupulous attention to remaining in the midline.*

The needle must either be perpendicular or preferably aiming 10–20° cephalad (i.e. away from the pelvis). Gently aspirate on the syringe as the needle is plunged in; thus urine will be retrieved as soon as the bladder is entered.

## 4.3 Subdural tap

Subdural collections most commonly occur after meningitis or trauma. A subdural puncture is indicated for diagnostic, or if the child is symptomatic, for therapeutic purposes.

### METHOD

1. Immobilize the child by wrapping him in a sheet.
2. Shave anterior two-thirds of scalp.
3. Put on mask and sterile gloves. Prepare the skin with alcohol iodine.
4. Use a 21 Fr.g. butterfly or 20 Fr.g. lumbar puncture needle with stylet. The insertion site is the lateral angle of the anterior fontanelle at least 3 cm from the midline, or through the coronal suture.

5. Pointing the needle anteriorly, enter the skin obliquely, remaining in the sagittal plane (i.e. in the line of the ipsilateral eye), then advance horizontally aiming for the underside of the anterior rim of the fontanelle. If the needle abuts against bone, one can step the needle down a little deeper. At a depth of 0.5–1 cm the dura is penetrated with a recognizable 'pop'. *Do not go deeper than this.*
6. Fluid should flow passively. The needle may be rotated but do not aspirate fluid.
7. Send fluid for microscopy, culture, protein.

Fifteen ml per side may be removed daily. Most collections resolve within 2 weeks.

## 4.4 Ketamine anaesthesia/analgesia

Ketamine is a profound analgesic/anaesthetic/amnesic which preserves airway reflexes and does not affect hypercarbic or hypoxic respiratory drive when used in appropriate doses.

### SIDE EFFECTS

Increased salivation; emergence delirium, hallucinations; hypertension; rarely – laryngospasm, aspiration of gastric contents.

### CONTRAINDICATIONS

Possible raised intracranial pressure; patient not fasted for >4 h (a relative contraindication); hypertension; stridor.

### USES

It may be of use for painful procedures or where a child is required to remain still, e.g. setting a fracture, manual faecal evacuation, bone marrow aspiration, renal biopsy.

### METHOD

#### *1 Prepare and check*

Suction catheter, $O_2$ source, bag and mask, intubation equipment.

#### *2 Inject ketamine*

1–2 mg/kg IV or 4–6 mg/kg IM. Give further 1 mg/kg aliquots IV as required. Many also give atropine 0.01 mg IV/IM with induction to reduce salivation.

### *3 Diazepam (optional)*

As the procedure finishes, administer diazepam 0.1 mg/kg IV (not IM). Minimizes emergence delirium.

### *4 Quiet recovery*

Allow recovery in a very quiet undisturbed environment, preferably with parent at the bedside.

---

# 4.5 Central venous cannulation

---

Insertion of a central venous catheter (CVC) is needed for measurement of right atrial pressure, administration of certain drugs (e.g. dopamine), or where peripheral venous access cannot be found. Ideally, all central venous cannulation should be done under strictly sterile conditions, by someone with experience in the endeavour. In dire situations one may have to attempt central cannulation before experienced help arrives and without the best possible cannula.

## *Possible sites*

### FEMORAL VEIN

This lies medial to the femoral artery (the femoral nerve lies lateral to the artery). It is a reliable and reasonably safe method, if the femoral arterial pulse can be palpated and used as a landmark.

#### *1 Complications*

**1.1 Faecal contamination** The sterility of inguinal skin is difficult to maintain.

**1.2 Septic arthritis of the hip** Small risk.

#### *2 Method*

Prepare skin with alcohol/iodine (wash it off later). Have hips in 30–45° of flexion and maximum abduction. Palpate the femoral artery, and leave finger on the pulse. Insert cannula 0.5–1 cm medial to the artery.

### INTERNAL JUGULAR VEIN

The following method is much safer and more successful than any of the approaches to the subclavian vein. It uses the Seldinger wire technique of venous cannulation. The technique should not be used in those with compromised haemostasis.

### *1 Preparation*

For children under 4 years some suggested catheters are: Vygon Leader Cath, 20 G 8 cm catheter, serial no. 115.09; Viggo Secalon Hydrocath SLR kit, 22 G 10 cm catheter, article no. 7520-0; Viggo Double Lumen Cath 18 G × 16 cm (20 G, 22 G), no. 7560-6.
Alcoholic iodine solution to skin (must be washed off later).
Gown and glove.
Sedation and/or local anaesthetic if child is conscious. Attempts at cannulation in a restless child are dangerous.
1 × 2 ml syringe – empty.
1 × 2 ml syringe – fill with normal or heparinized saline.

### *2 Method – sternomastoid triangle approach*

Position – 15° head-down tilt and have a rolled-up towel under the shoulders to extend the neck.
Attempt right side first, i.e. head turned to the left.
Find the triangle bounded by sternal and clavicular heads of sternomastoid and the clavicle (Figure 4.1).

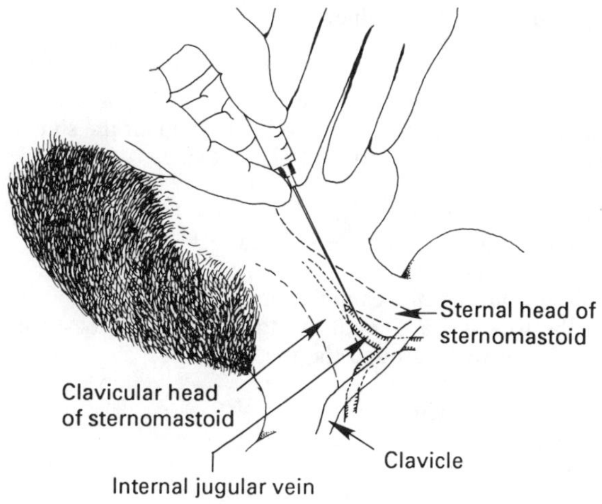


**Figure 4.1** Insertion of internal jugular venous catheter

Fix empty syringe onto the needle provided.
Insert needle into the *apex* of the triangle, at an angle of 20–40° to the surface.
While gently aspirating on the syringe, advance the needle caudally and laterally, aiming for the nipple, to puncture the internal jugular vein. *Do not advance more than 2 cm.*
When blood flashes back, take syringe off the needle and let blood dribble out.

Insert Seldinger wire (firm end).
Withdraw needle over the wire.
Insert cannula over the wire – you may first have to make a small nick in the skin.
Draw blood back and flush with saline.
Stitch the cannula at the skin insertion and then thread the stitch through the eye of the fixation wings of the cannula and tie that as well.
CXR – check CVC position.

*3 Complications*

There is a small risk of pneumothorax if one inserts the needle more than 1.5–2 cm. Inadvertent puncture of the carotid artery should be managed with firm pressure on only one side of the neck.

### EXTERNAL JUGULAR VEIN

*1 Preparation*

Central venous catheter – as for internal jugular vein.
Short 22 G IV cannula.
2 × 2 ml syringe, one filled with saline.
A syringe with local anaesthetic.

*2 Method*

Position – 15° head-down tilt, rolled-up towel placed under the shoulders so as to extend neck; head turned to contralateral side.
Gown and glove.
Alcoholic iodine skin preparation.
Local anaesthetic if child not otherwise sedated.
Insert short 22 G cannula into vein.
Insert Seldinger wire through the cannula, floppy end first.
Alternatively if the wire has a 'J' end, use that. This is the best way of negotiating the difficult route around the first rib.
Withdraw short cannula.
Insert CVC over Seldinger wire.
Withdraw Seldinger wire.
CXR – check CVC position.

## 4.6 Intraosseous fluids and drugs

In some circumstances it is impossible to get adequate venous access (e.g. burns, severe dehydration, cardiopulmonary resuscitation). Intraosseous (IO) fluids may be given until adequate venous access is secured. Drugs may be given at the same dose and fluids given at the same rate, as by the intravenous (IV) route. Drug concentrations achieved after IO injection are comparable to those after IV for adrenaline, atropine, bicarbonate, diazepam, phenobarbitone, calcium chloride and lignocaine.

### *1 Child<3 years*

Use a 20 G lumbar puncture (LP) needle and stylet.
Insert needle into the flat anteromedial aspect of upper third of tibia *or* lower and middle third of femur. Angle the needle away from the knee.

### *2 Child>3 years*

Use 16–18 G LP needle or any available bone marrow aspirate needle and stylet. Insert into posterior or anterior iliac crest.

Successful entry into the medullary cavity is suggested by: resistance suddenly overcome, signifying the needle passing through the cortex; the needle stands up without support; successful aspiration of bone marrow via the needle; and free flowing infusion without obvious subcutaneous swelling.

Disposable intraosseous infusion trocar and cannula are made by the Cook Group. Addresses: 12 Electronics St, Brisbane 4113, Australia (tel. 07 8411188); Sandet 6 DK4632, Bjaeverskov, Denmark (tel. 45 3-671133); POB 489 Bloomington IN 47402, USA (tel. 800 4574500).
Suggested specification: order number prefix C-DIN, gauge 14 or 18, length 4.0 cm, needle point T45 (written as order no. C-DIN 14-4.0-T45).

## Further reading

Andropoulos, D. B., Soifer, S. J. and Schreiber, M. D. (1990) Plasma epinephrine concentrations after intraosseous and central venous injection during cardiopulmonary resuscitation in the lamb. *J. Pediatr.*, **116**, 312–315

Orlowski, J. P., Porembka, D. T., Gallagher, J. M., Lockrem, J. D. and Van Lente, F. (1990) Comparison study of intraosseous, central intravenous and peripheral intravenous infusions of emergency drugs. *Am. J. Dis. Child.*, **144**, 112–115

Spivey, W. H. (1987) Intraosseous infusions. *J. Pediatr.*, **111**, 639–643

# 4.7 Intravenous puncture and cannulation

Venepuncture in children is similar to that in adults, but the child may need to be held more firmly. The usual sites are veins of the antecubital fossa, and dorsum of hand and foot. In difficult cases one can usually insert a broken-off bevelled needle into a small vein on the anterior aspect of the wrist, and allow blood to drip into the laboratory tube. Alternatively, puncturing the external jugular vein is relatively easy. The vein is usually found with ease if the child is crying and is laid flat or with slight head-down tilt, with head turned to one side. Femoral venepuncture carries a significant risk and should not be used.

Following venepuncture in the antecubital fossa, it is best to leave the arm extended (± raised above the head) and apply direct pressure with a cotton ball. Flexing the elbow increases bruising (Dyson, A. and Bogod, D. (1987) *Br. Med. J.*, **294**, 1659).

Insertion of intravenous catheters in children differs from that in adults in that the child is more likely to move at the time of insertion, and more likely to attempt to remove the catheter once it is in position. Using local anaesthetic for difficult insertions renders the child less likely to move at a crucial time. Firm strapping of the IV is important, and the terminal portion of the tubing should have a 'U' bend in it, so that in the event of the child tugging at the tubing the slack in the 'U' will be taken up in preference to the catheter being pulled out. In addition to the sites used in adults, consider veins of the dorsum of the foot and the scalp. If using the latter, shave a generous area of hair, be sure that the selected vessel has no palpable pulse, and immobilize the cannula with plaster of Paris or strapping secured to scalp which is treated with an application of tincture of benzine.

## 4.8 Local anaesthetic creams

Eutectic ('melting readily') lignocaine-prilocaine (EMLA) cream produces effective topical dermal anaesthesia for procedures such as arterial or venepuncture, lumbar puncture and split skin graft. The cream is applied under occlusive plastic dressing ('cling film'). It must usually be applied for 60 min to be effective, although in children aged 1–5 years, 30 min may be sufficient. Topical anaesthesia persists for at least 1 h after removing the cream.

### COMPLICATIONS

The total concentration of local anaesthetic is less than 5%. Systemic absorption of lignocaine and prilocaine is negligible when applied to intact skin. Local reactions are uncommon and include blanching, erythema and mild local oedema. Neither local nor systemic allergic reactions have been reported. There has been one report of methaemoglobinaemia in a 12-week-old infant who was also receiving cotrimoxazole.

### Further reading

Hanks, G. W. and White, I. (1988) Local anaesthetic creams. *Br. Med. J.*, **297**, 1215–1216

Chapter 5

# Poisoning

## 5.1 General concepts

In the UK it is always possible to obtain advice on known or unknown poisons from: National Poisons Centre, Guy's Hospital, London (tel. 071-635-9191 or 071-407-7600).

In Australia, advice is always available from: Poisons Information Centre, Royal Children's Hospital, Melbourne (tel. 03-345-5678 or 008-133-890).

Children under 5 yr account for 70% of cases of poison ingestion; however, the morbidity and mortality are low. In children, the ingestion is usually accidental and involves household products, over-the-counter medication, plants and cosmetics. In adolescents, the ingestion is frequently a suicide gesture or attempt and usually involves one or more prescription or non-prescription drugs.

### CLINICAL APPROACH TO THE POISONED CHILD

#### *1 Immediate evaluation*

Respiratory failure, hypotension and seizures are the most common life-threatening complications encountered. Assessment of these must precede any diagnostic or therapeutic endeavours.

**1.1 Respiratory** Maintain airway patency: extend the neck, pull the jaw forward, lie the child in the 'coma' position.
Hypoventilation or coma: endotracheal intubation by a skilled anaesthetist with 'crash induction' (preoxygenation, cricoid pressure, suxamethonium and atropine).

**1.2 Cardiovascular** Hypotension: usually due to hypovolaemia secondary to vasodilatation or capillary leak. Responds to IV normal saline 10–20 ml/kg bolus. Occasionally inotropic support is needed with dopamine 5–10 μg/kg/min.
Arrhythmias: detected by continuous cardiac monitoring which can be done in a general ward if the child is otherwise well.

**1.3 Neurological** Seizures: may be due to drug toxicity, hypotension, hypoglycaemia, hypoxia, or electrolyte disturbance.

### *2 Identify the poison*

It is often easy to elucidate from family and friends which poison a young child might have taken. An adolescent may falsify a history or be incoherent. The maximum possible amount of ingestion must be assiduously explored. In the absence of a satisfactory history, physical examination can provide valuable clues (Tables 5.1 and 5.2).

## RAPID LABORATORY AIDS TO DIAGNOSIS

### *1 Collect blood and first voided urine specimen* – for drug screen and quantitative analysis

Indicate time of collection and list all suspected poisons. Send to a drug assay laboratory and notify them personally.

### *2 Increased anion gap, metabolic acidosis*

Alcohols, ethylene glycol, salicylates, iron, cyanide, paraldehyde.

Anion gap = $Na^+ - (HCO_3^- + Cl^-)$. Normally <12 mmol/litre

### *3 Increased osmolar gap*

Alcohols, glycols.

$$\text{Calculated serum osmolality} = (2 \times Na^+) + \text{Urea} + \text{Glucose}$$

Osmolar gap is when there is a large difference between measured and calculated osmolality, indicating the presence of a significant amount of a small molecular weight osmotically active compound.

### *4 Blood sugar*

Hypoglycaemia – ethanol, paracetamol, salicylates, oral hypoglycaemic agents.
Hyperglycaemia – salicylates, organophosphates, iron.

### *5 Urinary ketones*

Ethanol, salicylates.

### *6 Decreased Hb saturation* (measured not calculated)

In the presence of normal measured $Pa_{O_2}$ it suggests CO poisoning, methaemoglobinaemia (nitrates, nitrites).

## TREATMENT

### *1 Removal of poison*

**1.1 Emesis** Used if child is alert and has intact gag reflex. Use it as soon as possible after the poisoning, but may be tried even 12 h or more

**Table 5.1 Common symptoms and signs of poisoning**

*1. Inspect*

1.1. Odour of breath:

| | |
|---|---|
| Bitter almond | Cyanide |
| Coal or gas | Carbon monoxide |
| Garlic | Organophosphates, arsenic |
| Alcohol | Ethanol, methanol |
| Pear | Chloral hydrate |
| Others – petrochemicals | |

1.2. Skin:

Cyanosis in 100% $O_2$ (methaemoglobinaemia) – nitrates, nitrobenzene, aniline dyes
Red flush – CO, cyanide, anticholinergics
Sweating – amphetamines, organophosphates, LSD, cocaine
Jaundice – paracetamol, $CCl_4$, iron
Purpura – aspirin, warfarin, snake bite

*2. Temperature*

Hypothermia – hypnotics, ethanol, CO, phenothiazines
Hyperthermia – anticholinergics, salicylates, TCA

*3. Mucous membranes*

Dry – anticholinergics (antimuscarinic), antihistamines
Excess salivation – organophosphates
Oral lesions – corrosives, paraquat

*4. Cardiovascular system*

Hypotension – opiates, hypnotics, TCA, phenothiazines, antihypertensives, iron
Hypertension – sympathomimetics (found in some cold remedies), organophosphates, amphetamine
Arrhythmia – digoxin, TCA
Bradycardia – digoxin, beta-blockers
Tachycardia – TCA, theophylline, sympathomimetics, cocaine, amphetamines

*5. Respiration*

Hypoventilation – most CNS depressants, e.g. narcotics, barbiturates, hypnotics
Hyperventilation – salicylates, CO
Kussmaul – salicylates
Wheezing – organophosphates
Pneumonia – inhalation, ?hydrocarbons
Pulmonary oedema – aspiration, salicylates

*6. CNS*

Coma – sedative/hypnotics, TCA, alcohol, anticholinergics, narcotics, CO, salicylates, organophosphates, anticonvulsant, phenothiazines
Seizures – TCA, amphetamines, organophosphates, lead, phenothiazines, salicylates, lignocaine
Hallucinations – anticholinergics, psychotropic drugs, amphetamines, camphor, TCA, psychoactive mushrooms
Pupil meiosis – narcotics (not lomotil), organophosphates, parasympathomimetics
Pupil mydriasis – anticholinergics, sympathomimetics, TCA
Hypertonicity, myoclonus, rigidity – phenothiazines/antiemetics, anticholinergics
Delirium – anticholinergics, phenothiazines, sympathomimetics, LSD, marijuana, cocaine, heavy metals
Weakness, paralysis – organophosphates, carbamates, heavy metals
Tinnitus – salicylates, quinines, ergot

*7. GIT*

Vomit, diarrhoea, abdominal pain – iron, organophosphates, heavy metals

TCA, tricyclic antidepressants.

**Table 5.2 Toxidromes (After Mofensen, N. C. and Greensher, J. (1974) *J. Pediatr.*, 54, 337, with permission)**

| *Drug involved* | *Clinical manifestations* |
|---|---|
| ANTICHOLINERGICS<br>Atropine, scopolamine, TCA, phenothiazines, antihistamines, hallucinogenic mushrooms | Agitation, hallucination, dystonic/ extrapyramidal movements, mydriasis, warm dry skin, dry mouth, tachycardia, decreased bowel sounds, urinary retention |
| CHOLINERGICS<br>Organophosphates and carbamate insecticides | Salivation, lacrimation, urination, defaecation, nausea and vomit, sweating, meiosis, wheezing, weakness, confusion, coma, fasciculation |
| SEDATIVE/HYPNOTICS | Coma, hypothermia, drowsiness, shallow breathing, hypotension |
| TRICYCLIC ANTIDEPRESSANTS | Coma, arrhythmia, convulsions, anticholinergic effects |
| OPIATES | Slow respiration, bradycardia, hypotension, meiosis, pulmonary oedema, seizures |
| SALICYLATES | Vomit, fever, hyperpnoea, lethargy, coma |
| PHENOTHIAZINES | Hypotension, tachycardia, dystonic reactions including oculogyric crisis and trismus, anticholinergic effects |
| SYMPATHOMIMETICS<br>Amphetamines, caffeine, ephedrine cocaine, aminophylline | Tachycardia, delirium, nausea, abdominal pain, pilo-erection. |

TCA, tricyclic antidepressants.

post-ingestion if there is a possibility of delayed gastric emptying (tricyclic antidepressants, opiates) or delayed gastric release of the substance (iron, salicylates, carbamazepine).

Syrup of ipecac (ipecacuanha)

*1.1.1 Dose* 6–12 months 10 ml (×1 only); 1–2 yr 15 ml; 2–3 yr 20 ml; 3–4 yr 25 ml; >4 yr 30 ml. Forcing additional fluids does not shorten the time to, nor increase the volume of, emesis (*J. Pediatr.* (1987) **110**, 970–972). Repeat dose if no emesis ensues after 30 min

*1.1.2 Contraindications* Caustic or hydrocarbon ingestion, seizures, coma.

*1.1.3 Side effects* None if used as above. Overdose causes severe vomiting, diarrhoea, hypotension, arrhythmias, tremor, seizures.

**1.2 Gastric lavage** Used when ipecac fails to induce emesis, where there is fear of a rapid decline in conscious state, or in the comatose patient (who must first have an endotracheal tube inserted).

*1.2.1 Method* Choose an orogastric tube with an internal diameter approximately that of the child's little finger (8–12 G). Measure the approximate distance from mouth to stomach. Insert orogastric tube, saving the first aspirate for toxicology. With child in left lateral position, and head down, aspirate stomach, and lavage with 10 ml/kg aliquots of tap water at body temperature, until aspirate is clear. On completion, leave first dose of activated charcoal in stomach (not in paracetamol poisoning) and remove the tube, having first clamped it to minimize risk of aspiration.

**1.3 Activated charcoal** Has a surface area of approximately 1000–2500 $m^2$/g. It forms a stable complex with the ingested poison, thus preventing absorption. It can also interrupt the enterohepatic and enterogastric circulation of drugs by holding onto the drugs secreted into the bowel lumen and forcing their excretion in faeces, and it may attract certain drugs from the circulation back into the gastrointestinal tract (GIT dialysis).

*1.3.1 Dose* 1 g/kg – usually via NGT. Wait 30–45 min following ipecac before giving it. It may subsequently be repeated hourly at 0.25 g/kg, especially for poisoning with digoxin, digitoxin, theophylline, phenobarbitone or carbamazepine.

*1.3.2 Contraindications* Ingestion of caustic agents, hydrocarbons, metals (iron, lead), alcohols. If an oral antidote is to be given (e.g. paracetamol poisoning), charcoal is relatively contraindicated, although giving a higher dose of antidote may compensate adequately.

*1.3.3 Indication* Almost all potentially serious overdoses except those mentioned above. A comprehensive list of its use against specific drugs and chemicals can be found in Boehnert *et al.* (1985).

*1.3.4 Side effects* Hypernatraemia – very rare (*J. Pediatr.* (1986) **109**, 719–722; also *Lancet* (1988) **i**, 1220). Charcoal may contain 18 mmol $Na^+$ per 5 g. Aspiration (*Ann. Emerg. Med.* (1981) **10**, 528) – this should not occur if the airway is protected (see above).

## 2 Enhanced excretion

**2.1 Activated charcoal** Gastrointestinal dialysis.

**2.2 Forced diuresis** Useful for drugs that are renally excreted if they are not highly protein bound.

**2.3 Altering urine pH** The pK of a drug and pH of a solution determine the proportion of ionized and un-ionized drug within that solution. An ionized drug can be 'trapped' in the urine and excreted, e.g. the pK of aspirin is 3. At a pH of 3, the ratio of ionized:un-ionized is 1:1. At pH 7.4, it is 25000:1. Drugs with a pK of 3–7.2 (salicylates, phenobarbitone, isoniazid) benefit from urinary alkalinization. Use 20–30 mmol of bicarbonate per 500 ml of IV fluid run at daily maintenance rates. Potassium supplements may be needed. Drugs with a pK of 7.2–9.5 (amphetamines, quinidine) benefit from urine acidification with oral ascorbic acid or oral/IV ammonium chloride (dangerous in renal or liver failure).

The following treatments have their uses, but will not be discussed:

1. Peritoneal dialysis and haemodialysis.
2. Exchange transfusion.
3. Plasmapheresis.
4. Drug antibodies (see Section 5.9).
5. Charcoal haemoperfusion.

### *3 Antidotes*

There is no universally accepted classification of antidotes. They may include agents that alter the biochemical impact of the poison such as *N*-acetylcysteine; pharmacological agonists or antagonists such as naloxone; substances that increase drug elimination such as fluids and bicarbonate in salicylate poisoning; chelating agents that bind toxins such as desferrioxamine for iron, EDTA for lead.

## DELIBERATE SELF-POISONING

The term 'parasuicide' has been applied to those with non-lethal motives who overdose in an attempt to attract the attention of and communicate with relatives and friends. A suicide attempt on the other hand implies deliberate lethal intent. In children, the distinction between the two is blurred and motives are often mixed. There is a strong association between deliberate self-poisoning and major family breakdown, psychiatric disorders in the individual or those around them, and sexual and physical abuse, such that many of these children would still need treatment even if they had never attempted to injure themselves. It makes sense to refer all cases of deliberate self-poisoning to counselling services.

## Further reading

Bateman, D. N. (1988) Adverse reactions to antidotes. *Adverse Dr. React. Bull.*, **133**, 496–499

Boehnert, M. T., Lewander, W. J., Gaudreault, P. and Lovejoy, F. H. (1985) Advances in clinical toxicology. *Pediatr. Clin. N. Am.*, **32**, 193–211

Clarke, C. F. (1988) Deliberate self poisoning in adolescents. *Arch. Dis. Child*, **63**, 1479–1483

Hepler, B., Sutheimer, C. and Sunshine, I. (1986) Role of the toxicology laboratory in suspected ingestions. *Pediatr. Clin. N. Am.*, **33**, 245–260

Rogers, G. C. and Matyunas, N. J. (1986) Gastrointestinal decontamination for acute poisoning. *Pediatr. Clin. N. Am.*, **33**, 261–286

Taylor, E. (1985) Physiological management of overdose in young people. *Arch. Dis. Child.*, **60**, 791–793

Vale, J. A., Meredith, T. J. and Proudfoot, A. T. (1986) Syrup of ipecacuanha: is it really useful? *Br. Med. J.*, **293**, 1321

## 5.2 Acute carbon monoxide (CO) poisoning

This is the main cause of paediatric death from poisoning in the UK. CO is a tasteless, colourless, odourless, non-irritating gas. Normal endogenous production saturates 0.4–0.7% of the body's haemoglobin and one's environment (urban dwellings, parents who smoke) may saturate up to 6%.

CO has a very high affinity for Hb and combines with it to form carboxyhaemoglobin, thus reducing the $O_2$ carrying capacity of the blood and shifting the oxygen dissociation curve to the left. CO also inhibits cellular respiration by reversibly binding to haem proteins, especially cytochrome oxidase. Hyperbaric oxygen therapy (HBOT) will replace carboxyhaemoglobin with oxy-Hb, increase the amount of dissolved plasma $O_2$ available to tissues, and reduce cerebral oedema. However, even in the presence of normal carboxy-Hb levels, there are numerous reports of dramatic resolution of neurological sequelae of CO poisoning with HBOT up to 3 weeks post-exposure. There is good evidence that HBOT reactivates the cytochrome oxygen system and thus prevents the formation of toxic free radicals which do harm long after the CO has been eliminated from the body. The traditional view that the pathophysiology of CO poisoning is solely related to low oxygen transport does not explain why symptoms, signs and outcome bear little relationship to the degree of CO saturation at the time of presentation, and why HBOT can result in dramatic resolution of symptoms long after carboxy-Hb levels have returned to normal.

### COMMON SOURCES OF POISONING

Car exhaust fumes, poorly ventilated heating systems, smoke from all types of fires, household gas (coal, not natural). Inhalation of methylene chloride (paint strippers).

## CLINICAL FEATURES

Headache, shortness of breath, diarrhoea, coma, convulsions, disorientation, weakness, cardiorespiratory arrest. Examination may show cutaneous erythema, oedema, blistering. Cherry red skin colour is uncommon.

## DIAGNOSIS

Inspect blood – chocolate brown colour. Measure percentage of carboxyhaemoglobin – this cannot be estimated by pulse oximetry or conventional blood gas analysis. Less than 10% is not usually associated with symptoms.

N.B. Fire victims should also have thiocyanate levels monitored because of the possibility of cyanide poisoning (Stevenson, R. N. *et al.* (1988) *Lancet,* **ii**, 1145).

## TREATMENT

### *1 100% $O_2$*

Use if the child is neurologically normal and if carboxy-Hb level is <40%. It will reduce the half-life of CO-Hb from 5–6 h to 1 h.

### *2 Hyperbaric oxygen*

The indications for *early* use are:

All who have been or are unconscious.
Any neurological features except headache or nausea.
Carboxy-Hb level of >40% at presentation.
Whenever CO poisoning symptoms recur.
N.B. *It should be used in comatose children even if they present late or if carboxyhaemoglobin levels are normal or approaching normality.*

Information about hyperbaric facilities in the UK can be obtained from Duty Diving Medical Officer (tel. 0705-822351 ext. 41769). After hours – Duty Staff Officer to Flag Officer (ext. 22008).

NHS hyperbaric facilities are found at Heatherwood Hospital, Ascot (tel. 0990-23333); Whipps Cross Hospital, London E11 (tel. 081-539-5522); Peterborough District Hospital, Peterborough (tel. 0733-67451); Royal Victoria Infirmary, Newcastle upon Tyne (tel. 091-232-5131); Monsall Hospital, Manchester (tel. 061 205-2393).

In Australia, contact the Hyperbaric Medicine Unit, Royal Adelaide Hospital.

## Further reading

Ekert, P., Tibbals, J. and Gorman, D. (1988) Three patients with carbon monoxide poisoning treated with hyperbaric oxygen therapy. *Aust. Paediatr. J.,* **24**, 194–196

Kindwall, E. P. (1985) Hyperbaric treatment of carbon monoxide poisoning. *Ann. Emerg. Med.*, **14**, 1233–1234
Langford, R. M. and Armstrong, R. F. (1989) Algorithm for managing injury from smoke inhalation. *Br. Med. J.*, **299**, 902–905
Meredith, T. and Vale, A. (1988) Carbon monoxide poisoning. *Br. Med. J.*, **296**, 77–78
Sanchez, R., Fosarelli, P., Felt, B. *et al.* (1988) Carbon monoxide poisoning due to automobile exposure: disparity between carboxyhemoglobin levels and symptoms of victims. *Pediatr.*, **82**, 663–666

## 5.3 Button (disc) battery ingestion

The growing use of these power cells in digital watches, hearing aids, calculators and cameras have made them a relatively new ingestion risk to children, often treated with undue alarm and occasionally unnecessary surgery. Button batteries are no exception to the general rule that ingested foreign bodies are exceedingly unlikely to do harm once they have passed through the oesophagus.

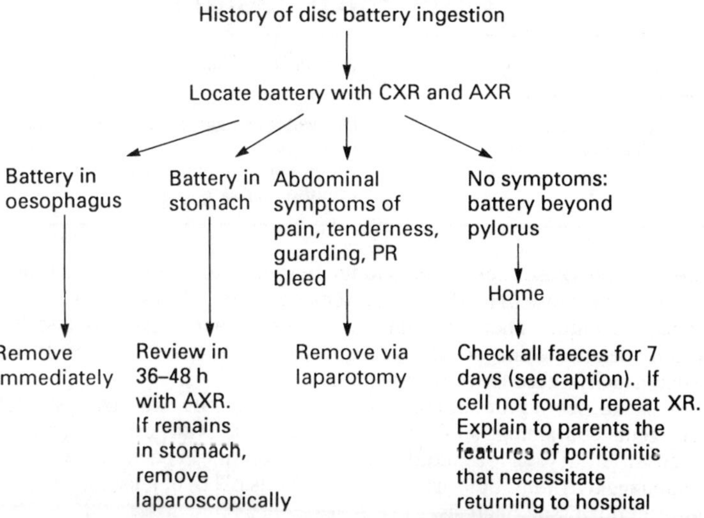


**Figure 5.1** Management of disc battery ingestion (After Bochnert, M. T. *et al.* (1985) *Pediatr. Clin. N. Am.* **32**; 198–199) To check faeces, give the parents wooden spatulae to take home, which can be used to break down the faeces. Collection of faeces is straightforward if the child is in nappies. Alternatively, stools can be collected by allowing the child to defaecate into a potty, or by covering the water of the toilet bowl with several layers of toilet paper prior to defaecation.

### MANAGEMENT

#### *1 Identify the type of cell swallowed*

Lithium and silver cells have never been known to cause problems. Mercury and alkaline manganese can provide a low voltage current or leak, rarely causing tissue injury (the older the battery, the less likely this is to happen) or very rarely causing mercury poisoning.

#### *2 Algorithm*

See Figure 5.1.

### Further reading

Boehnert, M. T. *et al*. (1985) Advances in clinical toxicology. *Pediatr. Clin. N. Am.*, **32**, 198–199

David, T. J. and Ferguson, A. P. (1986) Management of children who have swallowed button batteries. *Arch. Dis. Child.*, **61**, 321–322

Kuhns, D. W. and Dire, D. J. (1989) Button battery ingestions. *Ann. Emerg. Med.*, **18**, 293–300

## 5.4 Caustic ingestion

| *Typical household acids* | *Typical household alkalis* |
|---|---|
| Toilet bowl cleaners | Dishwater and laundry powder (not liquid) |
| Metal cleaners | Drain and oven cleaners |
| | Ammonia-containing compounds |
| | Clinitest tablets |

These agents cause caustic burns to the oesophagus. Acidic agents tend to be bitter and cause immediate pain, thus ensuring only a small quantity of ingestion. Liquid alkaline solutions are often odourless and tasteless. Alkalis penetrate the oesophageal mucosa more easily than acids, and hence usually cause more serious caustic injury.

Most household detergents are innocuous, but industrial strength detergent containing sodium tripolyphosphate can cause significant mucosal injury. Household bleach (sodium hypochlorite) is an oesophageal irritant, but fortunately, due to its pH of 6, it usually does not cause major tissue necrosis.

### CLINICAL FEATURES

Initial features may include vomiting, dysphagia, drooling, abdominal pain. Respiratory distress with stridor suggests extensive injury.

Examination of the mouth and pharynx may demonstrate oedema, ulceration or a white membrane over the soft palate, although 30% of children with significant oesophageal or gastric injury have no oropharyngeal burns (*Am. J. Dis. Child.* (1984) **138**, 863). Oesophageal perforation with mediastinitis or gastric perforation with peritonitis may occur. During the second week after ingestion, granulation tissue forms, while fibrosis begins during the third week.

## TREATMENT

### *1 Emesis and lavage*

Contraindicated.

### *2 Neutralization with acids or alkalis*

Contraindicated. A small amount of water or milk should be given to dilute and wash away the residual agent. If too much liquid is given, the child may vomit.

### *3 GI endoscopy*

To determine the presence and extent of oesophageal injury. Those with superficial oesophageal burns can be commenced on a normal diet immediately and no further treatment is necesary. For those more severely injured, the following treatments are used.

### *4 Prednisolone*

Controversial. 2 mg/kg/day may be of benefit. Begin within 48 h of the injury and continue for 3 weeks. Prophylactic antibiotics are not indicated.

### *5 Commence $H_2$ antagonists*

Alternatively, commence regular antacids to prevent secondary injury from reflux of gastric acid.

### *6 Other therapy*

Oesophageal strictures require repeated oesophageal dilatation (bouginage). Some experimental therapies are the placement of a rubber stent in the oesophagus, and the administration of 'lathyrogen' compounds.

## Further reading

Rothstein, F. C. (1986) Caustic injuries to the esophagus in children. *Pediatr. Clin. N. Am.*, **33**, 665–674.

# 5.5 Paracetamol (acetaminophen) overdose

Paracetamol is toxic to the liver, kidney and probably myocardium (*Br. Med. J.* (1987) **295**, 1097). In conventional doses it is mainly metabolized by conjugation with glucuronide and sulphate, while some is oxidized to an intermediary metabolite which is then conjugated with glutathione (Figure 5.2). In overdose, glutathione stores are used up. The intermediary metabolite accumulates and is toxic to liver and renal tubules. Treatment aims at raising intracellular glutathione, but it is of little value if administered more than 15 h after the ingestion.

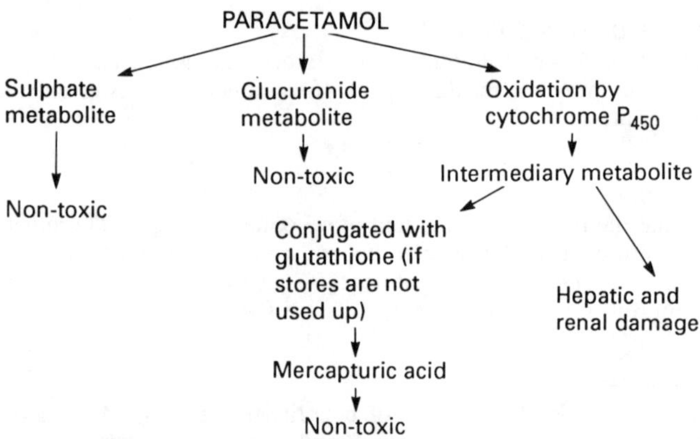


**Figure 5.2** Metabolism of paracetamol

## POTENTIAL TOXIC DOSE

Ingestion of 150 mg/kg can result in liver damage (>8 g in adolescents).

## CLINICAL FEATURES

0–24 h – may be asymptomatic; occasional vomiting.
24–36 h – occasional GIT symptoms.
36–72 h – onset of liver or renal failure.
72–120 h – jaundice, bleeding, encephalopathy, renal failure

## MANAGEMENT

### *1 General poisoning measures* – emesis or lavage

Activated charcoal is said to be contraindicated if oral antidote is to be used, although some advocate still giving one dose of charcoal for suspected toxic ingestion and 30% increase in oral antidote if levels are toxic.

### *2 Measure serum paracetamol at 4 h*

See Figure 5.3.

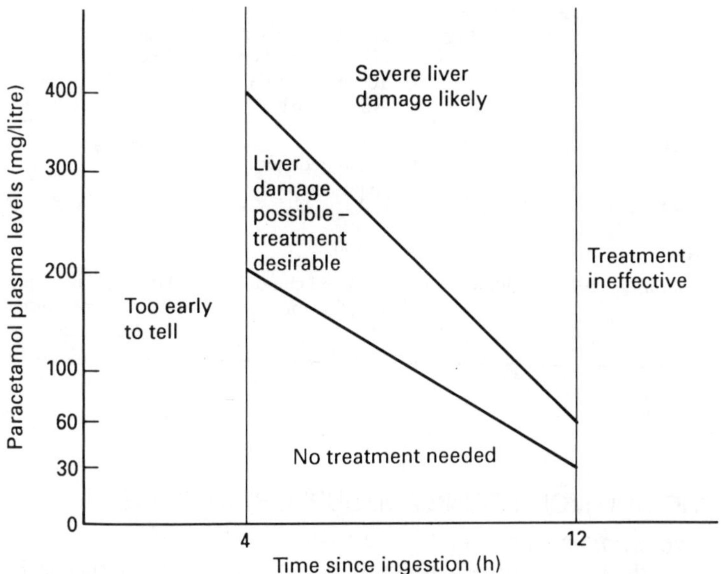


**Figure 5.3** Toxic range of plasma paracetamol against time (From Henry, J. and Volans, G. (1984) *ABC of Poisoning – Part 1: Drugs,* BMA, London, with permission)

### *3 Give antidote (Table 5.3) if:*

(a) 4–15 h level is toxic – see Figure 5.3. If level is non-toxic, the child can be discharged.

(b) Ingestion was 6–15 h ago and toxicity is possible but serum levels are as yet unavailable. Cease treatment if levels are below the toxic range. If more than 15 hours have elapsed since ingestion, antidote is unlikely to be helpful, although recent evidence suggests that it should nevertheless be given (*Lancet* (1990) **335**, 1572–1573).

### *4 Transfer to a specialist unit*

This should be effected at the first sign of encephalopathy, liver or renal failure, metabolic acidosis (pH <7.30) or hypotension.

**Table 5.3 Antidotes to paracetamol**

| | *Methionine* | *N-acetylcysteine (Mucomyst)* | *N-acetylcysteine (Mucomyst)* |
|---|---|---|---|
| *Route* | Oral | IV | Oral |
| *Dose* | 30 mg/kg/4 h for 4 doses; adult dose 2.5 g Q 4 h to 10 g | 150 mg/kg in 200 ml NS over 15 min, then 50 mg/kg in 500 ml NS over 4 h, then 100 mg/kg in 1000 ml NS over 16 h | 140 mg/kg stat<br>70 mg/kg/4 h for 17 doses |
| *Side effects* | Vomiting | Rash, angio-oedema, hypotension, bronchospasm | Vomiting |
| *Cost* | 80p | > £30 | |
| *Preparation* | 250 mg tablets | 2 g/10 ml ampoule (= 20% soln) | Use 20% soln diluted 1:4 with cola, orange juice or water |

NS, normal saline.

## ONGOING MONITORING AND SUPPORTIVE CARE

### *1 Prothrombin time (PT)*

This is the most sensitive indicator of liver damage. If it is normal at 72 h post-ingestion, the child can be discharged.

Encephalopathy is likely when PT exceeds 25 s at 48 h or 40 s at 72 h. Peak elevation occurs at 72–96 h. Treat any bleeding with fresh frozen plasma and add $H_2$ receptor antagonist for GI bleeding.

### *2 Hypoglycaemia*

Frequent monitoring of blood glucose is mandatory.

### *3 Renal function*

Plasma creatinine and urine volume should be measured daily. Dialysis should be started early (creatinine >400 µmol/litre) since delay makes cerebral oedema more likely.

### *4 Liver function*

Serum hepatic aminotransferases peak after 3–4 days, but are unreliable prognostic indicators of subsequent course.

## Further reading

Anon (1988) Management of serious paracetamol poisoning. *Drugs and Ther. Bull.*, **26**, 97–99

Ellenhorn, M. J. and Barceloux, D. G. (1988) *Medical Toxicology*, Elsevier, New York, pp. 156–166

Henry, J. and Volans, G. (1984) *ABC of Poisoning – Part 1: Drugs*, BMA, London

# 5.6 Salicylate poisoning

Serious accidental salicylate poisoning in children is now uncommon, due to the decreased use of aspirin in children and the use of child-resistant containers. It remains a problem in deliberate overdose in adolescents, and rarely children may accidentally ingest aspirin-containing adult cold remedies. The lethal acute dose in an adult is 20–25 g; in a small child 4 g; and considerably less than this in infants. Death from salicylate poisoning is due to CNS toxicity. Any factor causing a rise in tissue (including brain) salicylate levels is therefore dangerous.

## PHARMACOLOGICAL CONSIDERATIONS

1. Aspirin obeys zero-order kinetics (as do phenytoin and ethanol). Hence an increase in regular dose results in a greater than expected rise in serum level and tissue content of drug.
2. In overdose, salicylate shows an increase in apparent volume of distribution (decreased binding to plasma protein at higher doses) and therefore tissue levels (including brain) are higher.
3. The pKa of aspirin is 3.5, thus acidaemia favours the un-ionized form of the drug which diffuses easily into the brain.

## PATHOGENESIS

The toxic effects include direct stimulation of CNS respiratory centre, uncoupled oxidative phosphorylation, inhibition of Krebs' cycle enzymes, stimulation of gluconeogenesis, increased tissue glycolysis and inhibition of amino acid metabolism. These result in metabolic acidosis, respiratory alkalosis, hyper- or hypoglycaemia, fluid and electrolyte loss.

## POTENTIAL TOXIC DOSE

Acute ingestion of <150 mg/kg is safe. Moderate toxicity is expected with ingestion of 150–300 mg/kg. 300–500 mg/kg is serious, and ingestion of >500 mg/kg is potentially lethal (Temple, A. R. (1981) *Arch. Intern. Med.*, **141**, 364–369).

## CLINICAL FEATURES

Acute poisoning may resemble diabetic ketoacidosis. Features include:

- nausea, vomit, epigastric pain;
- tinnitus, deafness;
- sweating, fever;
- dehydration, shock;
- increased rate and depth of respiration, pulmonary oedema;
- agitation, altered conscious state, convulsions;
- hypokalaemia, hyper- and hyponatraemia, hyper- and hypoglycaemia;
- respiratory alkalosis followed by metabolic acidosis;
- hypoprothrombinaemia (decreased vitamin K dependent factor VII synthesis).

## INVESTIGATION

### *1 Plasma salicylate levels*

Should be done at presentation and at 6 h post-ingestion. If there is a suspicion of severe overdose the following tests should be performed and repeated often in the first 24–48 h.

### *2 Haematology*

Full blood count, packed volume, prothrombin time, partial thromboplastin time.

### *3 Biochemistry*

U + E, glucose, arterial gases, Ca, LFT.

## MANAGEMENT

### *1 General poisoning measures*

Emesis or gastric lavage may be used up to 24 h post-ingestion. Charcoal given in repeated doses may shorten elimination half-life (Hillman, R. J. and Prescott, L. F. (1985) *Br. Med. J.*, **291**, 1472).

### *2 Plasma salicylate level*

Obtained at presentation and at 6 h (Figure 5.4). If the 6 h sample is the higher of the two, admit and ? repeat gastric lavage. It is debatable whether to rely on plasma levels or rather proceed with the following measures only according to the child's clinical condition.

### *3 Hydration*

Restore circulating blood volume with 15–20 ml/kg normal saline + 5 mmol KCl/500 ml IV stat. May be repeated as required. Subsequent replacement depends on state of hydration. 0.45% NaCl + 2.5% dextrose + 15–20 mmol $NaHCO_3$ + 15 mmol KCl per 500 ml is a good starting fluid, initially at maintenance rates. A central venous catheter may be invaluable.

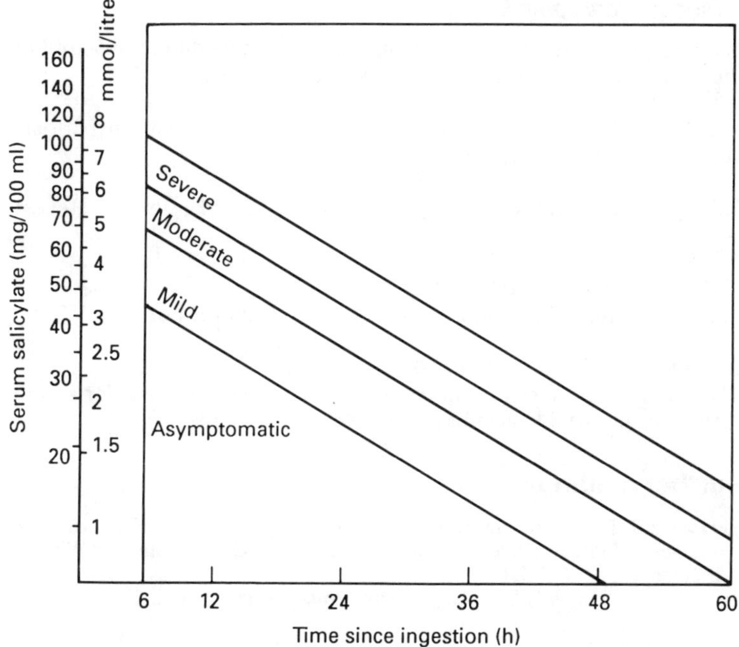


**Figure 5.4** Serum salicylate levels related to expected clinical severity of intoxication following a single dose of salicylate (After Done, A. K. (1960) *Pediatr.*, **26**, 800, with permission)

### *4 Correct acidosis*

To minimize CNS toxicity. $NaHCO_3$ is the drug of choice. Dose: 1–2 mmol/kg over 1–2 h. May be repeated to keep arterial pH >7.45. Complications of $NaHCO_3$ include worsening hypernatraemia, hypokalaemia, hypocalcaemia and pulmonary oedema. Tham is contraindicated (Dove, A. (1978) *Pediatr.*, **62**, 890).

### *5 Forced alkaline diuresis*

Dangerous and difficult, and according to many authorities should not be used (Bateman, D. N. (1988) Adverse reactions to antidotes. *Adv. Dr. Reaction Bull.*, **133**, 498). Aim for a urine output of >3 ml/kg/h with a urine pH of >7.5. Diuretics should not be employed unless one is certain of normo- or hypervolaemia. Use frusemide. Acetazolamide is contraindicated. Urine alkalinization is achieved with bicarbonate as above. Side effects of alkaline therapy are discussed above. The problems of hypokalaemia and hypovolaemia inherent in this condition make forced diuresis treacherous.

### *6 Biochemical complications*

**6.1 Hypokalaemia** KCl 15–20 mmol should be added to each 500 ml of the IV infusion at the outset, before serum $K^+$ drops.

**6.2 Hypoglycaemia** A common problem. Correct with hypertonic glucose infusion as necessary.

**6.3 Hypocalcaemia** Calcium gluconate 10%, 0.5 ml/kg slow IV. Repeat as necessary.

### *7 Vitamin K (phytomenadione)*

For hypoprothrombinaemia, 0.3 mg/kg (max. 10 mg) IM or slow IV.

### *8 Dialysis and haemoperfusion*

These efficiently remove salicylates from the blood. Reserve for severe toxicity or intractable acid-base and electrolyte disorders.

## Further reading

Berkowitz, I. D. and Rogers, M. C. (1987) Poisoning and the critically ill child. In *Textbook of Pediatric Intensive Care* (ed. Rogers, M. C.), Williams and Wilkins, Baltimore, pp. 1157–1164

Snodgras, W. R. (1986) Salicylate toxicity. *Pediatr. Clin. N. Am.,* **33**, 381–391

# 5.7 Potassium overdose/hyperkalaemia

Elevated serum potassium may be due to:

### *1 Factitious hyperkalaemia*

Haemolysed specimen, prolonged tourniquet time, thrombocytosis.

### *2 Excessive intake*

For example, overdose of $K^+$ supplements, IV supplements, massive transfusion of old blood.

### *3 Poor excretion*

Renal failure (hyperkalaemia is unusual until over 90% of renal function is lost), hypoadrenalism.

### *4 Release from cells*

Massive tissue injury, acidosis, use of suxamethonium in burns and crush injuries.

3.0 g of KCl supplies 40 mEq of potassium.

## IMMEDIATE INVESTIGATIONS

Serum potassium and ECG monitor.

## CLINICAL FEATURES

Diarrhoea, abdominal cramps, weakness.
Cardiac effects: rare below 6.5 mEq/litre and common above 8.0 mEq/litre.
Sequential ECG changes are roughly: peaked T-waves, depressed S–T segment, decreased amplitude of R- and P-waves, prolonged P–R interval, widened QRS complex, prolonged Q–T interval, ventricular fibrillation, asystole.

## MANAGEMENT

### *1 Drive $K^+$ intracellularly*

**1.1 Give glucose** 1 g/kg IV (2 ml/kg of 50% dextrose) + insulin 0.1 u/kg IV. *Monitor blood glucose levels.* Continue with glucose 0.5 g/kg/h (1 ml/kg of 50% dextrose) + insulin 0.1 u/kg/h.

**1.2 $NaHCO_3$** 8.4% 2 ml/kg stat, then 1 ml/kg aliquots to achieve metabolic alkalosis.

**1.3 Hyperventilation** To achieve respiratory alkalosis.

**1.4 Salbutamol** A potassium-lowering effect has been noted in asthmatics. 0.5 mg slowly IV has been successfully used in lowering $K^+$ in adults with chronic renal disease (*Arch. Intern. Med.* (1987) **147**, 713–717), as has inhaled salbutamol (*Ann. Intern. Med.* (1989) **110**, 426–429), although it is not yet conventional treatment.

### *2 Encourage loss of body $K^+$*

**2.1 Frusemide** 1 mg/kg/dose.

**2.2 Resonium exchange resin** 1 g/kg/dose 4 h via NGT (give lactulose) or rectal.

### *3 Protect the myocardium*

Ca gluconate 10% (0.22 mmol/ml), 0.5 ml/kg/dose (max. 20 ml) slowly over 20 min. Repeat as required for myocardial depression or significant ECG changes.

### *4 Peritoneal dialysis*

The best way of removing $K^+$ from the body if the child is anuric or for clinical features of hyperkalaemia refractory to the above treatment (see Section 13.7).

# 5.8 Iron poisoning

Iron tablets or iron-containing vitamins are often regarded as health-producing substances and not as dangerous drugs. The elemental iron content of ferrous gluconate, fumarate and sulphate salts in 12, 20 and 33%, respectively. Hence, 300 mg of ferrous gluconate contains 35 mg of elemental iron, and 200 mg of ferrous sulphate contains 60 mg. It is customary to express the amount of iron ingested as elemental iron.

## PATHOPHYSIOLOGY

Massive ingestion completely overwhelms the gut mucosal barrier to iron absorption. Once absorbed in the duodenum and jejunum in the ferrous form ($Fe^{2+}$) it is converted to ferric ($Fe^{3+}$) in mucosal cells and enters the blood, bound to transferrin which is normally only about 35% saturated. In acute intoxication, total iron binding capacity of transferrin is exceeded and toxic free iron circulates in the blood.

| *Clinical features* | *Pathogenesis* |
|---|---|
| Vomit, diarrhoea, abdominal pain, haemorrhage. | Direct corrosive effect |
| Shock | Increased venous pooling and capillary leak |
| Metabolic acidosis | Shock, mitochondrial damage, interference with Krebs' cycle |
| Prolonged PT and APTT | Diminished liver synthesis of clotting factors, alteration of clotting cascade, DIC, interference with activated thrombin and clotting proteases |

## POTENTIAL TOXIC DOSE

### *1 Assess maximum possible ingested dose*

For children < 5 yr:

<20 mg/kg – insignificant
20–60 mg/kg – treat with ipecac and send home
>60 mg/kg – admit
>180 mg/kg – potentially lethal

### *2 Other predictors of toxicity*

**2.1 Gastrointestinal symptoms** within the first 6 h, hypoglycaemia, and WCC >15 000/mm$^3$.

**2.2 Desferrioxamine challenge** 40 mg/kg (max. 1 g) deep IM injection (dilute 500 mg desferrioxamine in 2 ml sterile water). Those with free circulating iron will pass orange/red coloured urine. This suggests that further chelation may be needed.

## CLINICAL FEATURES

*Phase I*: 30–120 min post-ingestion, develop nausea, vomit, diarrhoea, abdominal pain. Rarely haematemesis and melana. Severe poisoning gives shock and encephalopathy.

*Phase II*: A period of apparent recovery lasting 6 h to several days. Some doubt the existence of this phase.

*Phase III*: Recurrence of GI symptoms (N.B. Black stools may be due to iron, or GI blood loss). Also metabolic acidosis, shock, CNS depression. Liver dysfunction may cause jaundice, elevated bilirubin and transaminases, hypoglycaemia and coagulopathy. Renal failure.

*Phase IV*: 2–6 weeks after ingestion may get pyloric, gastric or intestinal stenosis.

## INVESTIGATIONS

### *1 Serum iron, total iron binding capacity (TIBC), transferrin*

**1.1 Serum iron** Best assessed 2–4 h post-ingestion.

| *Iron level* (μmol/litre)* | *Potential severity* |
|---|---|
| <30 | No toxicity |
| 30–50 | Minimal toxicity |
| 50–100 | Moderate toxicity |
| >100 | Severe toxicity, aggressive therapy needed |

*1 μmol/litre of iron = 5.6 μg/dl.

**1.2 TIBC is the amount of unsaturated transferrin.** Serum Fe > TIBC = potentially serious ingestion.

1 g/litre of transferrin (normal range 1.9–2.5 g/litre) binds 22.75 μmol/litre of iron.

### *2 Other tests*

FBC, glucose, serum electrolytes, plain AXR (detects radio-opaque iron tablets), blood cross-match, prothrombin time, partial thromboplastin time.

## MANAGEMENT

### *1 Gastric emptying*

If maximum possible ingested dose is 20–60 mg/kg, use ipecac. If ingested dose >60 mg/kg, perform gastric lavage using a large-bore orogastric tube. A lavage solution containing 1–1.5% sodium bicarbonate (12 ml of 8.4% $NaHCO_3$ per 100 ml) will convert remaining gastric iron to relatively insoluble ferrous bicarbonate. Adding 2 g desferrioxamine to 1 litre of lavage fluid is controversial. Activated charcoal is not used.

If, in spite of vigorous lavage, tablets remain in stomach on AXR consider gastrotomy (Peterson, C. D. and Fifield, C. G. (1980) Emergency gastrotomy for acute iron poisoning. *Ann. Emerg. Med.*, **9**, 262). Alternatively, whole bowel irrigation with a polyethylene glycol electrolyte solution has been advocated (Tenenbein, M. (1987) *J. Pediatr.*, **111**, 142–145), but this is not widely available.

### *2 Chelation therapy*

Desferrioxamine 40 mg/kg (max. 1 g) IM – for moderate cases; repeat 6 hourly. In severe poisoning, give it IV (side effects – GIT symptoms, hypotension, tachycardia) 15 mg/kg/h (max. daily dose 6 g). End point of therapy is when the urine loses its orange/red (*vin rosé*) colour.

### *3 General supportive measures*

Anticipate shock and third space losses by giving liberal blood volume expansion. Correct acidosis, hypoglycaemia and electrolyte disturbance. Enteric losses may require blood transfusion.

### *4 Other treatments*

Peritoneal dialysis or haemodialysis will remove the desferrioxamine/iron complex, but not as well as functioning kidneys. Use only in renal failure. Exchange transfusion should be used in very severe intoxication (serum Fe > 800 µmol/litre).

## Further reading

Banner, W. and Tong, T. G. (1986) Iron poisoning. *Pediatr. Clin. N. Am.*, **33**, 393–409

Berkowitz, I. D. and Rogers, M. C. (1987) Poisoning and the critically ill child. In *Textbook of Pediatric Intensive Care* (ed. Rogers, M. C.), Williams and Wilkins, Baltimore, pp. 1164–1167

# 5.9 Digoxin poisoning

Poisoning with digoxin may result from chronic overuse or acute overdose. The toxicity resulting from the former typically is associated with a wide range of GIT, ocular and CNS manifestations, and also with hypokalaemia due to concomitant diuretic use. Acute poisoning is associated with nausea and vomiting. Other symptoms are uncommon.

Almost any arrhythmia or conduction abnormality can be seen with digitalis toxicity. In adults, bigeminy or multifocal ventricular ectopic beats are commonly seen. In children, these are uncommon; sinus bradycardia or heart block are often the earliest signs of toxicity, commonly followed by supraventricular tachycardia or atrial tachycardia with heart block.

## PREDICTION OF TOXICITY

Ingestion of 0.05 mg/kg would be expected to produce a digoxin blood level above the therapeutic limit of 2 ng/ml. Ingestion of doses higher than this should indicate gut decontamination, observation in a casualty department and measuring serum digoxin level 6 h post-ingestion. Therapeutic digoxin levels are 0.6–2 ng/ml (0.7–2.5 nmol/litre). Levels over 15 ng/ml indicate severe intoxication. Children without cardiovascular disease tolerate levels up to 10 ng/ml. Serum levels beyond that are not sensitive prognostic indicators of toxicity. In children with pre-existing heart disease, lower doses and levels may cause complications.

## MANAGEMENT

### *1 Chronic toxicity*

Usually no treatment is needed, apart from stopping the medication. The half-life of the drug is 36 h. About one-third of the drug is excreted per day, predominantly via the kidneys.

### *2 Acute overdose*

A narrow gap exists between optimal therapeutic doses and toxicity.

**2.1 Empty the stomach** Ipecac or gastric lavage.

**2.2 Activated charcoal** 1 g/kg via NGT.

**2.3 Correct electrolyte disturbance** Hypokalaemia (seen in those on diuretics) must be corrected. In acute overdose, hyperkalaemia may be seen and should be managed aggressively (see Section 5.7).

**2.4 Antiarrhythmics** Bradyarrhythmias – atropine, cardiac pacing. Ventricular arrhythmias – phenytoin (10–15 mg/kg over 2 h IV, then 2–4 mg/kg/12 h), lignocaine (1 mg/kg IV bolus, then 20–55 μg/kg/min). Supraventricular arrhythmias – phenytoin and/or propanolol (0.02–0.1 mg/kg slow IV).

Avoid drugs which may aggravate conduction disturbance (class I antiarrhythmics; quinidine, verapamil, procainamide), or drugs which increase plasma digoxin levels (e.g. quinidine, verapamil, amiodarone).

**2.5 Specific antidote** Digoxin-specific polyclonal Fab fragments from immunized sheep ('Digibind' – Wellcome). Used for life-threatening arrhythmias and/or hyperkalaemia > 6 mEq/litre caused by digoxin.
Dose – governed by digoxin body load. This can be estimated by:

(a) Estimated ingestion dose (mg) × 0.8 (because of incomplete absorption), *or*
(b) Plasma (serum) digoxin (nmol/litre) 6 h post-ingestion × 0.0044 × Weight = Estimated body load (mg)

(ng/ml × 1.28 = nmol/litre)

60 mg Fab fragment neutralizes 1 mg digoxin; therefore:

Dose of Fab (mg) = Digoxin body load (mg) × 60

The ampoules (40 mg) should be reconstituted with 4 ml sterile water and administered IV over 30 min through a 0.22 μm Millipore filter. Despite lacking the antigenic determinants of the Fc fragment, it still poses an antigenic threat to the child.

**2.6 Peritoneal dialysis, haemodialysis, exchange transfusion:** results are disappointing.

**2.7 Cardioversion** is relatively contraindicated because it may cause ventricular fibrillation refractory to further treatment. If used, administer prophylactic phenytoin or lignocaine before DC shock.

## Further reading

Ellenhorn, M. J. and Barceloux, D. G. (1988) *Medical Toxicology,* Elsevier, New York, pp. 200–207

Weinhous, E. *et al.* (1987) Digoxin toxicity in childhood: emphasis on recent advances. *Ped. Rev. Commun.,* **1**, 67–88

# 5.10 Tricyclic antidepressants

### COMMON TRICYCLICS

Imipramine, amitriptyline.

### RELATED COMPOUNDS

Butriptyline, dothiepin, doxepin, nortriptyline, protriptyline.

## PREDICTION OF TOXICITY

Ingestion of 10–20 mg/kg is serious, 35 mg/kg may be fatal. There is no correlation between serum drug levels and degree of toxicity.

## CLINICAL FEATURES OF POISONING

Death is usually due to cardiac toxicity or respiratory depression.

### *1 Anticholinergic*

Sinus tachycardia, mydriasis, dry mucous membranes, flushed warm skin without sweating, urinary retention.

### *2 CNS effects*

Drowsiness, hallucinations, delirium, coma, brisk tendon reflexes, extensor plantar reflexes, respiratory depression, convulsions.

### *3 Cardiac*

Sinus tachycardia, ECG changes – QRS > 100 msec (correlates well with major toxicity, but 25% of people have it as a normal phenomenon), atrioventricular block, ventricular arrhythmias, hypotension.

### *4 Metabolic*

Hypothermia, hypoxia, metabolic acidosis, hypokalaemia.

## MANAGEMENT

### *1 Gastric lavage*

Intubate first if conscious state is questionable. Lavage may be performed up to 12 h after ingestion because of delayed gastric emptying.

### *2 Activated charcoal via NGT*

1 g/kg/dose. May repeat hourly with 0.25 mg/kg/dose. Give cathartic, e.g. magnesium sulphate 250 mg/kg or lactulose 30 ml 4–8 h via NGT.

### *3 ECG monitoring for 24 h*

### *4 Correct metabolic problems*

Ventilate if hypoxic, correct acidosis and hypokalaemia.

### *5 Treat hypotension*

It usually responds to fluid replacement. Dopamine or dobutamine may be required.

### *6 Cardiac arrhythmias*

May respond to: bicarbonate bolus, phenytoin 15 mg/kg at max. rate of 0.5 mg/kg/min, propanolol 0.02–0.1 mg/kg/dose IV over 10 min, repeat as required, then 6 h, or direct current cardioversion. Physostigmine (see below) may be of use in intractable arrhythmias. Avoid lignocaine, quinidine, disopyramide and procainamide.

### *7 Convulsions*

Oxygenate, ± diazepam and phenytoin.

### *8 Physostigmine – controversial*

Should be avoided in the presence of intraventricular conduction delay. Intractable arrhythmias, hypotension or fits may respond to 0.02 mg/kg IV every 5 min till response (max. 0.1 mg/kg), then 0.5–2.0 μg/kg/min. Side effects include seizures, bradyarrhythmias, asystole, cholinergic crisis (vomit, diarrhoea, bronchospasm, increased oral and bronchial secretions).

Haemodialysis is of little use.

## Further reading

Berkowitz, I. D. and Rogers, M. C. (1987) Poisoning and the critically ill child. In *Textbook of Pediatric Intensive Care* (ed. Rogers, M. C.), Williams and Wilkins, Baltimore.

Henry, J. and Volans, G. (1984) *ABC of Poisoning, Part I: Drugs,* British Medical Association, London

# 5.11 Organophosphate poisoning

These compounds are mainly used as insecticides. Generally speaking, those used for commercial agriculture are more concentrated and more toxic than those in domestic use. Organophosphates are rapidly absorbed through the skin, GIT and lungs. Poisoning in children is by ingestion, skin contamination, or inhalation.

## PATHOPHYSIOLOGY

Organophosphates bind irreversibly to acetylcholinesterase, allowing unhydrolysed acetylcholine to accumulate, stimulating neourotransmission initially, but subsequently blocking the receptor.

The clinical features reflect stimulation of cholinergic muscarinic and nicotinic receptors, followed by paralysis of neurotransmission.

## CLINICAL MANIFESTATIONS

Death is due to a mixture of central and peripheral nervous system depression and cardiorespiratory involvement. Mild poisoning usually manifests as fatigue, headache, nausea, abdominal cramps and diarrhoea. A wide spectrum of presentation is encountered.

### *1 CNS*

Headache, restlessness, dizziness, confusion, coma, seizures, respiratory depression.

### *2 Muscarinic effects*

| | |
|---|---|
| Cardiac | – bradycardia, hypotension, heart block. |
| Respiratory | – wheezing, increased secretions. |
| GIT | – abdominal cramps, diarrhoea, nausea, vomit. |
| Eyes | – meiosis, lacrimation, blurred vision. |
| Salivary glands | – increased salivation. |
| Sweat glands | – increased sweating. |
| Bladder | – urinary incontinence. |

### *3 Nicotinic effects*

| | |
|---|---|
| Skeletal muscle | – weakness, cramps, fasciculation, paralysis. |
| Sympathetic ganglia | – tachycardia, hypertension, arrhythmia, mydriasis. |
| Others | – garlic odour, fever, pulmonary oedema. |

## INVESTIGATIONS

Serum pseudocholinesterase and red cell cholinesterase (the more specific test) activity can be assayed. Collect at least 2 ml blood in lithium heparin tube and send to biochemistry department. Clinical signs do not always reflect the degree of cholinesterase inactivation; however, mild poisoning is usually associated with $> 20\%$ activity and severe poisoning with $< 10\%$ activity.

## TREATMENT

### *1 Decontamination*

Remove all contaminated clothing and wash all contaminated skin. If the poison has been ingested, administer ipecac if the child is conscious or if not proceed to endotracheal intubation and gastric lavage (wash vomitus off skin).

### *2 Drugs*

Do not withhold treatment until laboratory confirmation of the diagnosis.

**2.1 Atropine** Antagonizes the central and muscarinic signs, but has no effect on muscle weakness (e.g. respiratory muscles) caused by nicotinic overstimulation. (N.B. large doses may be required.) Those unfamiliar with organophosphate toxicity tend only to use conventional doses, occasionally with disastrous results to the patient.

Dose: 0.05 mg/kg IV (max. 1 mg). Repeat using 0.02–0.05 mg/kg every 10 min until cholinergic signs are reversed or atropine side effects supervene (dry mouth, warm dry skin, dilated pupils, bradycardia).

Titrate frequency and dose to patient's signs. In an intubated child, control of bronchial secretions provides a useful dosage monitor. Once adequate atropinization has been achieved, repeat dose every 30–60 min because of short half-life of atropine.

**2.2 Pralidoxime (2-PAM)** A cholinesterase reactivator which hastens *de novo* synthesis of acetylcholine especially at the neuromuscular junction. It has no central effects.

Dose 25–50 mg/kg (max. 750 mg) IV over 20 min. Repeat × 1 after 2 h, then 12 hourly if cholinergic signs return. It is of no benefit if given >36 h after exposure. *Do not use in carbamate poisoning.*

**2.3 Contraindicated drugs** Parasympathomimetic drugs (physostigmine, suxamethonium), phenothiazines and antihistamines may all potentiate anticholinesterase activity and should be avoided. Opiates increase the likelihood of respiratory arrest.

### CARBAMATE INSECTICIDES

These differ from organophosphates in that they only temporarily inactivate anticholinesterase and penetrate the CNS poorly, resulting in few CNS signs and shorter lived cholinergic effects. Treatment is identical to that of organophosphate poisoning except that pralidoxime is contraindicated.

## Further reading

Berkowitz, I. D. and Rogers, M. C. (1987) Poisoning and the critically ill child. In *Textbook of Pediatric Intensive Care.* (ed. Rogers, M. C.), Williams and Wilkins, Baltimore, pp. 1126–1129

Mortenson, M. L. (1986) Management of acute childhood poisonings caused by selected insecticides and herbicides. *Pediatr. Clin. N. Am.,* **33**, 421–446

Chapter 6

# Immunization

## 6.1 Childhood immunization

Low immunization rates in the UK and many parts of the developed world remain low, often due to the inappropriate advice of health workers (*Br. Med. J.* (1989) **298**, 1687). A sound knowledge of vaccination is needed by all health professionals working with children.

### IMMUNIZATION PROCEDURES

#### *1 Cleaning the skin*

Allow alcohol to evaporate before injecting vaccine since it purportedly can inactivate live virus!

#### *2 Immunization by nurses*

This is an acceptable policy provided that the nurse is familiar with contraindications to and complications of vaccines (*Br. Med. J.* (1987) **294**, 423–424).

#### *3 Site*

For all injectable vaccines with the exception of BCG, the intramuscular or deep subcutaneous routes should be used. In infants, the anterolateral aspect of the thigh or upper arm are recommended. If the buttock is used, inject only into the upper outer quadrant, but bear in mind that injection into fatty tissue may reduce the efficacy of some vaccines. BCG is administered intradermally over the insertion of the left deltoid.

### *4 Routine vaccination schedule in the UK*

| *Vaccine* | *Age* | *Comments* |
|---|---|---|
| DTP and polio | (a) 3 mo<br>(b) 5 mo<br>(c) 8.5–11 mo | If the course is interrupted, it may be resumed. There is no need to start again |
| MMR | 12–18 mo | Given to boys and girls |
| DT and polio | 4–5 yr | Give MMR as well if missed earlier |
| Rubella | 10–14 yr | Only in those not immunized in childhood |
| BCG | 10–14 yr | At least 3 weeks between rubella and BCG |
| Tetanus and polio | 15–18 yr | Tetanus booster 10 yearly thereafter |

DTP, diphtheria, tetanus, pertussis; DT, combined diphtheria, tetanus; MMR, measles, mumps, rubella.

## GENERAL CONTRAINDICATIONS

### *1 Acute febrile illness*

Minor infections such as a cold, cough or runny nose without fever or systemic upset are *not* contraindications.

### *2 Live virus vaccines (MMR, polio)*

These should not be given to immune compromised children, e.g. malignancy, immunodeficiency syndromes, immunosuppressive drugs or radiation, high-dose steroids (>2 mg/kg/day of prednisolone). Children on alternate day steroids are not at risk.

### *3 Pregnant women*

The patients should not electively receive live vaccines (see later this chapter). If there is a significant risk of exposure to polio or yellow fever, the need for vaccination outweighs the risks to the fetus.

### *4 Children recovering from immunosuppressive disease/ treatment (e.g. leukaemia)*

Should not receive live virus vaccines until 6 months after ceasing all treatment. Siblings and close contacts of these children should be immunized against measles. Children who have been off high-dose steroids (prednisolone >2 mg/kg/day) for more than 3 months can be vaccinated without any restrictions.

### *5 Immunoglobulin in the preceding 3 months*

Prevents the uptake of all live virus vaccines except yellow fever (immunoglobulin in the UK will not contain antibodies to yellow fever).

## THE FOLLOWING ARE NOT CONTRAINDICATIONS TO ROUTINE IMMUNIZATION

1. Asthma, eczema, 'snuffles', hay fever.
2. Antibiotics or inhaled/topical steroids.
3. Mother of the child is pregnant.
4. Breast-fed baby.
5. Neonatal jaundice.
6. Prematurity/low birth weight.
7. Over the age specified in immunization schedule.
8. Past history of measles, rubella, pertussis infection.
9. Stable neurological conditions – cerebral palsy (CP), Down's.
10. History of convulsion in 2° relatives.
11. Sibling with sudden infant death syndrome (Griffin *et al.*, 1988).

## RELATIVE CONTRAINDICATIONS TO PERTUSSIS VACCINE – ?DEFERRING IMMUNIZATION

### *1 History of seizures*

The reasons for not vaccinating such a child are medicolegal rather than medical. Nevertheless, for the doctor's and parents' peace of mind pertussis vaccination should not be administered. Some parents in this situation may consent to pertussis immunization once the risk:benefit ratio is explained. If so, defer vaccination until a progressive neurological disorder is excluded and seizures are well controlled or resolved. A history of simple febrile convulsions is not a contraindication, although administering paracetamol 15 mg/kg/4 h × 3 doses after vaccination may diminish the anticipated fever. Atypical febrile seizures are a contraindication until a progressive neurological disorder is excluded.

### *2 Known or suspected neurological conditions*

Diseases such as tuberous sclerosis, or metabolic/degenerative diseases that predispose to seizures or neurological deficit, are relative contraindications.

### *3 Family history of seizures*

The American Academy of Pediatrics has decided that this is not a contraindication because the risks of neurological damage are heavily outweighed by the risks of the disease. It is likely that children whose parents or siblings have epilepsy are at increased risk of developing a similar condition irrespective of vaccination.

In all of the above relative contraindications, the risk:benefit ratio is still in favour of vaccinating the child. The reasons for not doing so are more for the benefit of parents or doctor but are nevertheless valid.

## ABSOLUTE CONTRAINDICATIONS TO PERTUSSIS VACCINE

A history of *any* of the following reactions to a preceding dose:

1. Extensive redness, swelling, induration: covering most of the anterolateral aspect of thigh or most of the upper arm circumference. These reactions become more severe with each injection.
2. Fever >39.5°C: within 48 h of vaccine.
3. Anaphylaxis: bronchospasm, laryngeal oedema, hypotension.
4. Prolonged unresponsiveness.
5. Prolonged inconsolable screaming: or unusual high-pitched cry.
6. Convulsions: within 72 h, or encephalopathy within 7 days.

## REACTIONS TO THE DTP VACCINE

Any reactions to the DTP vaccine are likely to be due to the pertussis component. Some common reactions are listed in Table 6.1.

**Table 6.1 Common reactions following 15 752 DTP and 784 DT immunizations (all have $p < 0.0001$): the UCLA study (After Cody, C. L. *et al.* (1981) *Pediatrics*, 68, 650–660)**

| | *Per cent DTP group* | *Per cent DT group* |
|---|---|---|
| *Local reaction* | | |
| redness | 37.4 | 7.6 |
| swelling | 40.7 | 7.6 |
| pain | 50.9 | 9.9 |
| *Systemic reaction* | | |
| fever >38°C | 46.5 | 9.3 |
| drowsiness | 31.5 | 14.9 |
| fretfulness | 53.4 | 22.6 |
| vomiting | 6.2 | 2.6 |
| anorexia | 20.9 | 7.0 |
| persistent crying | 3.1 | 0.7 |

DTP, diphtheria, tetanus, pertussis; DT, diphtheria, tetanus.

### Severe side effects of DTP

These include attacks of persistent unusual high-pitched crying, pallor, cyanosis, convulsions, encephalopathy which may be temporary or improbably result in permanent brain damage. An estimate of risk of a severe neurological event after pertussis vaccination is about 1:140 000. Persistent neurological damage 1 year later is estimated at 1:330 000. These estimates are unreliable. There is a case for claiming that DTP does not 'cause' permanent damage at all, but rather brings out something which is to occur anyway but is just moved forwards because of the immunization. Indeed, three recent controlled studies involving 230 000 children and 713 000 immunizations found no evidence whatsoever of a causal relationship between pertussis vaccine and permanent neurological illness (Cherry, 1990). The time is almost upon us when we should abandon the notion of pertussis vaccine causing irreversible neurological damage. The risk of fatal pertussis in an unimmunized population heavily outweighs the risk of immunization. Hypotension and anaphylaxis are rare.

### Acellular pertussis vaccines

These promise fewer severe side effects. They have been found to be effective in older children in extensive Japanese studies, and results in younger Swedish children are encouraging (*Lancet* (1988) **i**, 955–960). They are still experimental.

## MEASLES VACCINE/MMR VACCINE

It is given to all children older than 12 months of age. It has low immunogenicity if administered earlier because of residual circulating maternal anti-measles IgG. If immunization has been missed at 12–18 months, give it at any age. It may be given at the same time as polio or DTP if given at different sites. The vaccine induces antibody more rapidly than that following natural infection, hence it can be used for susceptible contacts within 3 days of exposure.

### Adverse reactions

Fever, rash, febrile convulsion, encephalitis (very rare) – all much less common than in the naturally acquired infection.

### Contraindications

1. Febrile or immunosuppressed children.
2. Child within 3 weeks of BCG vaccine.
3. Allergy to eggs, neomycin, kanamycin.

The American Academy of Pediatrics defines egg-allergic children as those with hypotension, generalized urticaria, shock, wheezing, laryngeal spasm or swelling of the mouth or throat resulting from egg ingestion. These children should not have egg-derived vaccines until they have been skin tested. The majority of children with 'egg allergy' do not conform to the above definition and may safely be given the vaccine without skin testing (*Pediatr Alert* (1988) **13**, 105).

Skin testing requires a single intradermal injection of 0.02 ml of 1:100 dilution of MMR vaccine in normal saline with simultaneous administration of a negative control of 0.02 ml normal saline. Antihistamines must not be taken for >3 days prior to testing. Those children with induration or erythema greater than the control after 20 min should be referred to an allergist. Those with a reaction less than or equal to control may be vaccinated. Have basic resuscitation equipment standing by (see Section 1.5).

### New developments

1. Since 1 October 1988, in the UK, the measles vaccine is given as part of the MMR vaccine.
2. A new vaccine (Edmonston–Zagreb measles vaccine) is undergoing trials and it may well be immunogenic when administered to infants >6 months old.

## SPECIAL CONSIDERATIONS

### *1 The child who has missed a DTP vaccine*

DTP can be given at any age. If one of the first 3 doses has been missed, it can be given at any time without having to recommence the whole course.

### *2 Premature infants*

There is no need to delay the start of immunization of preterm infants beyond 3 months from the actual date of birth. Early protection against pertussis in this population is clearly desirable. The normal vaccine dose should be administered (*Pediatrics* (1989) **83**, 471).

### *3 Rubella immunization in pregnancy*

The CDC-Atlanta have reports of 1176 pregnant women receiving live attenuated rubella vaccine within 3 months before or 3 months after date of conception: <2% of those tested had rubella-specific IgM in cord blood and no babies had features of congenital rubella syndrome (Anon., 1987). Pregnancy remains a contraindication to rubella vaccination, but the risks of congenital rubella syndrome are so exceedingly small as to not ordinarily have to consider termination of pregnancy.

### *4 Routine immunization for the immunosuppressed child*

**4.1 Live viruses** These are contraindicated, i.e. measles, mumps, rubella, oral polio (Sabin).

**4.2 Killed inactivated vaccines (diphtheria, tetanus, pertussis, inactivated polio – Salk)** These are safe, although the host response may be less than normal. Typhoid and hepatitis B (both inactivated) can be given.

**4.3 Immunosuppressive treatment (e.g. leukaemia)** If this treatment has been discontinued for at least 1 year (6 months in some centres) and the disease is in remission, live viruses may be administered.

**4.4 The child on steroids** A child on inhaled, alternate day, or low-dose daily steroids (<1 mg/kg/day of prednisolone) can receive live vaccines. Those receiving 2 mg/kg/day of prednisolone for more than 1 week should not be given live viruses until 3 months have elapsed after treatment has ceased.

## *5 Immunosuppressed children in contact with infectious disease*

**5.1 Measles** Give human normal immunoglobulin (HNI) as soon as possible after exposure. It may also be used to attenuate an established attack. Dosages of HNI:

| *Age* (yr) | *Dose* (mg) |
|---|---|
| <1 | 250 |
| 1–2.9 | 500 |
| >3 | 750 |

In Scotland, concentrated human measles immunoglobulin is available.

### 5.2 Varicella

*5.2.1 Prophylactic antivaricella zoster immune globulin (ZIG)* Best given within 24 h of exposure and will attenuate but not prevent an attack. It may be given within 10 days of exposure. There are only limited supplies of ZIG. Varicella fatalities have still been reported in those who have received it. Dosages of ZIG:

| *Age* (yr) | *Dose* (mg) |
|---|---|
| 0–5 | 250 |
| 6–10 | 500 |
| 11–14 | 750 |
| 15+ | 1000 |

*5.2.2 Prophylactic acyclovir* A good alternative to ZIG. Dosages of acyclovir:

| *Age* (yr) | *Dose* (mg) |
|---|---|
| 0–5 | 200 q.d.s. oral for 21 days |
| 5–10 | 400 q.d.s. |
| >10 | 800 q.d.s. |

Immunosuppressed or leukaemic children with a past history of chickenpox do not necessarily need prophylaxis if antibody titres taken before contact are high. If antibody status is in doubt, prophylaxis should be administered. Bone marrow transplant recipients should have ZIG or acyclovir prophylaxis regardless of past history of chickenpox.

*5.2.3 ZIG (at above doses)* Recommended for:

(a) Immunosuppressed or leukaemic contacts of people with chickenpox or zoster (alternatively, can use acyclovir).
(b) Neonates born 6 days or less after onset of maternal chickenpox.
(c) Neonates whose mothers develop chickenpox after delivery.
(d) Neonates who come into contact with chickenpox, but whose mothers have no history of chickenpox.

N.B. In neonates, fatal cases continue to be reported with ZIG prophylaxis alone. Most neonatologists would agree that IV acyclovir should also be used as prophylaxis (Carter, P. E. *et al.* (1986) *Lancet,* **ii**, 1459–1460)

(e) Pregnant contacts – fetal damage is rare. Prevents severe maternal infection.
(f) Serious acute attacks – no evidence that it is of value, but it is nevertheless tried in serious infections.

Immunocompromised children who actually develop chickenpox should receive high-dose acyclovir (see Section 2.1).

## 6 Siblings of immune compromised children

They should all receive live measles vaccine, preferably prior to the affected child returning home. If siblings are unimmunized against polio they should receive inactivated polio vaccine (Salk) rather than the live virus (Sabin).

## 7 School contacts of children with cancer

Children with cancer are encouraged to return to school as early as possible, although there is considerable risk from unimmunized playmates. High uptake of measles vaccine in the class is most desirable and cooperation of the other parents and the school should be sought in this endeavour (Eden, O.B. *et al.* (1988) *Lancet,* **ii**, 283–291). There have been rare cases of probable transmission of measles after MMR vaccination (Milson, S. (1989) *Lancet,* **i**, 271). School contacts should preferably be immunized well before the child with cancer returns to school.

## 8 HIV infection and immunization

HIV-positive individuals whether symptomatic or not *should* receive the following vaccines:

Live – MMR (Anon., 1988).
Inactivated – pertussis, diphtheria, tetanus, typhoid, cholera, hepatitis B.

Polio vaccine should probably be given as inactivated (Salk) vaccine if the child is symptomatic for HIV, but live (Sabin) vaccine may be given to those who are asymptomatic. Contacts of HIV-positive individuals should receive inactivated polio (Salk) vaccine.

BCG is contraindicated.

Yellow fever vaccine should not be given to children with HIV symptoms.

## Further reading


Anon. (1987) Rubella vaccination during pregnancy – United States 1971–86. *M. M. W. R.*, **36**, 457–461

Anon. (1988) Immunization of children infected with HIV – supplementary ACIP statement. *M. M. W. R.*, **37**, 181–183

Anon. (1990) Routine immunization of preterm infants. *Lancet*, **335**, 23–24

Bowie, C. (1990) Lessons from the pertussis vaccine court trial. *Lancet*, **335**, 397–399

Campbell, A. G. M. (1988) Immunisation for the immunosuppressed child. *Arch. Dis. Child.*, **63**, 113–114

Cherry, J. D. (1990) Pertussis vaccine encephalopathy: it is time to recognize the myth that it is. *J. Am. Med. Ass.*, **263**, 1679–1680

Cherry, J. D., Brunell, P. A., Golden, G. S. and Karzon, D. T. (1988) Report of the Task Force on pertussis and pertussis immunization. *Paediatr.*, **81**, 939–984 (suppl.)

Cody, C. L., Barraff, L. J., Cherry, J. D. *et al.* (1981) Nature and rates of adverse reactions associated with DTP and DT immunizations in infants and children. *Pediatr.*, **68**, 650–660

Convay, S. P., James, J. R., Smithells, R. W., Melville-Smith, M. and Magrath, D. (1987) Immunisation of the preterm baby. *Lancet*, **ii**, 1326

Griffin, M. R., Ray, W. A., Livengood, J. R. and Schaffner, W. (1988) Risk of sudden infant death syndrome after immunization with the diphtheria–tetanus–pertussis vaccine. *N. Engl. J. Med.*, **319**, 618–623

Holland, P., Isaacs, D. and Moxon, E. R. (1986) Fatal neonatal varicella infection. *Lancet*, **ii**, 1156

Ipp, M. M., Gold, R., Greenberg, S. *et al.* (1987) Acetaminophen prophylaxis of adverse reactions following vaccinations of infants with DTP/polio vaccine. *Pediatr. Inf. Dis.*, **6**, 721–725

Joint Committee on Vaccination and Immunisation (1988) *Immunisation Against Infectious Disease*, HMSO, London

Markowitz, L. E. and Bernier, R. H. (1987) Immunization of young infants with Edmonston–Zagreb measles vaccine. *Pediatr. Inf. Dis.*, **6**, 809–812

Rutledge, S. L. and Snead, O. C. (1986) Neurological complications of immunizations. *J. Pediatr.*, **109**, 917–924

# 6.2 Immunoprophylaxis against tetanus

## DEFINITION OF A TETANUS-PRONE WOUND

Compound fractures.
Wounds with extensive tissue damage – burns.
Wounds with foreign bodies.
Penetrating wounds.
Wounds contaminated with: soil, dust, horse manure in which there has been more than 6 h delay in receiving topical disinfection or surgical cleansing.
Pyogenic wounds.
Crush injuries including dog bite.

## MANAGEMENT OF TETANUS-PRONE WOUND

### *1 Thorough surgical toilet*

### *2 Not known to have ever been fully immunized against tetanus*

1. Give 250 iu antitetanus immunoglobulin IM in one limb (500 iu if more than 24 h have elapsed since injury).
2. Give the first of 3 injections of adsorbed tetanus toxoid 0.5 ml IM (can give DT if no prior diphtheria vaccination).

### *3 Last primary or booster vaccination more than 10 years ago*

Give antitetanus immunoglobulin 250 iu *and* adsorbed toxoid (in different limbs).

### *4 Last tetanus toxoid between 5 and 10 years ago*

Give 1 dose of adsorbed toxoid.

### *5 Last tetanus toxoid within 5 years*

No treatment required.

## MANAGEMENT OF A CLEAN (NOT TETANUS-PRONE) WOUND

If the last tetanus toxoid was given more than 5 years ago, then administer a booster dose. If the child has never been fully immunized, then complete the primary course. Do not give immunoglobulin for clean cuts.

## SPECIAL CONSIDERATIONS

1. Immunosuppressed children have uncertain immunity even if fully immunized and therefore may require immunoglobulin for tetanus-prone wounds.
2. HIV individuals should be immunized against tetanus.

Chapter 7

# Respiratory system

## 7.1 Sore throat, pharyngitis, tonsillitis

This common clinical condition continues to cause endless controversy about optimal diagnosis and management. Most cases are caused by viruses and need only symptomatic treatment. In 10–30% of acute sore throat a bacterial pathogen is responsible, almost always group A beta haemolytic streptococci (GABHS), although groups C or D are rarely implicated. In the second decade of life, *Corynebacterium haemolyticum* gives an illness indistinguishable from GABHS including a rash that resembles scarlet fever.

Doctors must be aware that rheumatic fever cannot be considered a disease of the past, and they must therefore be prepared to diagnose and treat GABHS infection.

### CLINICAL FEATURES

Clinical features that *suggest* bacterial pharyngitis include headache, anorexia, tender cervical nodes, tonsillar exudate and absence of cough (Platts, Manson and Finch, 1982). It should be noted that adenovirus and Epstein–Barr virus are also strongly associated with pharyngeal exudate. By contrast, features weakly associated with streptococcal pharyngitis are excoriated nares in children (not infants), coryza, conjunctivitis, hoarseness, cough and diarrhoea (Wannamaka, 1972). The best clinical assessment is, however, unreliable in differentiating bacterial from viral pharyngitis.

### INVESTIGATION

#### *1 Throat swab*

Taking a swab is the diagnostic gold standard for GABHS and is to be encouraged.

### 2 Rapid antigen detection tests

In some countries paediatricians routinely use rapid antigen detection kits for GABHS in any child presenting with a sore throat. This is neither routinely available nor advocated in the UK (Burke *et al.*, 1988). The latex agglutination technique has been most thoroughly evaluated and published work on the reliability of the tests varies greatly. The sensitivity (positive test/positive culture × 100) ranges from 55% to 95%, with positive predictive values of 58–96%. False-negative tests can occur in 40–45% of patients (*Pediatr. Inf. Dis. Newsletter* (1988) **14**, 19). Those with a positive test should be managed as having GABHS disease. Those with a negative test should have a throat culture performed.

Newer enzyme immunoassays offer the appeal of colour reactions rather than agglutination to signify a positive test, which makes them easier to interpret, and this may be reflected in higher sensitivity and positive predictive values. The Streptozyme test (Wampole Laboratories, Canbury, NJ, USA) is a rapid test that measures antibody to 5 extracellular antigens. It is comparable to antistrepsinolysin-O titre or antideoxyribonuclease B, but is much less expensive or time consuming. There are many variations in the test which result in inappropriate diagnoses.

## MANAGEMENT

### 1 To treat or not to treat

If a throat culture has been taken it will usually take 24–48 h to yield meaningful results. Delaying treatment for 2–3 days does not increase the small risk of rheumatic fever. Early treatment may reduce the duration of the illness (Nelson, 1984), but symptomatic improvement early in the illness is minimal (Middleton, D'Amico and Merenstein, 1988). Early treatment may also predispose to more frequent reinfection (Pichichero *et al.*, 1987). On balance, if the child has clinical features mentioned above that do not suggest bacterial illness, offer only symptomatic treatment until the throat culture result is available. If the child has the features that suggest bacterial illness, one can await culture results, although for sick children it is sensible to commence antibiotics and subsequently to desist if the culture is negative.

### 2 Antibiotics

Penicillin V 15 mg/kg/8 h orally. For a very sick child initial therapy may be with procaine penicillin 25–50 mg/kg IM × 1, then continue with penicillin V. Stop treatment if culture is negative. If culture is positive, continue for 10 days. Benzathine penicillin G is recommended by many on both sides of the Atlantic, but it is not readily available in the UK, injections are uncomfortable, and it provides only low penicillin levels. Twice daily penicillin V therapy has been shown to be effective (*Am. J. Dis. Child.* (1985) **139**, 1145–1148), and it may increase compliance over a 10-day course. There is nothing at present to recommend the admittedly effective alternative treatments of amoxycillin, erythromycin, cephalosporins or clindamycin as first-line drugs, since penicillin V is cheap, effective and narrow in its spectrum.

### RECURRENCE OF INFECTION

Children who become symptomatic immediately after completing an antibiotic course should be recultured. If they have GABHS infection they should receive erythromycin estolate or, if compliance is an issue, benzathine penicillin G. For frequent attacks or recurrences of GABHS-positive pharyngitis, rifampicin 15 mg/kg/12 h orally may be added to the last 4 days of a course of penicillin in order to rid the nasopharynx of GABHS colonization.

### CARRIERS OF GABHS

Asymptomatic carriers require no treatment. Exceptions include: an individual with rheumatic fever, close contact of the carrier with an individual who had rheumatic fever, carriers in a family with recurrent GABHS infection. Treatment is with rifampicin as above.

### TONSILLECTOMY

Recurrent tonsillitis is seldom regarded as an indication for tonsillectomy nowadays. The size of the tonsils is irrelevant in reaching such a decision (Barr and Crombie, 1989).

## Further reading

Anon. (1987) Bacterial pharyngitis. *Lancet,* **i**, 1241–1242

Barr, G. S. and Crombie, I. K. (1989) Comparison of size of tonsils in children with recurrent tonsillitis and in controls. *Br. Med. J.,* **298**, 804–805

Burke, P., Bain, J., Lowes, A. and Athersuch, R. (1988) Rational decisions in managing sore throat: evaluation of a rapid test. *Br. Med. J.,* **296**, 1646–1649

Denny, F. W. (1985) Effect of treatment on streptoccocal pharyngitis: is the issue really settled? *Pediatr. Inf. Dis.,* **4**, 352–354

McCracken, G. H. (1986) Diagnosis and management of children with streptococcal pharyngitis. *Pediatr. Inf. Dis.,* **5**, 754–759

Middleton, D. B., D'Amico, F. and Merenstein, J. H. (1988) Standardized symptomatic treatment versus penicillin as initial therapy for streptococcal pharyngitis. *J. Pediatr.,* **113**, 1089–1094

Nelson, J. D. (1984) The effect of penicillin therapy on the symptoms and signs of streptococcal pharyngitis. *Pediatr. Inf. Dis.,* **3**, 10–13

Pichichero, M. E., Disney, F. A., Talpey, W. B. *et al.* (1987) Adverse and beneficial effects of immediate treatment of Group A B hemolytic streptococcal pharyngitis with penicillin. *Pediatr. Inf. Dis.,* **6**, 635–643

Platts, P., Manson, P. G. C. and Finch, R. (1982) Acute pharyngitis: a symptom scorecard and microbiological diagnosis. *Br. Med. J.,* **284**, 387–388

Wannamaka, L. W. (1972) Perplexity and precision in the diagnosis of streptococcal pharyngitis. *Am. J. Dis. Child.,* **124**, 352–358

# 7.2 Recurrent/persistent cough

The presence of a cough indicates inflammation of or excess secretions in the larynx, trachea or bronchi. Cough receptors are not present in alveoli, but there are receptors in pleura and diaphragm which may initiate coughing. Asthma is an underdiagnosed cause of recurrent cough. Bronchodilators are more likely to be of therapeutic use than any other 'cough medicine'.

## AETIOLOGY

1. Asthma.
2. Viral bronchitis. Many doubt the existence of viral bronchitis in children with normal airways, and claim that it is all bronchial hyperreactivity or asthma. In either case, the only sensible treatment is to offer nothing or bronchodilator therapy. Smoking by the parents or child is also implicated.
3. Specific infections: pertussis, *Mycoplasma pneumoniae*, tuberculosis.
4. Suppurative lung disease: cystic fibrosis (CF), bronchiectasis.
5. Focal lesions: foreign body, mediastinal lymph nodes/tumours.
6. Chemical irritants – milk inhalation due to reflux, dyskinetic swallowing, overfeeding, H-shaped tracheo-oesophageal fistula (TOF). Active or passive smoking.
7. Congenital anomalies: tracheobronchomalacia ± aberrant great vessels, pulmonary sequestration, bronchogenic cyst, H-shaped TOF.
8. Heart failure.
9. Psychogenic.

## HISTORY

Cough commencing soon after birth suggests milk inhalation or CF. Spontaneous or exercise-induced cough with or without spontaneous or exercise-induced wheeze is likely to be due to asthma, especially if the cough is nocturnal. A child who is not thriving, has gastrointestinal symptoms or has delayed resolution of lung disease must have a sweat test to exclude CF. Inhaled foreign body may also cause delayed resolution of lung disease. With careful questioning, a history of a choking episode can often be elicited. School children with frequent recurrent bouts of coughing but who are otherwise well could have recurrent viral bronchitis. Weight loss and night sweats are features of TB (haemoptysis is uncommon in childhood TB). A family history of a similar illness should be sought. Paroxysmal coughing which results in the child going red or blue in the face and which may be terminated by vomiting is likely to be whooping cough or a viral pertussis-like illness. On examination the child looks remarkably well, despite the parents recounting dramatic symptoms. The 'whoop' may have gone, leaving only a chronic cough in its wake. Infants with pertussis may never whoop, but may merely cough and/or have apnoeic attacks.

### EXAMINATION

Nutritional status, growth and finger clubbing should be assessed, along with evaluation of upper airways and general chest examination. Examination after a period of forced exercise may elicit cough or wheeze that suggest asthma.

### POSSIBLE INVESTIGATION

1. Chest X-ray. If foreign body is suspected, perform inspiratory/expiratory films or fluoroscopic screening of diaphragm.
2. Barium swallow. Useful in suspected vascular malformation or suspected milk inhalation. Also consider oesophageal pH monitor or radiolabelled milk/lung scan.
3. Sputum. Difficult to collect. Do not bother.
4. Lung function tests. Difficult in children under 7–8 years.
5. Bronchial provocation tests. Can be performed even in very young children (Avital, A. *et al.* (1988) *J. Pediatr.*, **112**, 591–594).
6. Bronchoscopy. See Section 7.13.
7. CT scan of chest. Useful for suspected bronchiectasis or when considering surgery for congenital malformation. Bronchoscopy is an alternative.
8. Mantoux test. 0.1 ml of 1:1000, intradermal purified protein derivative (PPD).

### TREATMENT

Treatment depends on the underlying cause. The most common cause of acute or recurrent cough is asthma or a viral illness. 'Cough medicines' and antibiotics are often unnecessarily prescribed (see Section 7.3).

## Further reading

Morgan, W. J. and Taussig, L. M. (1987) The child with persistent cough. *Pediatr. in Rev.*, **8**, 249–253

## 7.3 Practical use of antitussive medication

The only 'cough medicine' likely to have a significant effect is a bronchodilator in the case of the unsuspected asthmatic. The fact that a child coughs does not imply a need for treatment. Most coughs are viral and self-limiting in nature. Cough suppressants are counter-productive for moist coughs, and there is no effective expectorant for dry cough apart from adequate hydration. Parents should be informed that there is little objective benefit to cough mixtures. Symptomatic relief may well be obtained from simple linctus or other demulcents which are cheap and safe. A dry irritating cough may occasionally warrant a suppressant. In general, if one feels the need to prescribe a cough mixture, demulcents make the most sense, and if there is even a faint suspicion of asthma, bronchodilators should be tried.

## CLASSIFICATION OF ANTITUSSIVES

### *1 Cough expectorants*

Ammonium chloride, potassium iodine, ipecacuanha, guaiphenesin. All irritate gastric mucosa and may act by reflex stimulation of secretory glands of lower respiratory tract. These agents have not been shown to work better than placebo. Good hydration is probably the best expectorant.

### *2 Cough suppressants*

Pholcodine, codeine, dextromethorphan – all are effective. Controlled trials as to their value in viral bronchitis are lacking. Do not use in children less than 2 years, if at all.

### *3 Demulcents*

Substances which coat the irritated pharyngeal mucosa include glycerine, honey, liquorice and simple linctus. They are cheap, harmless and do not need prescription.

### *4 Antihistamines*

For example, diphenhydramine. Probably has mild antitussive and topical anaesthetic effect. N.B. Danger of sedation.

### *5 Antibiotics*

Bacterial bronchitis in a young child with normal airways is rare. Under normal circumstances, antibiotics should not be prescribed.

# 7.4 Pertussis/whooping cough

Whooping cough is caused by *Bordatella pertussis* by a mechanism that is almost certainly toxin mediated. Especially in infancy, several viruses as well as *B. parapertussis* may give a pertussis-like illness (whooping cough syndrome, parapertussis), but it is usually (not always) milder and shorter than true pertussis. Britain has unfortunately led the world in demonstrating how decreased vaccination rates result in increased mortality from pertussis. The only reservoir of pertussis is man. Vaccination of more than 80% of the population gives herd immunity. It is possible that with universal vaccine compliance, the disease might be eradicated (Kendrick, P. L. (1985) *J. Infect. Dis.*, **132,** 709–712).

## INCUBATION PERIOD

Seven to 14 days.

## CLINICAL FEATURES

### *1 Catarrhal or coryzal phase*

The most infectious phase. Lasts 1 week, with dry cough and watery nasal discharge. Similar to the common cold.

### *2 Paroxysmal or spasmodic phase*

The cough typically occurs in bursts of short paroxysms which gradually lengthen. During coughing, the child goes red or blue in the face and tears stream from the eyes. The spasm may end with an inspiratory 'whoop'. Paroxysms are often terminated by vomiting. Infants often do not whoop and may sometimes become apnoeic with no or a trivial cough. This period lasts from 4 to 8 weeks. Between paroxysms the child looks well; hence the typical presentation is that of a well child with a tired anxious mother who fears that her child will choke with any coughing episode and therefore maintains a sleepless bedside vigil. The temptation is for the doctor to assume neurotic anxiety in the mother and prescribe several unnecessary series of antibiotics for the child. Frequent vomiting may result in temporary weight loss.

### *3 Convalescent phase*

Begins when a chronic cough replaces paroxysms. Usually lasts 3–4 weeks. However, it may persist for months. A new respiratory infection in the ensuing months may result in a short illness resembling whooping cough.

## COMPLICATIONS

Hypoxia – causes fitting and CNS damage.

Pressure effects – epistaxis, subconjunctival haemorrhage, cerebral haemorrhage.

Bronchopneumonia – usually secondary to infection with *Streptococcus pneumoniae*, *Staphylococcus aureus*, or *Haemophilus influenzae*.

Lobar/segmental collapse – usually resolves without treatment or physiotherapy.

## DIAGNOSIS

### 1 Per nasal and post-nasal swabs

Must be plated immediately on Bordet–Gengou medium to which penicillin has been added to inhibit growth of other organisms.

### 2 Immunofluorescence

Fluorescent antibody staining of post-nasal or pharyngeal specimens may provide a rapid specific diagnosis.

### 3 Blood lymphocyte count

Absolute lymphocyte count of $>20\,000/\text{mm}^3$ is suggestive of pertussis.

## PREVENTION

### 1 *Vaccination* (see Section 6.1)

Confers high (but not complete) protection for about 3 years, declining thereafter. Immunized children who develop pertussis have milder shorter illnesses with markedly decreased infectivity. Acellular vaccines currently on trial promise fewer side effects.

### 2 Antibiotics

Erythromycin 30–50 mg/kg/day for 14 days decreases infectivity but does not modify the illness if given after the coryzal phase. It may prevent illness if given to susceptible contacts. The estolate ester is best.

### 3 Isolation

Mandatory if child is to be admitted.

## TREATMENT

### 1 Admission

Admit all suspected cases under 6 months and any older child who has cyanotic or apnoeic spells. If one does not admit a child with pertussis, explain the natural history to the parents to reduce their expectation of a rapid recovery.

### 2 Antibiotics – see above

All children admitted to hospital should be started on erythromycin to minimize infectivity. Secondary bacterial pneumonia does occasionally occur and should be treated on its merits.

### 3 Supportive care

**3.1 Attention to fluid and nutritional status** This is important because of the frequent vomiting seen in pertussis. One can try giving feeds immediately after a coughing burst or small regular feeds.

**3.2 Apnoeic or cyanotic turns** Managed with suction and gentle stimulation ± head box $O_2$. An apnoea alarm or cardiac monitor is useful in an infant with frequent episodes.

**3.3 Sympathomimetics** Numerous anecdotal and small controlled trials suggest these to be of benefit. Oral salbutamol can be given at 0.1–0.15 mg/kg/6 h (*Lancet* (1977) **i**, 150–151; (1977) **ii**, 1083; (1982) **i**, 310–312; (1986) **ii**, 282) or it can be nebulized.

**3.4 Corticosteroids** Only one controlled trial performed (*Arch. Dis. Child.* (1973) **48**, 51). It supports the use of steroids in severely ill infants. Use hydrocortisone 30 mg/kg/day IM/IV or prednisolone 6 mg/kg/day oral.

**3.5 Nasal continuous positive airway pressure (CPAP)/ ventilation** CPAP has been tried successfully in a 3-week-old infant (*Anaesthesia* (1979) **34**, 1028–1031). One group advocates early intervention with intubation ventilation and morphine sedation (Gillis *et al.* (1988) *Arch. Dis. Child.*, **63**, 364–367), but they do not appear to have first considered CPAP.

**3.6 Other care** Physiotherapy, cough suppressants, expectorants, mucolytic agents and mist therapy are not helpful. Sedation is regarded by many as being dangerous, but there are sporadic reports that barbiturate sedation may be worth trying (Davis, J. A., personal communication).

## Further reading

Anon. (1986) Antibiotics in whooping cough. *Drug Ther. Bull.*, **24**, 91–92

Anon. (1988) Whooping cough in infants. *Lancet*, **ii**, 946

Bass, J. W. (1985) Pertussis: current status of prevention and treatment. *Pediatr. Inf. Dis.*, **4**, 614–619

Broomhall, J. H. and Herxheimer, A. (1984) Treatment of whooping cough: the facts. *Arch. Dis. Child.*, **59**, 185–187

# 7.5 Stridor

Stridor is a high-pitched noise heard predominantly during inspiration, which is usually louder with higher inspiratory flow rates, i.e. in a crying or agitated child. It suggests blockage of the upper airway (which may include the extrathoracic trachea and upward). Acute stridor in children is most commonly due to croup, whereas chronic or congenital stridor in infants is usually due to infantile larynx. It is axiomatic that other causes of stridor must be considered.

## CAUSES OF STRIDOR

| *Acute* | *Persistent/chronic* |
|---|---|
| Croup | Infantile larynx |
| Acute epiglottitis | Subglottic stenosis |
| Laryngeal foreign body | Vocal cord palsy |
| Diphtheria | Laryngeal web, cleft, cysts, warts |
| Angioneurotic oedema | Tracheal stenosis |
| Retropharyngeal abscess | Vascular ring |
| Tetany | Tracheomalacia |

Some causes of acute and chronic stridor will be discussed in detail. Angioneurotic oedema is discussed in Section 1.5.

# 7.6 Acute laryngotracheobronchitis (croup)

## INTRODUCTION

Croup is the most common cause of acute stridor in childhood.

## AETIOLOGY

Parainfluenza viruses account for most cases.

Other viruses – RSV, influenza A + B, rhinovirus, adenovirus, EBV, measles, varicella.

Bacteria – rarely cause croup. Consider *Staphylococcus aureus, Corynebacterium diphtheriae*, Group A beta haemolytic streptococci.

## CLINICAL FEATURES

Coryzal prodrome.

Harsh barking (croupy) cough ± hoarse voice.

Inspiratory stridor ± chest indrawing.

Symptoms are usually worse at night or when agitated

Fever is variable but rarely more than 39°C.

## SIGNS OF SEVERE OBSTRUCTION

Hypoxia – restlessness, tachycardia, cyanosis.

Physical exhaustion – stridor and indrawing may decrease, lethargy.

## DIAGNOSIS AND DIFFERENTIAL DIAGNOSIS

### *1 Croup*

Gives a characteristic cough and usually has a coryzal prodrome. The stridor may fluctuate from hour to hour.

### *2 Epiglottitis*

The parents usually first notice the very rapid onset of fever and lethargy. Over 2–3 h, the child develops snoring-like breathing, drooling of saliva and seldom coughs (if he does, the cough is never barking). The child looks ill, pale and toxic, and prefers sitting to lying down.

### *3 Laryngeal foreign body*

The child is usually not febrile or ill. A history of a choking episode is common (but not essential), followed by symptoms of stridor, cough and hoarse voice.

### *4 Others*

Diphtheria, acute anaphylaxis.

## MANAGEMENT

### *1 At home*

A child with no stridor at rest when seen in hospital can be managed at home.

**1.1 A moist atmosphere** This is (anecdotally) helpful. This is best done by running hot taps in the bathroom. Steam inhalations from boiling water on the stove are forbidden because of the risk of spillage and burns. Sedation is contraindicated.

**1.2 Alternatively,** taking the child to an open window, promenading the child outside in a pram or taking the child for a drive may all be of use.

**1.3 Explain to the parents** that the stridor will last 2–3 days and be worse at night. The cough may persist for several weeks. Stress that the parents may freely bring the child back to hospital if they are concerned or if the child develops stridor at rest.

### *2 In hospital*

**2.1 Admit,** if the child has stridor at rest.

**2.2 Avoid increasing the child's anxiety and irritability**. Therefore:

(a) A parent should remain with the child.
(b) Do not examine the pharynx. It is particularly distressing and may precipitate obstruction.
(c) As few 'hands on' observations as possible.

(d) Blood gas analysis has little role. The decision to intubate a child is made on clinical grounds. Performing a painful arterial stab in a child with severe stridor might precipitate total obstruction.

**2.3 Observation** Pulse and respiratory rates, degree of chest indrawing and irritability of the child are useful monitors of hypoxia. Frequent measurement of temperature is of little use and may unnecessarily distress the child. Measuring $O_2$ saturation with pulse oximetry does not distress the child, gives useful information, provides a method of continuous monitoring and is advised.

**2.4 Humidification** This is traditional but not of proven value (Bourchier *et al.*, 1984). Its use may be justified if the child can still be observed and if it does not distress him. If the child clearly objects to being in a steam tent, it is far better to promenade him up and down the ward than have him struggling and held in the tent against his will.

**2.5 Drugs**

*2.5.1 Nebulized adrenaline* This is of greatest use in facilitating the safe transport of a child from a smaller centre to one with better facilities for managing the paediatric airway. All children unwell enough to receive it in an emergency department should be admitted for close observation because it will mask the underlying severity of the illness and there is a theoretical risk of rebound obstruction as the drug effect wears off.

Dose: adrenaline 0.1% (1:1000) – 0.25 ml/kg/dose (max. 5 ml); racemic adrenaline 1% or 2.25% – 0.05 ml/kg/dose.

*2.5.2 Corticosteroids* Their use is controversial, and as yet there are no satisfactory trials to recommend them, although side effects if any are rare. The issue is not yet resolved. Articles by Tunnessen and Kairys and colleagues, cited below, cover the topic well.

**2.6 Intubation/tracheostomy** Intubate using inhalational anaesthesia, as in Section 7.7. Use ETT one-half size smaller than predicted, i.e. (Age/4 + 4) – 1/2. Expect copious secretions immediately post-intubation, which will require very frequent suction by diligent nurses. In the first instance, approximately 5 days' intubation is needed.

## Further reading

Anon. (1989) Steroids and croup. *Lancet*, **ii**, 1134–1136

Bourchier, D. *et al.* (1984) Humidification in viral croup – a controlled trial. *Aust. Paediatr. J.*, **20**, 289–291

Henry, R. (1983) Moist air in the treatment of laryngotracheitis. *Arch. Dis. Child.*, **58**, 577

Kairys, S. W., Olmstead, E. M. and O'Connor, G. T. (1989) Steroid treatment of laryngotracheitis: a meta-analysis of the evidence from randomized trials. *Pediatr.*, **83**, 693

Phelan, P. D., Landau, L. I. and Olinsky, A. (1982) *Respiratory Illness in Children*. Blackwell, Melbourne, pp. 59–67

Tunnessen, W. W. and Feinstein, A. R. (1980) The steroid croup controversy – an analytic review of methodological problems. *J. Pediatr.*, **96**, 751

# 7.7 Acute epiglottitis

This is a most serious form of acute laryngeal obstruction requiring prompt recognition and treatment. The obstruction is caused by gross oedema of the epiglottis and aryepiglottic folds and is almost always due to infection with *Haemophilus influenzae* type B. Peak age incidence is 3 years, but the range is wide and extends into adulthood.

## CLINICAL FEATURES

Rapid onset of symptoms over 3–4 h.
Snoring, inspiratory and expiratory noises.
Toxic, pale, febrile.
Drooling saliva.
Prefers to sit up.
Refusing to eat or drink.
Absence of or unremarkable cough.

## DIAGNOSIS AND MANAGEMENT

- *Do not inspect the pharynx.*
- *Keep the child propped up and undisturbed.*
- *Notify an anaesthetist (paediatric).*
- *Do not put in an IV line.*
- *Do not perform a lateral neck x-ray.*

### *1 Severe obstruction*

Direct laryngoscopy and intubation should be performed by a skilled paediatrician or anaesthetist, if possible with an ENT surgeon at the bedside should a tracheostomy be needed. The child can be anaesthetized by inhaling gradually increasing concentrations of halothane (up to 4%). A nasotracheal tube is most easily managed. After intubation, splint the child's arms aggressively. Apply a condenser humidifier (Thermal Humidifying Filter, Portex, Hythe, Kent) to the ETT. Transfer the child to intensive care. Sedation or paralysis may be considered if the risk of self-extubation is thought to be high and if there is no one on hand for the first 3–5 h capable of reintubating the child should the need arise.

Extubation is indicated when the child looks better and the temperature drops. This is usually within 24 h of intubation.

### *2 Mild or atypical cases*

Lateral neck x-ray may help in making the diagnosis but may precipitate obstruction, hence it should only be performed in the intensive care unit (ICU) setting (James, I. (1986) *Lancet,* **i**, 112) with someone capable of emergency intubation at hand. Direct laryngoscopy by an anaesthetist in theatre or the ICU is usually more appropriate. Alternatively, one can treat with antibiotics and observe in the ICU (at least 13% of cases managed in large centres do not require intubation).

### INVESTIGATION

Epiglottic swab at the time of intubation.
Blood culture only after the airway has been stabilized.

### TREATMENT

Chloramphenicol 40 mg/kg IV or IM, followed by 25 mg/kg/6 h IV or NGT. Treatment is continued for a total of 4 days. After extubation, oral treatment is acceptable. Alternative therapy is cefotaxime 50 mg/kg/6 h.

### PROPHYLAXIS FOR CONTACTS

See *H. influenzae* meningitis – Section 8.2.

## Further reading

Butt, W., Shann, F., Walker, C. *et al.* (1988) Acute epiglottitis: a different approach to management. *Crit. Care. Med.*, **16**, 43–47

Davis, H. W., Gartner, J. C. and Galvis, A. G. (1981) Acute upper airway obstruction: croup and epiglottitis. *Pediatr. Clin. N. Am.*, **28**, 869–879.

## 7.8 Laryngeal foreign body (FB)

### CLINICAL FEATURES

### *1 If the child is stable and pink*

Calm the child down
Laryngoscopy under controlled conditions.

### *2 If the child is conscious but actively choking*

Put the child prone over an attendant's knees and deliver 4 back blows. If unsuccessful, administer 4 chest thrusts as for external cardiac massage.

Heimlich manoeuvre (abdominal thrusts) is not advised for young children because of the risk of damage to abdominal organs. Lift jaw and open mouth in an attempt to see and hopefully remove the FB.

*3 If the child is unconscious with inadequate respiration*
Attempt a quick laryngoscopy and removal of FB. If not immediately successful, proceed to tracheostomy or cricothyroid puncture with the largest bore needle available (see Section 1.3).

## 7.9 Chronic stridor/infantile larynx

Infantile larynx (laryngomalacia) is the most common cause of chronic stridor in infants, and it is due to inspiratory laryngeal collapse. The glottic region in particular may be disproportionately small for the child's size, especially so in those with Down's syndrome. The pathological basis of the lesion is not known.

### CLINICAL FEATURES

Stridor is the presenting feature, often not present at birth but developing within the first 4 weeks of life, although a respiratory infection may unmask a mild case several weeks later. Classically the stridor changes with posture and is usually mildest in the prone or sitting positions.

### DIAGNOSIS

A presumptive clinical diagnosis is usually made. Direct laryngoscopy is important and in young infants can be done in the ward without anaesthesia or sedation. The larynx is small and anterior; the epiglottis is long and curled up on itself (omega shape). During inspiration, the structures of the larynx collapse in on themselves, leaving a slit-like opening through which air must pass.

Digital palpation of the tongue to the level of the epiglottis should be attempted, to exclude cysts at the base of the tongue (*Arch. Dis. Child.* (1987) **62**, 1173–1174). Cutaneous haemangiomata may provide a clue to laryngeal or tracheal haemangiomata. If there is doubt about the diagnosis of infantile larynx, the child should have a barium swallow to exclude a vascular ring, and consideration should be given to bronchoscopy.

### TREATMENT

Posturing the child in the prone position may be of some use. Beyond that, the management is expectant. The natural history should be explained to the parents, accompanied by abundant reassurance if the child is thriving.

### NATURAL HISTORY

Major improvements occur by 1 year of age and stridor has usually resolved by 3 years. Until then, the child is at greater risk of symptomatic croup than his peers.

## Further reading

McSwiney, P. F., Cavanagh, P. C. and Languth, P. (1977) Outcome in congenital stridor (laryngomalacia). *Arch. Dis. Child.*, **52**, 215–218

# 7.10 Wheezing

This is a moist musical continuous sound heard mainly (although not solely) during expiration associated with prolonged expiratory time. It indicates obstruction in medium or smaller airways, although it is occasionally due to narrowing of a major bronchus or the trachea. It is important to differentiate between acute, recurrent and persistent wheeze, as their aetiologies and managements differ.

**Axioms** All that wheezes is not asthma. By far the commonest cause of wheeze is asthma.

### CAUSES OF WHEEZE

See Table 7.1.

#### *1 Infants*

Bronchiolitis is by far the commonest cause of acute wheeze, although aspiration should be considered in infants with persistent or recurrent wheeze. Children with gastro-oesophageal reflux may have acute or recurrent wheeze. Incoordinate swallowing seen in children with severe CNS disease predisposes to inhalation of milk and wheezing. Children surviving hyaline membrane disease as premature babies may wheeze and are prone to respiratory syncytial virus (RSV) bronchiolitis. Airway

**Table 7.1 Causes of wheeze according to age**

| *Infants* | *Toddlers* | *Children/adolescents* |
|---|---|---|
| Bronchiolitis | Asthma | Asthma |
| GOR | Bronchiolitis | *Mycoplasma* |
| Milk inhalation | CF | Bronchiectasis |
| BPD | IFB | Mediastinal mass |
| Asthma | Bronchiectasis | A1AT deficiency |
| CF | Mediastinal mass | |
| Airway malformation | | |
| Vascular malformation | | |
| Mediastinal cyst | | |

GOR, gastro-esophageal reflux; BPD, bronchopulmonary dysplasia; CF, cystic fibrosis; IFB, inhaled/ingested foreign body; A1AT, alpha-1 antitrypsin.

malformations that cause wheezing are rare and include tracheo/bronchomalacia, congenital lobar emphysema, subglottic haemangioma. Vascular malformations include vascular rings and large left to right cardiac shunts. Mediastinal cysts may be cystic hygromata (usually in the neck) or bronchogenic cysts.

### *2 Toddlers and older children*

Wheeze in this age group is commonly due to asthma. Suppurative lung disease, especially cystic fibrosis, must be considered, although cough is a more prominent feature than wheezing. As children develop greater ambulatory and manual dexterity, they are increasingly vulnerable to inhaling a foreign body. Mediastinal masses (mainly hilar lymphadenopathy including reticuloendothelial malignancy) can cause extrinsic compression of the main bronchi. A history of weight loss, cough, fever and night sweats, in addition to wheeze, suggests tuberculosis or lymphoma. Alpha 1 antitrypsin deficiency usually causes liver disease rather than overt respiratory disease in childhood.

## 7.11 Acute viral bronchiolitis

Bronchiolitis is an illness with inflammation of bronchioles of the calibre 300 μm to 75 μm, resulting in increased airway resistance and lung hyperinflation. It occurs primarily in children under 1 year of age and usually during the winter months, usually as a result of RSV infection.

## CLINICAL FEATURES

Usually begins as coryza progressing over 1–2 days to irritating cough, wheeze, distressed rapid breathing and difficulty in feeding. Examination reveals chest indrawing, widespread (end) inspiratory crepitations and dense expiratory rhonchi. Chest is barrel shaped and liver is displaced downwards due to hyperinflated lungs (high functional residual capacity).

In more severe disease or when exhaustion supervenes, cyanosis in air and $CO_2$ retention occur. Apnoea is a common complication in those born prematurely.

## INVESTIGATIONS

### *1 CXR*

Hyperinflation, peribronchial thickening and 35% have areas of consolidation and segmental or lobar collapse.

### *2 Arterial gases*

Usually not necessary. $P\text{aco}_2$ may be low, normal or raised. Respiratory rate parallels the degree of hypoxia.

### *3 Nasal mucus aspirate*

Immunofluorescence of RSV or other viruses if available.

## DIFFERENTIAL DIAGNOSIS

### *1. Acute asthma*

The distinction is almost arbitrary. The first attack of wheezing in an infant is called bronchiolitis. Recurrent wheezing is asthma.

### *2 Pneumonia*

Typically causes higher fever, more constitutional disturbance and no hyperinflation.

### *3* Chlamydia *pneumonia*

May occur in or soon after the neonatal period. A history of neonatal conjunctivitis is occasionally elicited. Cough is more prominent than wheeze.

### *4 Heart failure*

Often has heart murmur, extra heart sounds, and a large heart on CXR.

## MANAGEMENT

Most can be managed at home with no treatment.

### *1 Admit*

If child has difficulty feeding (a good sign of respiratory distress).

### *2 $O_2$ – via head box or oxygen cot*

May need up to 70% $O_2$.

### *3 Fluids*

IV or NGT (usually the former if unwell).

### *4 Monitoring*

An apnoea alarm, bedside ECG or pulse oximeter.

### *5 Assisted ventilation*

Needed in approx. 1% of hospital admissions. There is no absolute value of $P\text{co}_2$ that indicates the need for positive pressure ventilation (*Arch. Dis. Child.* (1974) **49**, 143–148). The decision is a clinical one, not one based on blood gases. Nasal CPAP is effective treatment, relatively free of complications. Endotracheal intubation with CPAP alone should be tried next, followed by intermittent positive pressure ventilation (IPPV), probably with high end expiratory pressure (see Section 7.12).

### *6 Others*

Bronchodilators and/or steroids – not for routine use. There is some evidence that inhaled beta agonists are of use in a small percentage of children. It makes sense to try several doses and desist if there is no clear improvement.
Ribavirin – rarely indicated except in children with CF, cyanotic congenital heart disease, bronchopulmonary dysplasia, or those needing ventilator support.
Antibiotics – should not be used routinely.
Small particle water vapour – of no use.

## PROGNOSIS

The overwhelming majority recover within 7–10 days.

## Further reading

Beasley, J. M. and Jones, E. F. (1981) Continuous positive pressure in bronchiolitis. *Br. Med. J.*, **283,** 1506–1508

Milner, A. D. (1988) Ribavarin and acute bronchiolitis in infants. *Br. Med. J.*, **297**, 998–999

Phelan, P. D., Landau, L. I. and Olinsky, A. (1982) *Respiratory Illness in Children*, Blackwell, Melbourne

# 7.12 Asthma

Asthma is generally an underdiagnosed, undertreated condition. Although deaths are rare, there have been suggestions of increased mortality in recent years. The main reasons are a lack of appreciation of the severity of the problem by the family and doctor, coupled with inadequate treatment.

## DEFINITION

### *1 Clinical*

Recurrent cough, wheeze, or shortness of breath, especially at night, or with exercise, which reverse spontaneously or with bronchodilator therapy.

### *2 Pathophysiological*

Hyperreactive airways, especially to stresses such as histamine, methacholine, cold, smoke and exercise.

### *3 Pathological*

Narrowing of bronchi and bronchioles by smooth muscle spasm, mucosal oedema and mucus production.

## CLASSIFICATION (FAIRLY ARBITRARY)

### *1 According to the severity of acute attacks*

**1.1 Mild attack** One that is readily reversed by oral or inhaled $\beta_2$ agonists alone.

**1.2 Moderate attack** One requiring both inhaled $\beta_2$ agonists and methyl xanthines.

**1.3 Severe attack** As above, plus requiring steroids.

### *2 According to the pattern of the attacks*

**2.1 Mild (episodic) asthmatic** Infrequent attacks occurring less often than once a month or just seasonally such that they do not substantially affect the everyday activities of the child.

**2.2 Moderate (chronic) asthmatic** Attacks occurring every 2–4 weeks or more often, of sufficient severity that were treatment not to be offered, they would disturb the everyday life of the child, but which respond well to non-steroid prophylaxis.

**2.3 Severe (chronic) asthmatic** Frequent or continuous attacks requiring steroid prophylaxis.

Mild asthmatics tend to have mild attacks, moderate asthmatics tend to have moderate attacks, and so on; however, this is by no means always the case.

## NATURAL HISTORY

Seventy-five per cent of asthmatic children are mild asthmatics. Virtually all of these either become symptom free before puberty, or else continue into adulthood with trivial infrequent symptoms, usually associated with exercise or intercurrent infections. About 16% of affected children are moderate asthmatics requiring non-steroid prophylaxis either from the start or after a period of mild asthma. About half of these are symptom free before puberty. About 9% of asthmatics fall into the steroid-dependent severe group from the start or after a number of years of milder disease. Most of these also improve, but it usually occurs after puberty, and the improvement is usually incomplete.

By age 21 years some 44% of asthmatics will have become symptom free, 41% will have mild symptoms, and only 15% will still have troublesome disease, mostly those from the severe group.

## EVALUATING THE KNOWN OR SUSPECTED ASTHMATIC

### *1 During an acute attack*

Cough, wheeze, hyperinflated chest, chest indrawing.
Signs of severity include:

(a) pulsus parodoxus – if absent, this does not exclude severe disease;
(b) poor air entry;
(c) shortness of breath while speaking or difficulty in feeding;
(d) cyanosis.

### *2 The moderate–severe (chronic) asthmatic*

History of nocturnal cough or exercise-induced asthma are helpful clues. Examine for chest deformity (Harrison's sulcus) and growth failure. At each visit, compliance with and understanding of the treatment should be verified. Clubbing, increased anteroposterior diameter of the chest or failure to thrive suggest other disorders such as cystic fibrosis, bronchiectasis or immunodeficiency.

### *3 Lung function tests*

After age 7 years or thereabout, a child will often cooperate in lung function testing, which can be helpful in either establishing the diagnosis or following the progress of the asthma. If a child is wheezy, then simple spirometry should show at least a 20% decrease in the forced expired volume in 1 second ($FEV_1$) and maximum mid-expiratory flow rate

($MEF_{50}$). A marked (>20%) improvement after correct administration of a $\beta_2$ agonist makes the diagnosis of asthma virtually certain.

Peak flow readings (Figure 7.1): the peak expiratory flow rate (PEFR) which is easy to measure will be low unless the asthma is very mild and only affects the smaller airways. It is lowest in the morning. A fall of more than 15% after exercise or a similar rise after bronchodilator therapy is suggestive of asthma. Regular PEFR readings are helpful in monitoring the daily progress of asthma, the severity of an attack, and the resolution with treatment.

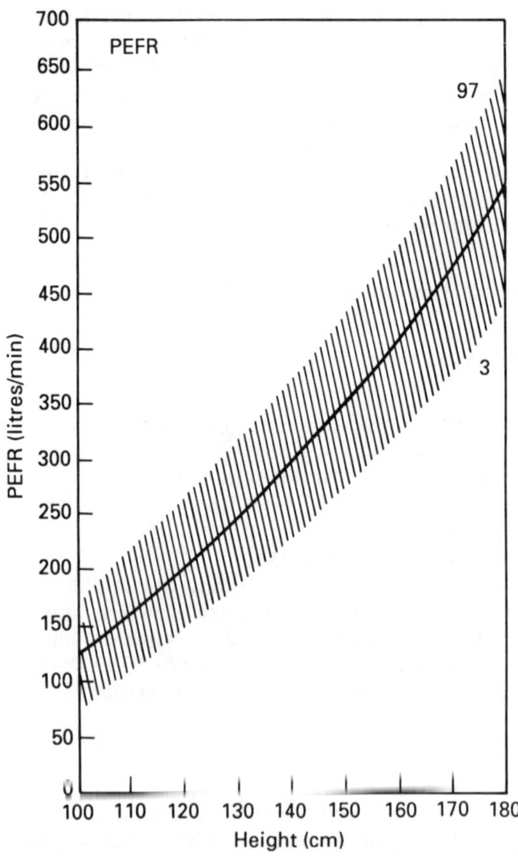


**Figure 7.1** Peak expiratory flow rate (PEFR) according to height (Redrawn by Professor S. Godfrey, from Godfrey, S. *et al.* (1970) *Br. J. Dis. Chest.*, **64**, 15, with permission of the author)

### *4 Bronchial provocation tests*

Used if the diagnosis is uncertain either because of an atypical clinical picture or because the child is well at the time of testing. The provocation of an asthmatic child results in bronchial hyperreactivity.

**4.1 Exercise challenge** Hard exercise for 6 min (Godfrey, 1983).

**4.2 Methacholine or histamine challenge** (Cockcroft, D. *et al.* (1977) *Clin. Allergy,* **7**, 235–243).

**4.3 Methacholine challenge with tracheal auscultation** This recently described method can be used in young children unable to perform lung function tests (Avital, A. *et al.* (1988) *J. Pediatr.,* **112**, 591–594).

## PRECIPITANTS OF ACUTE ATTACK

Viral upper respiratory tract infection is by far the commonest. A careful history should be taken for obvious allergic triggers (e.g. child wheezes every time the cat walks in or floor is swept) and these allergens avoided. Other triggers include cold air, exercise, dust, smoke, chemicals (notably aspirin, particularly in children with nasal polyps and sinus disease) and emotional factors.

## OUTPATIENT MANAGEMENT GUIDELINES

### *1 Drug treatment* (Table 7.2)

**1.1 Infrequent acute mild attacks** Require intermittent treatment with bronchodilators using $\beta_2$ agonists. Nebulized inhalation is best, but in children older than 8 years a metered aerosol may be tried if proper technique is used. Children between 4 and 8 years can avoid the need for perfect technique by using an aerosol with spacing chamber (Table 7.3). Continue treatment for several days after clinical resolution of an attack. Oral treatment is seldom used because of frequent side effects and poor efficacy.

**1.2 Infrequent acute moderate attacks** Use nebulized $\beta_2$ agonist and slow-release theophylline (SRT). Increasingly, a short (3-day) course of prednisolone 1–2 mg/kg/day is being given at home as curative treatment or at the onset of wheezing as preventative treatment (Brunette, M. G. (1988) *Pediatr.,* **81**, 624–629).

**1.3 Prophylaxis for the moderate asthmatic** Use either cromoglycate or SRT. There appears little benefit in using both together. Cromoglycate can be given by nebulized inhalation to young children, by spinhaler to children beyond 4 years of age, or by metered aerosol. It is cheap, safe and does not require blood tests. SRT has the advantage of twice daily administration in an oral form, but has more side effects. Pre-dose blood

**Table 7.2 Bronchodilator doses**

| *Drug* | *Preparation* | *Dose* | *Notes* |
|---|---|---|---|
| $\beta_2$ AGONISTS<br>Salbutamol sulphate<br>(Ventolin) | *Oral*:<br>Mixt. 2 mg/5 ml<br>Tab. 2 mg, 4 mg | 0.1–0.15 mg/kg/6 h | S/E tremor, hyperexcitability, tachycardia |
| | *Inhaled*:<br>Rotacaps 200 µg, 400 µg | 1 q.i.d. | Respirator soln and nebules may be used more frequently in ward, and continuously in ICU |
| | Inh. 100 µg/puff | 1–2 puffs 4–6 times daily | |
| | Nebules 2 mg/2.5 ml | 1 neb. 3–6 h | |
| | Resp. soln 5 mg/ml | 0.05 ml/kg to max. 1 ml diluted to 2 ml 3–6 h | In moderate–severe asthma nebulize with $O_2$ |
| | *Intravenous*:<br>Amp. 500 µg/ml | 5–10 µg/kg/min | |
| Terbutaline sulphate<br>(Bricanyl) | Mixt. 300 µg/ml<br>Tab. 5 mg | 75–125 µg/kg/6 h | |
| | Inh. 250 µg/puff | 1–2 puffs 4–6 h | |
| | Resp. soln 10 mg/ml | 0.25–0.5 ml diluted to 2 ml 3–6 h | |
| | Amp. 500 µg/ml | 5 µg/kg/dose subcut. | Useful for GP home visit to a severe asthmatic when no nebulizer is available |
| XANTHINE DERIVATIVES<br>Theophylline | Tab. 125 mg<br>Mixt. 60 mg/5 ml | 5 mg/kg/6 h | S/E nausea, vomit, abdominal pain. In toxic doses, cardiac arrhythmias and convulsions occur. SR tabs are scored and may be broken in two but not crushed or chewed. Capsules may be opened and contents sprinkled on food or fed on a spoon. Level 55–110 µmol/litre (10–20 µg/ml). Irritability, school and learning difficulties may be a problem |
| | Slow-release tabs 175, 200, 250, 400 mg<br>Cap. (slophylline) 60, 125, 200 mg | 8–10 mg/kg/12 h | |

| | | | |
|---|---|---|---|
| XANTHINE DERIVATIVES contd. | | | |
| Aminophylline (25 mg is equivalent to 20 mg theophylline) | Amp. 25 mg/ml | IV loading dose 5 mg/kg over 20 min, then 6 mg/kg/6 h over 20 min *or* 1 mg/kg/h infusion | N.B. Bolus doses are potentially cardiotoxic |
| CROMOGLYCATE | | | |
| Sodium cromoglycate | Inh. cap. 20 mg<br>Resp. soln 20 mg/2 ml | 3–4 caps/24 h<br>2 ml 3–4 times/24 h | |
| STEROIDS | | | |
| Beclomethasone diproprionate | Rotacap 100 μg | <8 yr 1 cap. 2–4 times/24 h | May adversely affect height development (*Lancet* (1988), **i**, 115 and 475–476; also *Lancet* (1986), **i**, 942 and 1393) |
| | Inh. 50 μg/dose | >8 yr 1–4 puffs 2–4 times/24 h | |
| | Resp soln. 50 μg/ml | <1 yr 50 μg 2–4 times daily<br>1–12 yr 100 μg 2–4 times daily | |
| Prednisolone | Tab. 1 mg, 5 mg | 2 mg/kg/day for 3–4 days, then stop abruptly | |
| Methylprednisolone | Amp. 40 mg, 125 mg, 1 g, 2 g | 1 mg/kg/6 h IV | |
| Hydrocortisone | 100 mg, 500 mg | 3–5 mg/kg/6 h IV | |
| ANTICHOLINERGICS | | | |
| Ipratropium bromide | Inh. 18 μg/dose | 2–4 puffs 4 times/24 h | |
| | Resp. soln 250 μg/ml | 0.25–1 ml diluted to 2 ml, 4–6 h | May be mixed with salbutamol |

S/E, side effects; ICU, intensive care unit; GP, general practitioner; SR, slow release.

**Table 7.3 Delivery methods and relevant ages for inhaled bronchodilators**

| *Mode of administration*: | Nebulized inhalation | Powder preparation (rotahaler, spinhaler) | Metered aerosol | Metered aerosol with spacing chamber |
|---|---|---|---|---|
| *Age* (yr): | Any | Over 3–4 | Over 8 | 4–8 |

levels should be monitored. Acute asthma attacks should be treated with inhaled $\beta_2$ agonist, with or without the addition of a 3–4-day course of oral steroids.

**1.4 Prophylaxis for the severe asthmatic** Establish that the asthma cannot be controlled without steroids. This involves checking technique of metered aerosol inhalation and measuring theophylline levels. Steroids should preferably be given by metered aerosol because inhalation of the respirator solution provides only very low doses. Oral steroids are to be avoided, but if used should be given on an alternate day basis (cataracts can still occur).

Prophylaxis with SRT or cromoglycate may not be necessary in a child on inhaled steroids.

**1.5 Exercise-induced asthma** A pre-exercise dose of $\beta_2$ agonist will usually prevent it. Inhaled cromoglycate may also be effective.

### *2 Antibiotics*

These have no part to play in the routine management of asthmatics. It is likely that the asthmatic who is not responding needs more aggressive bronchodilator therapy, not antibiotics.

### *3 CXR*

Indicated perhaps on the first presentation with asthma. Thereafter, x-rays are of no help except in the rare case of suspected pneumothorax.

**Axiom** Asthmatics earn themselves one x-ray.

### *4 Additional therapy*

Dietary treatment and exercise training are of little value, although exercise in general and swimming in particular are to be encouraged. Physiotherapists are of help in teaching inhaler techniques. Avoiding obvious trigger factors is desirable, but pursuing ones such as house dust mite is difficult. Skin tests and radioallergosorbent tests (RAST) may well indicate atopy, but they do not implicate the allergen as a cause of the child's asthma and they are therefore of little use. Desensitization is of dubious value and may be dangerous.

Asthma may be exacerbated by emotional disturbance, which may also make stabilizing the disease difficult. Psychotherapy usually only involves careful, gentle explanation of the condition, but occasionally more formal approaches may be needed as a therapeutic adjunct.

## ADMISSION TO HOSPITAL

### *1 Admit*

If the child is not responding to his usual home treatment or if signs of increasing severity have developed (see below).

### *2 Nebulized $\beta_2$ agonist*

Can be given in any age group. If asthma is moderate–severe, nebulize it with $O_2$ because beta agonists may cause transient hypoxia.

### *3 Methyl xanthines*

Commence slow-release theophylline 10 mg/kg/12 h, but if the child is deteriorating or is seriously ill, IV aminophylline should be used (see below).

### *4 Steroids – oral or IV*

A useful adjunct to the above therapies. Use prednisolone oral 1–2 mg/kg/day *or* IV hydrocortisone 3 mg/kg/6 h *or* IV methylprednisolone 1 mg/kg/6 h. In the UK there is a strong move towards the early use of a short (3–4-day) sharp burst of steroids for acute asthma.

## DETERIORATING ASTHMA

### *1 IV fluids*

Administer at normal maintenance fluid rate.

### *2 $\beta_2$ agonist*

Nebulize salbutamol more frequently (with $O_2$). The child who needs nebulizers more than half-hourly should be transferred to an intensive care unit.

### *3 Aminophylline*

5 mg/kg over 15 min loading dose (N.B. A bolus is cardiotoxic). Then 5 mg/kg over 15 min every 6 h *or* commence infusion at 1 mg/kg/h. If slow-release theophylline has been administered within the past 8 h, do not give a loading dose. Monitoring serum levels is desirable.

### *4 Hydrocortisone*

As above.

### *5 Ipratropium bromide (Atrovent)*

0.4–1.0 ml of 0.25% solution diluted to 2 ml/2–4 h nebulized. It may be mixed with salbutamol.

### *6 IV salbutamol infusion – at 5 μg/kg/min*

Used if continuous nebulized β agonists are not working. Isoprenaline at 0.1–1.0 μg/kg/min is an alternative.

### *7 Arterial gases*

These provide little more information than one can glean from good clinical examination and judgement. Use them only in severe asthma.

### *8 Artificial ventilation*

The decision to ventilate is a clinical one, not pegged to any level of $P\text{CO}_2$. Ventilation is hazardous in asthmatics because of the high pressures needed. Use high PEEP (6–8 $\text{cmH}_2\text{O}$) rather than low to mimic the pursed lips of the asthmatic. This will paradoxically improve minute ventilation and decrease functional residual capacity (FRC) (Quist, J. *et al.* (1982) *N. Engl. J. Med.*, **307**, 1347–1348). Halothane or ether are good bronchodilators, but they are only to be used by those skilled in managing the paediatric airway.

## Further reading

Anon. (1988) Asthma in the preschool child. *Drug Ther. Bull.*, **26**, 21–24

Anon. (1989) Delivery systems for inhaled drugs in asthma. *Drugs Ther. Bull.*, **27**, 66–68

Asthma Mortality Task Force (1987) Recommendations of Asthma Mortality Task Force. *J. Allergy Clin. Immunol.*, **80**, 364–366

Godfrey, S. (1983) Exercise induced asthma. In *Asthma* (eds Clark, T. J. H. and Godfrey, S.), Chapman and Hall, London

Stead, R. J. and Cooke, N. J. (1989) Adverse effects of inhaled steroids. *Br. Med. J.*, **298**, 403–404

Valman, H. B. (1987) ABC of 1 to 7 (revised). *Br. Med. J.*, **294**, 753–757

Warner, J. O., Gotz, M., Landau, L. I. *et al.* (1989) Management of asthma: a consensus statement. *Arch. Dis. Child.*, **64**, 1065–1079

# 7.13 Intrabronchial foreign body (IFB)

Edible nuts account for half the paediatric cases of inhaled foreign bodies. Alternative culprits include other foods, small pieces of plastic, nails, pins, seeds, cork. Most lodge in a main or stem bronchus, the right side being more commonly involved than the left. Eighty per cent of patients are under 4 years old. Classically, the IFB has a ball valve effect, resulting in air trapping and hyperinflation on the affected side.

## CLINICAL FEATURES

A high index of suspicion of IFB in a child with any of the following features will serve the clinician in good stead.

### *1 Acute presentation*

The child has a cough of sudden onset as if choking. Wheeze or a clicking sound with breathing may be noted.

### *2 Delayed presentation*

This is usually due to the inhalation episode not being seen by parent or being discounted by the doctor. Features are 'wheezy bronchitis', failed resolution of acute respiratory infection, chronic cough with haemoptysis and/or lung collapse, recurrent or persistent radiological features of pneumonia.

### *3 Examination findings*

Classically the affected side demonstrates: hyperinflation; hyperresonance; diminished breath sounds; flat diaphragm (ptosed liver); trachea deviated to the contralateral side, more pronounced on expiration.

In practice, the examination is often only abnormal in retrospect.

## INVESTIGATION

### *1 CXR*

Look for radio-opaque FB (uncommon), hyperinflation or collapse. Inspiratory and expiratory films may show hyperinflation and decreased diaphragmatic movement on the affected side, and tracheal deviation to the unaffected side, more pronounced on expiration.

### *2 Fluoroscopic screening of the diaphragm*

With image intensifier, may show similar features.

## MANAGEMENT

### *Rigid bronchoscopy*

A useful (but not invariable) rule is that if a child has two out of either a history, examination or x-ray that suggest IFB, then bronchoscopy must be considered for diagnostic and therapeutic purposes.

## Further reading

Phelan, P. D., Landau, L. I. and Olinsky, A. (1982) *Respiratory Illness in Children*, 2nd edn, Blackwell, Oxford

# 7.14 Pneumonia

Pneumonia accounts for over 3 million of the estimated 15 million deaths annually in children under 5 years of age (Leowski, J. (1986) *Wld Hlth Statist. Q.*, **39**, 138–144). Most of these are in developing countries; however, it is nevertheless a cause of significant morbidity and uncommon mortality in the more developed countries.

## AETIOLOGY

The clinical, laboratory and radiographic findings usually do not distinguish bacterial infection from viral (Turner *et al.*, 1987). Although viruses are the most common cause of pneumonia, antibiotics are always indicated unless the viral cause is readily apparent.

| *Treatable pathogen* | *Comment/drug of choice* |
|---|---|
| *Streptococcus pneumoniae* (pneumococcus) | Penicillin |
| *Haemophilus influenzae* | Amoxycillin/cefuroxime/3rd gen. cephalosporins, chloramphenicol |
| *Staphylococcus aureus* | Flucloxacillin |
| *Mycoplasma* and *Chlamydia* | Erythromycin |
| *Legionella pneumophila* | Erythromycin |
| *Branhamella catarrhalis* | Penicillin |
| Group B streptococci (neonates) | Penicillin and gentamicin |
| Immunocompromised | |
| Fungi – *Aspergillus* spp. | Amphotericin, steroids |
| Pneumocystis | Cotrimoxazole |
| Gram negatives | A penicillin and an aminoglycoside |

## AETIOLOGICAL SUBGROUPS

### *1 Neonates*

Gram-positive cocci, especially group B streptococci and occasionally *S. aureus*. Gram-negative enteric bacilli.

### *2 Children 1 month–5 years of age*

Respiratory viruses probably account for more than a half of paediatric pneumonias. RSV is the commonest, but parainfluenza, influenza, adenovirus, measles, varicella, EBV are important. The major bacterial pathogens are pneumococcus and *H. influenzae* (type b and possibly non-serotypable). *S. aureus* is rare and causes an aggressive pneumonia with empyema, lobular ectasia and pneumotoceles; however, even in an extremely ill child, the initial CXR may show only faint mottling. *Chlamydia trachomatis* causes an afebrile pneumonia in the first 4 months of life, often associated with neonatal conjunctivitis, eosinophilia and radiological changes of hyperinflation and diffuse interstitial infiltrates.

### *3 Children > 5 years of age*

Pneumococcus is the major bacterial pathogen. *Mycoplasma* is common in school children and young adults.

### *4 The immunocompromised child*

Susceptible to any organism, especially Gram-negative bacilli, *Pneumocystis carinii* and fungi.

### *5 Inhalation pneumonia*

Usually sterile (i.e. a chemical pneumonitis). Occasionally caused by penicillin-sensitive oral anaerobes.

### *6 Others*

Tuberculosis should be considered when pneumonia is slow to resolve, or there is a history of TB contact, weight loss or night sweats.

## CLINICAL FEATURES

Children with mild pneumonia usually have cough, fever and tachypnoea. Features of increasing severity include chest indrawing, nasal flaring, grunting respiration and difficulty in feeding. Crepitations are unreliable predictors of pneumonia, with unacceptably high false-positive and false-negative rates.

*Mycoplasma* characteristically causes insidious onset fever, headache and abdominal pain, followed by cough and crepitations, also associated with skin rashes and arthralgia in an older child – these features are all too commonly seen with other bacterial pneumonias to be regarded as reliable distinguishing features (*Paediatr. Inf. Dis.* (1986) **5**, 71–85).

*Chlamydia trachomatis* typically causes an afebrile pneumonia with dry staccato cough in the first 4 months of life, usually associated with neonatal conjunctivitis. Several viruses mimic this picture.

In general, symptoms, signs and white cell count cannot distinguish viral pneumonia from bacterial (Turner *et al.*, 1987).

## INVESTIGATIONS

### *1 Initial tests*

CXR and blood culture.

Sputum or nasopharyngeal bacterial cultures are of no help and are often misleading.

Viral culture and immunofluorescence of mucus aspirate may be helpful – they are rarely positive in asymptomatic individuals.

Total and differential white cell count cannot differentiate bacterial from viral (Turner *et al.*, 1987). Low WCC is associated with a worse prognosis.

### *2 Later tests*

If there is unsatisfactory response to treatment, consider the following:

Diagnostic thoracocentesis if there is pleural fluid.

Antibody serology – *Mycoplasma, Chlamydia* (also high vaginal swab of mother), respiratory viruses (adenovirus, parainfluenza, influenza, RSV) and legionella.

*Mycoplasma* complement fixation test.

Cold agglutinins – present in 75% of those with *Mycoplasma* infection. A simple bedside technique is to add 4 drops of whole blood to an oxalate or sodium citrate tube. Place on ice for 30 s, then hold tube up to the light while tilting it and observing for agglutination, which should disappear after warming the tube in one's hand. Formal testing should be done in the laboratory because of the large number of bedside false positives.

Investigation for inhaled FB (see Section 7.13).

Mantoux test: 0.1 ml of 1:1000 given intradermally.

Pneumococcal or *H. influenzae* rapid antigen detection in urine.

Needle aspiration of affected part of the lung – only if very sick.

Tracheal aspirate or broncho-alveolar lavage.

Open lung biopsy.

## TREATMENT

Depends on child's age. In this section, the immune competence of the child is assumed.

All cases of pneumonia should receive antibiotics unless a viral cause is apparent.

### *1 Neonates*

Crystalline penicillin 60 mg (100 000 u)/kg/6 h and gentamicin 2.5 mg/kg/8 h.

### *2 Infants*

**2.1 Not severely ill** Amoxycillin 10–20 mg/kg/8 h. A first dose of procaine penicillin 30 000–50 000 u/kg IM is optional.

**2.2 Moderate–severely ill** IV ampicillin 25 mg/kg/6 h. For worsening disease use cefuroxine 35 mg/kg/8 h IV. This will cover pneumococcus, resistant *Haemophilus* and staphylococcus. Erythromycin 10 mg/kg/6 h oral is given for suspected *Chlamydia*.

### 3 1–5 years

Amoxycillin 10–20 mg/kg/8 h oral, or ampicillin 25 mg/kg/6 h IV. These cover about 75% of *H. influenzae* in most Western societies. For those commencing oral therapy there is the option of a single starting dose of procaine penicillin 30 000–50 000 u IM. (In communities where *H. pneumoniae* is not recognized, penicillin alone is used as a first-line drug.) If there is no response to treatment within 48 hours, cover resistant *H. influenzae* with cefuroxime 35 mg/kg/8 h IV or chloramphenicol or a third-generation cephalosporin. These second-line treatments will also cover *Staphylococcus aureus*.

### 4 >5 years

Pneumococcus is the most common pathogen. *Haemophilus* disease is uncommon and the incidence of *Mycoplasma* begins to rise. Use penicillin V 10–15 mg/kg/6 h oral or benzyl penicillin 30–60 mg (50 000–100 000 u)/kg/6 h IV. The option exists for a starting dose of procaine penicillin as above. If there is no response to treatment, cover *Mycoplasma* with erythromycin and consider covering *Haemophilus* and *S. aureus* as above.

## OTHER TREATMENTS

Mask or intranasal $O_2$ as necessary – may need to be humidified.

Empyema – needs large-bore needle aspiration or insertion of large intercostal catheter.

Physiotherapy or postural drainage is of help in those with underlying lung disease (bronchiectasis, CF), but otherwise is useless at best in the routine management of uncomplicated pneumonia (*Br. Med. J.* (1985) **290**, 1703–1704; *New Engl. J. Med.* (1979) **300**, 1155–1157 and correspondence; *New Engl. J. Med.* (1978) **299**, 624–627 and correspondence; *Lancet* (1978) **ii**, 228–230 and correspondence; *Br. Med. J.* (1989) **298**, 541–542).

In RSV pneumonia, ribavirin has a very limited role to play primarily in cases complicating CF (see Section 7.11).

## Further reading

Anon. (1988) Pneumonia in childhood. *Lancet,* **i**, 741–743

Isaacs, D. *et al.* (1988) Ribavirin in respiratory syncytial infection. *Arch. Dis. Child.,* **63**, 986–990

Leventhal, J. M. (1982) Clinical predictors of pneumonia. *Clin. Pediatr.,* **21**, 730–734

MacFarlane, J. T. (1987) Treatment of lower respiratory infection. *Lancet,* **ii**, 1446

Shann, F. (1986) Etiology of severe pneumonia in developing countries. *Pediatr. Inf. Dis.,* **5**, 247–252

Turner, R. B. *et al.* (1987) Pneumonia in paediatric outpatients. *J. Pediatr.,* **111**, 194–200

# 7.15 Cystic fibrosis (CF)

CF is one of the most common inherited disorders and the most frequent cause of suppurative lung disease in Caucasian children and young adults. It occurs in about 1:2000 live births, i.e. 450 babies annually in the UK. It is in the best interests of all children with CF to be managed primarily in a specialized centre where there is integrated management by physiotherapists, social workers, nurses, pharmacists, dietitians and doctors.

## PATHOGENESIS

There is abnormal concentration of organic ions in serous gland secretions (e.g. increased $Na^+$ in sweat) and increased viscosity of secretions from mucus-secreting glands with undue susceptibility to specific bacterial infection of the bronchi. At a cellular level, there is an increased transepithelial potential difference, probably due to a block in chloride transport, but this may be a secondary abnormality. Abnormal mucus glycoproteins are also found.

## GENETICS

The inheritance is autosomal recessive: 1 in 22 people in our society carries the gene (?heterozygote advantage). The defect lies on chromosome 7. Usually both parents of affected children are carriers (very few new mutations). It is possible to identify which chromosome 7 an affected child has inherited from each parent. This allows fairly accurate antenatal diagnosis of affected fetuses with chorionic villus sampling, but is only possible if DNA is available from an affected member of the family. Almost all couples who have a child with CF are fully informative in this way, enabling them to foretell antenatally whether a subsequent pregnancy is affected. Previously many couples felt that a 1:4 chance of another affected child was too high.

At time of writing the announcement of the discovery of the actual CF gene had just been made (Scrambler, 1989).

## PRESENTATION

The major ways in which CF presents are:

### *1 Meconium ileus (also jejunal/ileal atresia)*

10–15% of CF babies present in this way. All cases of meconium ileus should have a sweat test.

### *2 Failure to thrive (FTT)*

Due to fat malabsorption with steatorrhoea. Licking the skin of a child with FTT is a useful part of the clinical assessment, as the child with CF may taste salty (prior explanation to the parents is prudent).

### *3 Recurrent chest infections, nasal polyps*

### *4 Rectal prolapse – due to bulky stools*

### *5 Positive neonatal screening test*

About 6:1000 babies have high immunoreactive trypsin on neonatal dried blood spot sample assay (taken with PKU screen). One in 10 of those will be positive when repeated at 28 days. Most of these will prove to have CF when a sweat test is then performed. It is of diminished use after 1 month or after surgery. The value of neonatal screening is controversial.

### *6 Positive family history*

All siblings of a newly diagnosed case should have a sweat test.

## DIAGNOSIS

### *1 Sweat test*

Any of the above should lead to confirmation with a sweat test which is still the key to diagnosis. This is done with pilocarpine iontophoresis, collecting preferably more than 100 mg of sweat. A positive diagnosis is made if:

(a) $Cl^- > 60$ mmol/litre;
(b) $Na^+ > 60$ mmol/litre;
(c) Osmolarity > 200 mosm/litre.

Infants are increasingly being tested due to use of neonatal screening. A lower sweat $Na^+$ in this group is still compatible with CF and it should be rechecked when older.

## CLINICAL FEATURES

### *1 General features*

Most cases are recognized because of recurrent or persisting pulmonary infections or failure to thrive. The onset may be obvious or insidious. Chronic or recurrent cough is common, although there may be initial confusion with asthma or whooping cough. Dyspnoea and lack of general well-being are later features. Physical signs are unimpressive early in the disease. Thick secretions in small airways cause adventitious sounds on auscultation. Later, emphysema, chest deformity and eventually features of cor pulmonale will develop. Finger clubbing is often an early sign.

### *2 Features of acute exacerbation of respiratory tract infection*

Worsening cough; change in volume, appearance or colour of sputum; tachypnoea or dyspnoea; progressive findings on chest auscultation; new infiltrates on CXR; decreased appetite and weight loss; fever; decreased exercise tolerance.

## COMPLICATIONS AND MANAGEMENT

With optimal management, children with CF can remain relatively well and many now survive beyond 30 years of age. Infertility in males is absolute, but in females is only relative. The mainstays of treatment are:

### *1 GI tract*

**1.1 Pancreatic enzyme supplementation** 'Creon' is a capsule containing enteric-coated pH-resistant pancreatic enzyme granules (Pancrease has similar properties). A lower dosage can be used than for the old uncoated preparations which were denatured in the stomach. It can be administered to infants by opening the capsules; however, post-prandial gum cleansing is important to prevent ulceration. Infants start off with half a capsule with meals. Adults often taken from 3 to 8 capsules with meals. Inadequate dosage results in foul-smelling stools and poor weight gain. The dose should be increased until the stool character is normal. Cimetidine is occasionally given to raise upper jejunal pH, resulting in improved effectiveness of the treatment. With these enzymes, a 'free diet' can usually be tolerated.

**1.2 Nutrition** There is a high caloric requirement due to residual steatorrhoea, increased work of breathing, and chronic or recurrent infection. Options for increasing caloric intake include: oral supplements to the diet, nocturnal nasogastric feeding, gastrostomy feeding, or parenteral nutrition. Suitable food supplements include Polycal, Fortical, Ensure Liquid, Build Up. Supplements of all vitamins, especially the fat-soluble vitamins A, D, K and E, should be given ('Ketovite' is a good choice).

**1.3 Hepatobiliary problems** Abdominal pain is common in CF and can be due to biliary disease or meconium ileus equivalent. Cirrhosis occurs in 2–5% of cases and cannot be prevented. Portal hypertension and its attendant problems is a serious complication.

**1.4 Meconium ileus equivalent** This is a distal bowel obstruction due to bulky stools and chronic faecal stasis. *N*-acetylcysteine (Parvolex) may disperse the secretions. A typical regimen involves: rectal *N*-acetylcysteine, 30 ml of a 20% solution added to 120 ml enema solution (e.g. Fletcher's phosphate enema) t.d.s.; oral *N*-acetylcysteine 10 ml of a 20% solution diluted with or followed by 100 ml of water or orange juice, t.d.s.; IV fluids. Gastrographin enema 50–100 ml may also be given.

**1.5 Diabetes** Occurs in 1% and is treated on its merits. Impaired GTT is seen in 40%.

**1.6 Others** Pancreatitis, intussusception, rectal prolapse.

## *2 Respiratory*

**2.1 Prophylaxis** A controversial topic. The value of long-term prophylaxis is unknown, but many children are taking one of amoxycillin, cotrimoxazole or flucloxacillin in the first year of life, or inhaled anti-pseudomonal agents for this purpose (e.g. gentamicin or tobramycin 40–80 mg b.d.). Characteristic organisms are:

*Staphylococcus aureus* – most commonly in the first year of life.
*Pseudomonas.*
*Haemophilus influenzae.*
*Klebsiella.*

Other efforts aimed at maintaining lung function include:

physiotherapy;
inhalations of Mucomyst and/or $\beta_2$ agonist;
exercise programmes;
steroids – may reduce immune complex injury but may make the child less eligible for eventual heart–lung transplant.

**2.2 Exacerbations** Aggressive management with IV antibiotics is indicated. Home treatment is possible for some families if the child is well enough. Exacerbations are often due to *Pseudomonas*, so that combinations of ceftazidime or an antipseudomonal penicillin with an aminoglycoside are often used. Higher than usual doses of aminoglycosides may be needed because of a higher volume of distribution due to a relative increase in extracellular fluid volume per kg because of a lack of adipose tissue. Ciprofloxacin may prove useful. Very high doses are needed as sputum penetration is poor and it is not as yet recommended for children < 12 yr because of possible damage to articular cartilage. Some typical regimens are:

(a) ticarcillin 75 mg/kg/6 h + tobramycin 2.5 mg/kg/8 h;
(b) azlocillin 75–100 mg/kg/6 h + gentamicin 2.5 mg/kg/6–8 h;
(c) ceftazidime 50 mg/kg/6–8 h + gentamicin 2.5 mg/kg/6–8 h.

*Aspergillus* and allergic aspergillosis may require steroids and/or inhaled amphotericin.

**2.3 Asthma** Many CF patients have bronchospasm and are helped by bronchodilators. N.B. *Aspergillus* must be considered.

**2.4 Pneumothorax**

**2.5 Haemoptysis** Can be severe and may require interventional radiology.

### *3 Psychosocial difficulties*

As with the general management of CF, these are best prevented or addressed by the coordinated efforts of community and hospital-based social workers and nurses, physiotherapist, paediatrician, and occasionally psychiatrist.

## MONITORING

### *1 Regular monitoring of (often 3 monthly):*

height and weight;
CXR;
lung function – first abnormality is increased RV/TLC, then FEF,
– bronchodilator response;
sputum microscopy and culture;
FBC and eosinophil count;
Liver function tests/clotting studies;
blood sugar;
immunoglobulins.

### *2 Other investigations to consider*

**2.1 For splenomegaly** Hepatic ultrasound; barium swallow and endoscopy (for varices); alpha 1 antitrypsin phenotype.

**2.2 For abdominal pain** US; plain abdominal x-ray.

## THE FUTURE

Even though the basic gene defect has recently been identified, it is quite likely that in the short term there will be no fundamental change in the current approach to management. Heart–lung transplant is still experimental. There is about 25% early postoperative mortality, and the transplanted lungs become colonized with *Pseudomonas aeruginosa* and are at risk of progressive obliterative bronchiolitis; however, CF-type lung disease does not seem to occur.

## Further reading

Carter, E. *et al.* (1984) Improved sweat test method in diagnosis of cystic fibrosis. *Arch. Dis. Child.*, **59**, 919–922

Daniels, L. A. and Davidson, G. P. (1989) Current issues in the nutritional management of children with cystic fibrosis. *Aust. Paediatr. J.*, **25**, 261–266

David, T. J. (1990) Cystic fibrosis. *Arch. Dis. Child.*, **65**, 152–157

Dodge, J. A. (1988) Implications of the new genetics for screening for cystic fibrosis. *Lancet,* **ii**, 672–675

Goodchild, M. C. and Dodge, J. A. (1985) Cystic fibrosis. In *Manual of Diagnosis and Management,* Baillière Tindall, London

Marshall, J. M. (1989) Drugs in the management of cystic fibrosis. *Pharm. J.*, 3 June: 642–645

Scrambler, P. J. (1989) The cystic fibrosis gene. *Arch Dis. Child.*, **64**, 1647–1648

Chapter 8

# Neurology

## 8.1 Cerebrospinal fluid (CSF) – normal and abnormal

Always examine CSF within 1 h of collection for cells and Gram stain.

### NORMAL VALUES

#### White cell count

Neonate 8.2/$mm^3$ (0–22/$mm^3$).
> 1 month 0–7.

#### Glucose

Normal = two-thirds blood glucose. Take blood before CSF.

#### Protein

Full-term neonate: < 100 mg/100 ml (1.0 g/litre).
> 1 month: < 30 mg/100 ml (0.3 g/litre).

#### CSF pressure

Normally: < 180 mm$H_2O$.
Neonates: < 120 mm$H_2O$.

#### Traumatic tap

This usually manifests as blood-stained CSF which clears as the collection progresses. For each 1000 RBC/$mm^3$ allow:

1 mg/100 ml protein (0.01 g/litre).
1–2 white cells.

#### Chloride

Normal = 120–128 mmol/litre.
Not a routine test. Of value in suspected TB meningitis, when it is usually decreased (? because of inappropriate ADH syndrome).

## CSF ABNORMALITIES

### Colour

True CSF bleeding will give a xanthochromic supernatant. A traumatic tap will usually have a clear supernatant.

### Cloudy

100–200 white cells/$mm^3$ will cause cloudiness. Polymorphs suggest bacterial infection or early viral disease. Lymphocytes suggest viral or chronic inflammatory process. Atypical lymphocytes are seen with EBV. Eosinophils suggest parasitic infection. Many organic diseases of the CNS produce a mild pleocytosis.

### Glucose

Increased levels reflect hyperglycaemia. Decreased levels are seen in bacterial, tuberculous and fungal meningitis. It is usually (but not always) normal in viral meningitis.

### Protein

Raised levels reflect damage to the blood brain barrier. Purulent meningitis will raise the level regardless of the cause. Brain tumours often give levels of 1–2 g/litre (not so in brain stem gliomata).

Spinal cord tumours, especially when obstructing CSF flow, give very high levels (7.5–10 g/litre). Infectious polyneuritis (Guillain–Barré) characteristically causes a modest rise after the first week of illness. Other conditions that cause CNS degeneration may elevate it as may lead intoxication (LP is dangerous in lead poisoning, but if one is reading this with a high CSF protein in hand, the horse has no doubt already bolted).

### Gamma-globulin

Normally $< 15\%$ of CSF protein. Dramatically raised in subacute sclerosing panencephalitis (SSPE), herpes encephalitis, Schilder's disease.

### Fungal disease

An India ink preparation must be specifically requested in most laboratories. Amateurs may wish to try it by placing a coverslip over 1 drop of CSF. Place 1 drop of India ink next to the coverslip and allow it to seep under. *Cryptococcus* is best seen at the interface.

## Further reading

Weiner, H. L., Bresnan, M. J. and Levitt, L. P. (1982) *Pediatric Neurology for the House Officer,* Williams and Wilkins, Baltimore

# 8.2 Meningitis

## INTRODUCTION

This is a condition where early presentation by the parents, early referral by the GP and rapid diagnosis and treatment by hospital doctors are of paramount importance. In this section, the aetiology of meningitis in general is presented, but thereafter only bacterial meningitis is addressed.

## AETIOLOGY

*Haemophilus influenzae*
*Streptococcus pneumoniae* } > 95% of non-neonatal bacterial meningitis
*Neisseria meningitidis*

Viral – Coxsackie, echo, mumps, polio, herpes simplex.
Fungal (rare) – *Candida, Cryptococcus, Histoplasma.*
Protozoal (rare) – amoeba, *Toxoplasma.*
Tuberculosis.

Neonates – above + group B streptococci, *Listeria, Escherichia coli, Streptococcus faecalis*, other Gram negatives (*Klebsiella, Proteus, Pseudomonas*).

## PREDISPOSITIONS

Usually none – the pathogen is usually acquired from nasopharyngeal carriage, although an association with otitis media is recognized. Uncommonly – compound skull fracture, orbital/facial cellulitis, neural tube defects, cyanotic heart disease, infected ventriculoperitoneal (VP). shunt, immune deficiency. Premature babies are relatively immune deficient and have an undeveloped blood brain barrier.

## CLINICAL FEATURES

### *1 Neonates – no specific signs*

The child may have fever, pallor, vomiting, lethargy, apnoea, poor feeding, bulging fontanelle, convulsions.

### *2 Infants*

Classical features such as headache, neck stiffness, photophobia are seldom reliably elicited in this age group. The child is usually pale, unwell, febrile, lethargic, and if asked, the mother will often testify to the child being 'distant'.

### 3 Older children

Variable signs. Headache, neck stiffness and photophobia are the typical features. Neck stiffness is best elicited by interesting the child in an object that he will follow through the full range of neck flexion and extension, or by 'knee kissing'. Other features include irritability, lethargy, fever, purpuric rash (usually but not invariably meningococcus), convulsions.

Examination must include an assessment of conscious state and adequacy of ventilation, pulse, BP, head circumference, fundoscopy, and general neurological evaluation.

## DIAGNOSIS

### 1 Lumbar puncture (LP)

See Section 8.1 for normal values and Table 8.1 for CSF changes in meningitis.

**Table 8.1 CSF characteristics in meningitis**

| | *Bacterial* | *Viral* |
|---|---|---|
| WHITE CELLS* | | |
| Lymphocytes | ↑ | ↑ |
| Neutrophils | ↑ ↑ ↑ | ↑ |
| PROTEIN | ↑ | normal |
| GLUCOSE† | ↓ | normal |
| CHLORIDE | normal ( ↓ in TB) | normal |

* If specimen has blood contamination allow 1–2 white cells/1000 red.
† Normal CSF sugar is > two-thirds that of plasma. Macroscopically cloudy CSF occurs with > 100 cells/$mm^3$.
For normal CSF data see Section 8.1.

- *Always suspect meningitis in an unwell child.*

Do not rely on the physical signs, especially in neonates and infants. LP is the only way to diagnose it, and doctors young and old are advised to err on the side of doing too many, rather than run the risk of missing a single case. Check fontanelle and fundi first. If there is a suspicion of raised intracranial pressure, take a blood culture, commence treatment and do a CT scan *before* attempting the LP. If the child is too sick to tolerate an LP, it is preferable to defer the LP, take a blood culture and commence treatment, rather than risking the child's life for the sake of the test.

### 2 Blood

Culture, glucose, $Na^+$, FBC.

### 3 Urine

Rapid antigen detection (latex agglutination or CIE). Useful diagnostic aid if the child has had recent antibiotics or if one is unable to perform a LP, but the tests have variable reliability and are not a substitute for LP.

## TREATMENT

### 1 Antibiotics

**1.1 Children <2 months of age** Cefotaxime 50 mg/kg/6 h IV + ampicillin 50 mg/kg/4–6 h (for *Listeria* and *S. faecalis*) IV. Continue treatment for 3 weeks.

**1.2 Children >2 months of age** Chloramphenicol 40 mg/kg loading dose, then 25 mg/kg/6 h IV. Continue until the organism and its sensitivities are known, after which single drug therapy with chloramphenicol, penicillin 60 mg (100 000 u)/kg/4 h or ampicillin 50 mg/kg/4 h is given.

*1.2.1 Duration of treatment* *H. influenzae* – chloramphenicol for 10 days. Oral chloramphenicol suspension (palmitate) or capsules (base) may be given under inpatient supervision as soon as a child is well, with no vomiting or diarrhoea. Ampicillin may be used if the organism is fully sensitive. *Pneumococcus* – crystalline penicillin IV for 10–14 days. *N. meningitidis* – crystalline penicillin for 7–10 days.

*1.2.2 Alternative treatment* In a community with a significant prevalence of chloramphenicol-resistant *H. influenzae*, consider cefotaxime 50 mg/kg/6 h or ceftriaxone 100 mg IV/IM once daily as first-line treatment beyond the neonatal period. There is evidence to suggest that third-generation cephalosporins sterilize CSF more quickly and more reliably than chloramphenicol (Peltola, Anttila and Renkonen, 1989), although the clinical significance of this is unclear. Cefuroxime should not be used (*J. Pediatr.* (1989) **114**, 1049–1054).

### 2 Fluids

The principle is to maintain cerebral perfusion pressure (Mean arterial BP – ICP > 40 mmHg); see Section 8.7. In the rare situation of the child in shock (usually meningococcal septicaemia), plasma expansion and restoration of BP take priority over all else. If, however, BP is well maintained, there is no need for IV fluids. Give 0–30 ml/kg/day while the child is unable to drink. IV fluid should be regarded as a dangerous drug, because of the likelihood of syndrome of inappropriate ADH and cerebral oedema. It is usually only with IV fluids that ADH release seen commonly in meningitis becomes inappropriate. Frequent monitoring of serum osmolarity and urea or creatinine will provide early warning of dehydration.

### *3 Biochemistry*

Monitor serum $Na^+$, and serum and urine osmolarity 1–2 times daily while conscious state is impaired. If using chloramphenicol, measure serum levels every 2 days.

### *4 Weight and head circumference*

Measure daily.

### *5 CT scan*

Indicated before LP if raised ICP is thought possible. After treatment has commenced, it is indicated in those with persistent neurological dysfunction, persistent positive CSF cultures, new neurological signs after a period of apparent recovery, or recurrent meningitis. It is of little value as a routine test in meningitis or in those with persistent fever alone (Kline, M. W. (1988), *Pediatr. Inf. Dis., J.*, **7**, 855–857).

### *6 Dexamethasone*

A dose of 0.15 mg/kg/6 h IV for 4 days reduces the meningeal inflammatory response and may improve outcome (especially hearing) in *H. influenzae* meningitis. It is, however, by no means proved and given the possible complications of dexamethasone, recommending this treatment is as yet premature. If one does decide to give it, there are theoretical reasons for its administration prior to the first dose of antibiotic. Further studies are in progress and should resolve the issue in the near future (see Further reading for excellent discussions).

## ACUTE COMPLICATIONS

### *1 Syndrome of inappropriate antidiuretic hormone (SIADH)*

Diagnosed by a low serum osmolarity (< 275 mosm/litre) in the presence of high urine osmolarity. Presumptive evidence is low serum $Na^+$ (<135 mmol/litre), weight gain, oliguria.

Treatment: cease all fluid input. Once urine flow is established, restrict fluid input strictly to urine output.

### *2 Convulsions*

Treat them aggressively with diazepam/paraldehyde, phenobarbitone or phenytoin (see Section 8.4). Early intervention with thiopentone and mechanical ventilation is much less hazardous than allowing frequent or uncontrolled fits.

N.B. Some relevant drug interactions:

(a) diazepam + phenobarbitone = potent respiratory suppression (*New Engl. J. Med.* (1982) **306**, 1337–1340).
(b) chloramphenicol + phenobarbitone = decreased chloramphenicol levels (*Pediatr. Inf. Dis.* (1982) **1**, 232–235).
(c) chloramphenicol + phenytoin = increased chloramphenicol levels (*Pediatr. Inf. Dis.* (1982) **1**, 232–235).

### 3 Raised intracranial pressure

Restrict fluids but *maintain cerebral perfusion pressure* – see Section 8.7.
Elevate head of bed to 20°.
Low threshold for intubation and ventilation to a $P\text{CO}_2$ of 30 mmHg (4 kPa).
Mannitol 0.5 g/kg IV × 1 only.
Strict control of seizures – may need thiopentone infusion.
Keep head in midline.

### 4 Subdural collection

May give new focal neurological signs or unexplained halt in clinical improvement. Diagnosed with CT scan (US is unreliable). Large collections are treated with subdural taps (see Section 4.3) or burr holes. Small or asymptomatic collections require no treatment.

## PROGNOSIS AND LONG-TERM SEQUELAE

Case fatality rates are > 40% for neonates and 5–10% for older children. Sequelae from meningitis occur in > 25% of survivors and include:

behaviour problems;
learning difficulties;
mental retardation (10%);
motor abnormalities (3–7%);
hearing impairment (4–10%) – survivors should have hearing tested;
language disorders (15%);
seizures (2–7%).

## CHEMOPROPHYLAXIS FOR CONTACTS

### 1 *H. influenzae*

Causes a low secondary attack rate in the UK and hence prophylaxis is controversial, although it is widely accepted in the USA. May be of use if given to household contacts under 4 yr. Use rifampicin 10 mg/kg/12 h orally for 4 days.

### 2 Meningococcus

Administer prophylaxis to all adult and child household contacts, close school contacts but not the whole class, nurses in constant close contact and perhaps medical staff. Seventy per cent of secondary cases occur within 1 week of the index case. Use oral rifampicin for 2 days – neonates, 5 mg/kg/12 h; children, 10 mg/kg/12 h, adults, 600 mg/12 h. Ceftriaxone 125 mg IM × 1 has also been shown to be effective (*Lancet* (1988) **i**, 1240–1242). N.B. Meningitis can still occur in those who have received prophylaxis.

### 3 Pneumococcus

None.

## Further reading

Kaplan, S. L. (1989) Dexamethasone for children with bacterial meningitis. *Am. J. Dis. Child.*, **143**, 290–291

Kaplan, S. L. and Fishman, M. A. (1987) Supportive therapy for bacterial meningitis. *Pediatr. Infect. Dis.*, **6**, 670–677

Klein, J. O., Feigin, R. D. and McCracken, G. H. (1986) Report of the task force on diagnosis and management of meningitis. *Pediatr.*, **78**, 959–982

McCracken, G. H. and Lebel, M. H. (1989) Dexamethasone therapy for bacterial meningitis in infants and children. *Am. J. Dis. Child.*, **143**, 287–289

McCracken, G. H. and Nelson, J. D. (1983) *Antimicrobial Therapy for Newborns*, Grune and Stratton, New York, pp. 119–127

Peltola, H., Anttila, M. and Renkonen, O. V. (1989) Randomised comparison of chloramphenicol, ampicillin, cefotaxime, and ceftriaxone for childhood bacterial meningitis. *Lancet*, **i**, 1281–1287

Smith, A. L. and Weber, B. S. (1983) Pharmacology of chloramphenicol. *Pediatr. Clin. N. Am.*, **30**, 209–234

Smith, H. (1986) Chemoprophylaxis of meningitis. *Arch. Dis. Child.*, **61**, 4–5

Stutman, H. R. and Marks, M. I. (1987) Therapy for bacterial meningitis. *J. Pediatr.*, **110**, 812–814

Tauber, M. G. and Sande, M. A. (1989) Dexamethasone in bacterial meningitis: increasing evidence for a beneficial effect. *Pediatr. Inf. Dis. J.*, **8**, 842–844

# 8.3 Convulsions

The most common cause of seizures is simple febrile convulsions (see Section 8.5). A recurrent seizure disorder is called epilepsy (which is a description, not a diagnosis), of which idiopathic epilepsy is the most common subgroup. There are many different seizure disorders with varied aetiologies, treatments and prognoses.

A seizure is only a symptom of cerebral dysfunction. One must decide whether it is a sign of fixed non-progressive deficit, a progressive intracranial disorder or idiopathic epilepsy.

## SOME HELPFUL CLINICAL FEATURES

### *1 History*

**1.1 A good description** of the seizure from a witness is mandatory. This should include events precipitating the seizure, such as lights or watching TV, focal features, duration, position of head and eyes, tonic/clonic activity and post-ictal state. Some children may give a history of an aura.

**1.2 Past history** of prematurity, perinatal asphyxia, birth trauma, or other neurological insult (meningitis, head injury).

**1.3 History** of abdominal pain, dizziness, behavioural disturbance, automatism (features of complex partial seizures).

**1.4 Have there been brief staring spells** with no loss of postural control (absence seizures)?

### *2 Examination*

**2.1 General examination** – including BP, neurological state, fundi.

**2.2 Post-ictal (Todd's) paralysis.**

**2.3 Tonic deviation of the eyes.**

**2.4 Asymmetry** of finger- and toe-nails, digits or limbs suggests long-standing damage to contralateral hemisphere.

**2.5 ?Cranial bruit** – arteriovenous malformation.

**2.6 Skin examination** – phakomatoses (neurocutaneous syndromes).

**2.7 Hyperventilation** for 3 min can precipitate a petit mal seizure ('blow away a piece of paper').

**2.8 Head circumference.**

## SPECIFIC SEIZURE TYPES

*Anticonvulsants are mentioned in order of preference.* Doses are listed in Table 8.2.

### *1 Grand mal seizures*

May have preceding aura, followed by a fall and tonic and clonic movements of all extremities. Urine or faecal incontinence is common as is post-ictal drowsiness. Use carbamazepine, valproate, phenobarbitone (phenytoin).

### *2 Petit mal/absence seizures*

Staring spells with mild ptosis or eye fluttering, that last a few seconds. May have hundreds per day. Initially the child may seem to be day-dreaming. Postural control is maintained. Classical EEG findings are 3 per second spike and wave discharges. In an untreated child, hyperventilation (see above) often produces an absence. Use ethosuximide or valproate.

### *3 Complex partial seizures (temporal lobe/psychomotor epilepsy)*

May have:

Preceding aura (abdominal pains, 'butterflies', and various illusions).
Automatic semi-purposeful movements – swallowing, lip smacking, picking at one's clothes.

**Table 8.2 Anticonvulsants**

| *Drug* | *Major indication* GM | PM | Focal | *Dose* | *Therapeutic range* | *Major* (S/E) | $T_{1/2}$ (h) |
|---|---|---|---|---|---|---|---|
| Carbamazepine | +++ | – | +++ | 2 mg/kg/8 h oral inc. over 2 wk to max. 10 mg/kg/dose | 20–50 µmol/litre (4–10 mg/litre) | Leucopenia<br>Rashes<br>Liver dysfunction | 15–30 |
| Valproic acid | +++ | +++ | ++ | Grade up to 15 mg/kg/12 h | 350–700 µmol/litre (50–100 mg/litre) | Weight gain<br>GIT upset<br>Liver toxicity<br>Sedation, alopecia<br>Thrombocytopenia | 6–15 |
| Phenobarbitone | +++ (mainly in infants) | + | +++ | 20 mg/kg/emerg. load. dose<br>3–5 mg/kg/day maint. IV/IM/oral | 50–170 µmol/litre (10–40 mg/litre) | Hyperactivity<br>Transient sedation | 48–96 |
| Phenytoin | +++ (2nd-line drug) | – | +++ | 3–4 mg/kg/12 h IV/oral<br>Emerg. load. dose 15–20 mg/kg over 30 min | 40–80 µmol/litre (10–20 mg/litre) | Ataxia, nystagmus<br>Rash, hirsutism<br>Blood dyscrasias | 5–30 |
| Ethosuximide | – | ++ | – | 2.5 mg/kg/8 h<br>Inc. by 50% weekly to max. 12.5 mg/kg/8 h | 280–700 µmol/litre (40–100 mg/litre) | GI disturbance<br>Thrombocytopenia | |

OTHER DRUGS

ACTH: for infantile spasms 150 u/m$^2$/day IM for 4 wk, then decrease over 4 wk
Prednisolone: 2 mg/kg/day. For infantile spasms
Acetazolamide: 2nd line in petit mal, myoclonic or seizures related to menstruation

GM, grand mal; PM, petit mal; TLE, temporal lobe epilepsy = complex partial seizures; GIT, gastrointestinal tract; ACTH, adrenocorticotrophic hormone.

Behaviour abnormalities – walking to another part of the room.
Post-ictal confusion and drowsiness.
An EEG or sleep EEG may demonstrate temporal lobe discharges.
Use carbamazepine, valproate, phenobarbitone (phenytoin).

### *4 Infantile spasms (hypsarrhythmia/salaam spasms)*

Usually begin at 3–9 months. Truncal spasms may be flexor, extensor, or just involve neck flexion. Tuberous sclerosis (look for pale or pigmented skin patches), various inborn errors of metabolism and most major causes of CNS damage in infancy are recognized aetiologies. In over 50%, no cause is found. EEG often shows chaotic high-voltage slow waves and spikes (hypsarrhythmia). More than 90% are ultimately severely mentally handicapped. Use ACTH or prednisolone.

### *5 Myoclonic/akinetic seizures*

Brief jerks of limbs or sudden loss of tone. Often associated with neurodegenerative or structural CNS lesions. Use valproate, benzodiazepines.

### *6 Benign focal epilepsy of childhood (Rolandic/Sylvian spike seizures)*

Preceding sensory aura related to the mouth, followed by difficulty speaking, facial twitching. Often occurs just after going to sleep or just prior to waking. EEG shows mid-temporal or central (Rolandic/Sylvian) spike focus. Excellent prognosis with spontaneous resolution usually by mid-teen years. Treatment is not always necessary. Carbamazepine or phenytoin readily prevent seizures.

### *7 Breath-holding attacks – not really epilepsy*

Characteristically occur as follows: provocation of the child is followed by crying for a few seconds, apnoea, change of colour (blue or white), rigidity, convulsions, stupor. Usually occurs between 6 months and 2 years. Disappears by age 4. No treatment necessary. Parents need much reassurance.

## INVESTIGATION

EEG – awake, asleep, 24 h. In grand mal seizures, excessive emphasis is placed on the EEG. Epilepsy is diagnosed on clinical grounds, *not EEG*. The EEG may be helpful in diagnosing the type of epilepsy, and therefore may help in optimum drug selection.
CT scan – if there is a suspicion of focal or progressive disorder.

## MANAGEMENT

Acute seizures – see Section 8.4.
Prophylaxis – see Table 8.2.

In general, treat the child, not the EEG.
Avoid polypharmacy.
One drug is often as good as two, and has fewer complications.
When changing a medication, make one gradual change at a time.
It takes 5 half-lives of any drug to reach a steady state after each change in dosage.
Parents initially need to be allotted much time for explanation and reassurance and frequent review.
Children who are well controlled should be encouraged to normalize their lives by participating fully in the activities of their peer group. Cycling is allowed, provided that a helmet is worn. Swimming is permissible if there is adequate supervision by an adult.
Parents of epileptics may wish to contact the British Epilepsy Association. Head Office: Anstey House, 40 Hanover Square, Leeds LS3 1BE (tel. 0532-439 393). South East Region: 92–94 Tooley Street, London SE1 9SH (tel. 071-403 4111).

## MONITORING ANTICONVULSANT LEVELS AND SIDE EFFECTS

As a rule, the dose of anticonvulsant is adjusted according to seizure control and clinical state of the child, not the interpretation by a biochemistry laboratory of the clinical relevance of a drug level. If a child is well controlled and free of side effects, monitoring of drug levels is of modest use. The predictive value of drug level regarding effect and toxicity is good with phenytoin, intermediate with carbamazepine, and poor with ethosuximide, phenobarbitone and valproate. Chadwick (1987) advocates drug monitoring for:

1. Those on phenytoin or multiple anticonvulsants in whom dosage adjustment is necessary because of possible toxicity or poor seizure control.
2. Mentally retarded patients in whom signs of toxicity may be masked.
3. Children with renal or hepatic disease.
4. Suspected poor compliance.

The measurement of most anticonvulsant levels must be interpreted with caution. Random valproate levels may represent unpredictable peak, trough or intermediate concentrations. Carbamazepine has active metabolites that are not measured. Phenytoin, carbamazepine and valproate are heavily protein bound, but only the free drug is pharmacologically active.

### Suggested protocol

1. Phenytoin – all children need regular anticonvulsant levels.
2. Carbamazepine – check FBC after 6 weeks because of possible neutropenia. If there is poor seizure control, check the drug level at the same time. Routine monitoring of levels is not required.

3. Valproate – check liver function tests (LFT) and platelets prior to starting and after 6 weeks. Liver toxicity is rare but is most likely in the first 6 months of use and in infants or young children receiving more than one anticonvulsant. The interpretation of the drug level is difficult and is not routinely recommended in the well child. If a child on valproate is unwell, especially with vomiting, drowsiness or deteriorating seizure control, then:
   (a) Stop the valproate.
   (b) Check liver transaminases and ammonia. If normal, then the drug may be resumed (a small rise in transaminase is allowed in any child on valproate).

## Further reading

Anon. (1988) Sodium valproate. *Lancet,* **i**, 1229–1231

Anon. (1989) Carbamazepine update. *Lancet*, **ii**, 595–597

Brodie, M. J. and Feely, J. (1988) Practical clinical pharmacology. Therapeutic drug monitoring and clinical trials. *Br. Med. J.,* **296**, 1110–1114

Camfield, C. S., Camfield, P. R., Smith, E. and Dooley, J. M. (1989) Home use of rectal diazepam to prevent status epilepticus in children with convulsive disorders. *J. Child Neurol.,* **4**, 125–126

Chadwick, D. W. (1987) Overuse of monitoring of blood concentration of antiepileptic drugs. *Br. Med. J.,* **294**, 723–724

Chadwick, D. and Usiskin, S. (1987) *Living with Epilepsy*, Macdonald Optima, London

# 8.4 Status epilepticus

Usually defined as unremitting or repetitive seizures where the child does not regain usual neurological state between seizures. It may increase the brain's requirements for glucose and $O_2$ by the brain, and cause hypoxia, hypoglycaemia, high temperature, low blood pressure, lactic acidosis, all of which contribute to neurological damage.

Nevertheless, over-zealous attempts at stopping seizures may result in respiratory depression, and the iatrogenic morbidity that ensues.

Assuming that ventilation, oxygenation and circulation are adequately maintained, the risk of CNS damage from a short or prolonged seizure appears very small. Therefore, the philosophy of treatment should be to take slow, small, graded steps towards terminating the convulsion.

## CAUSES

Inadequate anticonvulsant levels.
Idiopathic.
Poisons/drugs.
CNS tumour.
Metabolic disorder – e.g. renal failure, inborn errors of metabolism.
Sudden withdrawal of anticonvulsant.
Trauma.
Meningitis, encephalitis.
Hypertension.

## INVESTIGATIONS

Glucose, Na, Ca, LFT, $NH_3$ (Reye's syndrome).
Urine and serum drug levels.
LP – relatively contraindicated because status epilepticus may cause raised ICP.
Arterial gases.
Consider CT scan.

## TREATMENT

The treatment must first be aimed at providing CNS needs ($O_2$, glucose, blood pressure), and only then stopping the fits – be prepared to ventilate the child.

### *1 Airway*

Coma position, suck out oropharynx, $O_2$, ?bag and mask ventilation or endotracheal intubation if underventilating.

### *2 IV fluids*

10% dextrose 1 ml (100 mg)/kg/h. If hypoglycaemic, use 50% dextrose 1–1.5 ml (0.5–0.75 g)/kg of 50% dextrose and then provide 8–12 mg/kg/min. If blood pressure is well maintained, fluid restriction (25–40 ml/kg/day) is vital.

### *3 Drugs*

**3.1 Diazepam** 0.2 mg/kg/dose IV (0.2–0.5 mg/kg/dose PR). Never give it IM. Be prepared to support respiration. May be repeated once. If this fails, try paraldehyde.

**3.2 Paraldehyde** Rectal 0.25 ml/kg diluted in arachis oil 1:1, *or* 0.2 ml/kg deep IM.

**3.3 Phenobarbitone** 15–20 mg/kg IV or IM – potent respiratory suppressant when used with diazepam.

**3.4 Phenytoin** 15–20 mg/kg IV over 20 min.

**3.5 Clonazepam** 25–40 μg/kg/dose IV, may be repeated p.r.n. Typical doses: neonates, 0.25 mg; children, 0.5 mg, adults, 1 mg IV.

**3.6 Thiopentone** Very useful for intractable seizures, but patient must be ventilated. Loading dose: 4–5 mg/kg over 5 min (N.B. Hypotension is common and responds well to 10–20 ml/kg stat of normal saline), then 1–3 mg/kg/h infusion. The higher dose is needed until the fat stores are saturated, after which dose should be reduced. Continue IPPV after ceasing thiopentone until patient can protect his own airway and breath adequately.

*4 Empty stomach – NG tube*

*5 Treat any underlying condition*

For example, antibiotics, electrolyte correction, bicarbonate, dialysis.

*6 Keep temperature between 36.5 and 37.5°C rectal*

## Further reading

Maytal, J., Shinnar, S., Moshe, S. L. and Alvarez, L. A. (1989) Low morbidity and mortality of status epilepticus in children. *Pediatr.*, **83,** 323–331 (and editorial in same issue)

# 8.5 Simple febrile convulsions (SFC)

Convulsions of many varieties may be precipitated or unmasked by fever. To be regarded as simple (or true) febrile convulsions they must conform to a fairly strict definition. Approximately 4% of children will have at least one SFC. Febrile seizures that do not conform to the definition are called atypical or complex febrile seizures.

### DEFINITION

Fever > 38°C – in practice, the fever may first be detected after the seizure because a convulsion often occurs during the rapid ascent phase of the fever.
Age 4 months – 5 years.
Duration of < 15 min.
Minimal post-ictal drowsiness and no other post-ictal neurological signs.
No focal features.

No past history of afebrile seizures.
No past history of CNS damage.
No evidence of meningitis or metabolic cause.

## INVESTIGATION

Consider performing a lumbar puncture (LP) if meningitis cannot be clinically excluded with confidence, especially in children under 1 year. EEG is not indicated for SFC – it contributes nothing to the diagnosis, treatment or prognosis.

Laboratory tests such as blood count, serum electrolytes, calcium, skull x-ray are unhelpful.

## TREATMENT

### *1 Consider admission*

If meningitis is not excluded or for parental reassurance. If the child is not admitted, the parents need much reassurance and explanation about this highly benign but nevertheless frightening disorder.

### *2 Control fever*

Paracetamol, remove some clothes, tepid sponging or bathing in lukewarm water. Do not allow child to shiver.

### *3 Treat any infection*

## RECURRENT SIMPLE FEBRILE CONVULSIONS

### *1 Rectal diazepam*

Parents can be taught to administer a single dose of rectal diazepam (0.3–0.5 mg/kg) at home during a seizure or occasionally at the onset of fever.

### *2 Prophylactic anticonvulsants*

Controversial. Indicated for frequent recurrent seizures or if parents, despite repeated reassurance, unable to cope. Valproate 20–30 mg/kg/day or phenobarbitone 4 mg/kg/day can be used, but both have significant undesirable side effects. A better alternative is rectal diazepam as above, given at the onset of a fever.

## PROGNOSIS

Two per cent will have another seizure within 24 h.
One-third of those with SFC will have another attack at some stage.
Ten per cent of those with SFC have more than two attacks. The risk factors for recurrence are age < 1 yr, family history of febrile seizures, complex seizures. 2.2% of those having SFC subsequently are shown to

have epilepsy (0.6–1% of children who have not had febrile convulsions develop epilepsy). The risk of death or permanent neurological damage resulting from SFC is negligible.

SFCs have no effect on subsequent neurodevelopmental progress. There is no evidence that prophylaxis prevents subsequent epilepsy.

## Further reading


Camfield, C. S., Camfield, P. R., Smith, E. and Dooley, J. M. (1989) Home use of rectal diazepam to prevent status epilepticus in children with convulsive disorders. *J. Child Neurol.*, **4**, 125–126

Hirtz, D. G. (1989) Generalized tonic–clonic and febrile seizures. *Pediatr. Clin. N. Am.*, **36**, 365–382

Lorber, J. and Sunderland, R. (1980) Lumbar puncture in children with convulsions associated with fever. *Lancet*, **i**, 785–786

Nelson, K. B. and Ellenberg, J. H. (1976) Predictors of epilepsy in children who have experienced febrile seizures. *N. Engl. J. Med.*, **295**, 1029–1030

Nelson, K. B. and Ellenberg, J. H. (1978) Prognosis in children with febrile seizures. *Pediatr.*, **61**, 720–727

Rossman, N. P. (1987) Febrile seizures. *Emerg. Med. Clin. N. Am.*, **5**, 719–737

Verity, C. M., Butler, N. R. and Golding, J. (1985) Febrile convulsions in a national cohort followed up from birth. I and II. *Br. Med. J.*, **290**, 1307–1315


# 8.6 Brain stem death

The implication of diagnosing 'brain stem death' in a human being is that irreversible damage to the brain stem has occurred such that it is ethical and legal to withdraw treatment that is supporting life in other body organs. If one continues to 'ventilate till asystole', morale among staff decreases, others are denied facilities that are being used for hopeless life support, the cost-effectiveness equation is heavily unbalanced, relatives miss an opportunity of converting their anguish into positive action by consenting to organ donation, and a potential recipient may die or suffer unnecessary ongoing morbidity.

## DIAGNOSIS OF BRAIN DEATH

### *1 Preconditions*

The patient must be comatose and on a ventilator. A positive diagnosis of cause of coma must be reached and an understanding of how it causes irremediable brain damage is vital. The reasonable (but undefined) passage of time is an essential component in determining that a lesion is irremediable and it gives the relatives a chance to come to an understanding of the predicament. The criteria do not apply to neonates.

### *2 Exclusions*

Brain stem death cannot be considered in the presence of:

(a) possible drug influence;
(b) hypothermia;
(c) metabolic, biochemical or endocrine disturbance.

If the influence of drugs is suspected, it is useful to bear in mind the approximate plasma half-life of the drugs in question. Serum concentrations of such drugs are frequently required. Doubts about the influence of the neuromuscular blockade can be resolved by time, reversal of the blockade with neostigmine and atropine, nerve stimulation, the presence of knee or ankle jerks.

## TESTS OF BRAIN STEM DEATH

### *1 Who performs the test?*

Two medical practitioners with skill in this matter and who have understood the preconditions should perform the tests. One should be a consultant and the other a consultant or senior registrar. The second test should follow the first by 2 or 3 h (a period many times that which brain stem neurons can survive total ischaemia), although it is customary to wait at least 24 h.

### *2 Signs of brain stem death*

**2.1 Deep coma**

**2.2 No abnormal postures**, i.e. decerebrate or decorticate.

**2.3 No seizures.**

**2.4 No brain stem reflexes** – see below.

**2.5 No spontaneous respiration** (apnoea) – see below.

### *3 Brain stem reflexes*

**3.1 Pupillary response** to light.

**3.2 Corneal reflex** Use a throat swab. Apply firm pressure.

**3.3 Vestibulo-ocular reflex/caloric testing** Inspect tympanic membrane. Install 20 ml of ice-cold water into the ear via a small feeding tube. Any eye movement whatsoever suggests that part of the brain stem is alive.

**3.4 Grimacing in response to** (a) firm supra-orbital pressure; (b) painful stimulus of limbs, e.g. push the side of a pencil on patient's finger-nail. Do not use repeated pinpricking.

**Table 8.3 Checklist for brain stem death (After standard form at Children's Hospital, Boston, USA: *J. Pediatr.* (1987) 110, 16–17)**

**Date, time of examination:**
**Diagnosis:**
**Cause of coma:**
**Vital signs**
BP:
Temperature (rectal):

**Biochemistry**
Serum:
$Na^+$ ______ mmol/litre
$K^+$ ______
urea + creatinine ______ ______
osmalarity ______ mosm/litre

Urine:
osmolarity ______

Drugs:
barbiturate level ______ (phenobarbitone ther. range 45–170 μmol/litre or 10–40 mg/litre. Thiopentone ther. range 150–200 μmol/litre or 35–50 mg/litre)
other relevant drugs ______

**Drugs**
Relevant drugs used within the last 3 days ____________
Neuromuscular blockers:
Which?
Last used?
Reversal? Y/N
Nerve stimulation? Y/N
Tendon reflexes? Y/N

**Inspection**
Abnormal posturing? Y/N
Evidence of seizures? Y/N

**Coma**
Response to verbal commands? Y/N
Response to noxious stimuli? Y/N

**Brain stem tests**

| | | |
|---|---|---|
| Pupillary reaction | R ______ | L ______ |
| Corneal reflex | R ______ | L ______ |
| Ice-water caloric test | R ______ | L ______ |

(20 ml in each ear, check tympanic membrane)
Grimace response to supra-orbital pressure? Y/N
Gag, cough? Y/N
Doll's eyes? Y/N

**Table 8.3** (*Continued*)

| |
|---|
| **Apnoea**<br>Pre-test $Paco_2$ ______<br>100% $O_2$ for 10 min. Then turn off ventilator leaving continuous flow of 100% $O_2$ (apnoeic oxygenation)<br>Post-test $Paco_2$ ______<br>Any respiratory effort? Y/N |
| **Supplementary laboratory tests**<br>CT scan:-<br>date/time ______________<br>result ______________ |
| $99^m$ Tc brain scan:<br>date/time ______________<br>result ______________ |
| **Organ donation**<br>Have relatives been asked? Y/N<br>Permission Granted/refused.<br>Which organs (if any) were specified ______________ |
| Signed ______________________ Date/time |

**3.5 Gagging or coughing** Suction catheter down ETT.

**3.6 Oculocephalic reflex/'doll's eye' reflex** Not specifically mentioned in UK code. From the head of the bed, hold patient's eyes open with your thumbs. Rotate patient's head to one side, holding it there for 4 s and then through 180° to the other side. In brain stem death, the head and eyes move together, i.e. absent 'doll's eyes'.

### *4 Test for apnoea – 'apnoeic oxygenation'*

Pre-oxygenate with 100% $O_2$ for 10 min.
Have the patient's $Paco_2$ at 30–38 mmHg (4–5 kPa) before the test.
Stop ventilating the patient for 10 min (leave a flow of $O_2$ into the ETT).
This results in a minimum rise in $Paco_2$ of 2 mmHg/min (0.27 kPa/min).
Record the $Paco_2$ at the beginning and end of the test: it should reach at least 50 mmHg (6.65 kPa).

## DECLARATION OF DEATH

A checklist can be filled out to document the finding of brain stem death. Table 8.3 is a modified version of the form used at the Children's Hospital, Boston, USA (*J. Pediatr.* (1987) **110,** 16–17).

## Further reading

Freeman, J. M. (1988) New brain death guidelines in children: further confusion. *Pediatr.*, **81**, 301–313

Pallis, C. (1983) *ABC of Brain Stem Death.* British Medical Journal, London

Task Force for Determination of Brain Death in Children (1987) Guidelines for the determination of brain death in children. *Neurology,* **37**, 1077–1078

Taylor, R. M. R. and Salaman, J. R. (1988) The obligation to ask for organs. *Lancet,* **i**, 985–987 (an interesting discussion on organ donation; see also subsequent correspondence, *Lancet* (1988) **i**, 1229–1230)

# 8.7 Head injuries

The care of the child with hypoxic–ischaemic (near-drowning, near-miss SIDS) or inflammatory CNS injury has much in common with traumatic head injury. The latter is taken as the prototype for understanding neuro-intensive care.

### PATHOPHYSIOLOGY

The major causes of brain damage are:

1. Mechanical injury.
2. Haemorrhage into brain parenchyma or into subdural or extradural spaces.
3. Oedema around contusion or haematoma.
4. Ischaemia produced by expanding mass, brain swelling or hypotension.
5. Systemic complications of the injury including hypoxia, hypercarbia, poor cardiac output, acidosis, inappropriate ADH syndrome.

- *In CNS trauma always consider the possibility of associated visceral organ and cervical spine damage.*

### PREVENTION

Children (and adults) who cycle should wear protective helmets. The time has come for this to be a major public health priority. In motor cars, infants should be harnessed in child restrainers, and children (and adults) should wear seat belts.

### HISTORY

Obtain a clear outline of the nature of the injury, loss of consciousness with or without a lucid interval, and the time course prior to consultation. Mild blows to the side of the head are potentially serious and should be considered with extraordinary caution.

## EXAMINATION

Findings must be accurately documented as they may be of use as a baseline for further assessment. Important things to consider:

(a) Is there a possibility of cervical cord injury? If so, apply a soft collar and avoid moving the neck.
(b) Are there other hidden injuries, e.g. ruptured abdominal viscus?
(c) Are the airway, breathing, pulse and BP adequately maintained?

## MILD HEAD INJURY

A child with loss of consciousness (LOC) for less than 5 min in whom there are no neurological signs and no scalp haematomas or CSF leak does not need a skull x-ray (SXR). After a 4 h observation period, the child may go home if:

1. The parents feel reassured, they live close by, and have access to transport back to the hospital should it be required.
2. Written instructions are given to parents advising them to gently rouse their child 2 hourly for 12 h and to bring their child back if he becomes more difficult to rouse, confused, irrational, convulses, vomits repeatedly, or has blood or watery discharge from ear or nose. Many hospitals have a printed list of instructions to give to parents.

## MODERATE AND SEVERE INJURY

Admit and take a SXR of any child with any of the following features (a neurosurgeon must be involved):

### *1 History*

Age <1 yr.
LOC for >5 min, or fluctuating conscious state.
High-velocity or penetrating injury (as opposed to blunt trauma).

### *2 Examination*

Palpable scalp haematoma.
Skull depression – palpable or probed in scalp laceration.
CSF discharge from ear or nose.
Blood behind tympanic membrane.
Battle sign (bruising over the mastoid).
Periorbital haematoma (racoon's eyes).
Lethargy, coma, stupor.
Focal neurological signs.

### *3 Assess Glasgow Coma Scale* (see Table 8.4)

The Glasgow Coma Scale (GCS) aims to identify high-risk patients for more invasive therapies, and is a useful epidemiological tool. It is not an aid to deciding from whom to withhold or withdraw therapy, nor is it a substitute for a good neurological assessment.

**Table 8.4 The Glasgow Coma Scale**

| | *Age >1 yr* | *Age <1 yr* |
|---|---|---|
| *Eyes opening* | | |
| 4 | Spontaneously | Spontaneously |
| 3 | To verbal command | To shout |
| 2 | To pain | To pain |
| 1 | No response | No response |
| *Best motor response* | | |
| 6 | Obeys | Normal spontaneous movements |
| 5 | Localizes pain | Localizes pain |
| 4 | Flexion withdrawal | Flexion withdrawal |
| 3 | Flexor posturing | Flexor posturing (decorticate) |
| 2 | Extensor posturing | Extensor posturing (decerebrate) |
| 1 | None | None |
| *Best verbal response* | | |
| | (>2 yr) | (<2 yr) |
| 5 | Orientated, converses | Coos and babbles |
| 4 | Disorientated, converses | Irritable cries |
| 3 | Inappropriate words | Cries to pain |
| 2 | Incomprehensible sounds | Grunts |
| 1 | None | None |
| Total score = 3–15 | | |

Scores less than 8 on admission are suggestive of severe injury; children with such scores should have airway support and aggressive therapy to decrease ICP.

## MEDICAL MANAGEMENT OF SEVERE HEAD INJURY

Intensive care admission is mandatory if the child is fitting, has a compromised cardiorespiratory system or diminished conscious state such that the ability to protect his airway is in doubt.

Some or all of the following may be required.

### *1 Maintain airway*

Endotracheal tube, size = Age/4 + 4 mm.

### *2 Controlled hyperventilation*

Intermittent positive pressure ventilation (IPPV) is the cornerstone of management. In children more than about 1 year of age, one will usually use a volume cycled ventilator. On the Servo 900-C, for example, one sets a minute volume and a rate. Tidal volume = Minute volume/Rate. The machine will ventilate with whatever pressure is required to deliver this predetermined tidal volume. A child needs a minute volume of 200–250 ml/kg (tidal volume 15–20 ml/kg). Nevertheless one must look at the chest wall to see if there is adequate respiratory excursion. If there is a large air leak around the ETT, either set a higher minute volume or change to a larger ETT. The need for involving someone skilled in airway management (usually an anaesthetist) is self-evident. Ventilate to a $P\text{co}_2$ of 28–35 mmHg (3.5–4.5 kPa). Keep $P\text{ao}_2 > 75$ mmHg (10 kPa). Avoid high end expiratory pressures.

### *3 Maintain cerebral perfusion pressure (mean BP – ICP > 40 mmHg)*

**3.1 Keep BP high** Hypotension should be treated aggressively with dopamine 5–10 μg/kg/min and plasma expanders (whole blood/albumin) 10–20 ml/kg. Ongoing hypotension or need for transfusion is a warning of unsuspected visceral injury.

**3.2 Keep ICP low** In practice, many hospitals cannot or do not measure ICP. Nevertheless, one must constantly review the means of keeping it low in someone who is presumed to have raised ICP. Presumed raised ICP can be treated with additional hyperventilation, mannitol, control of seizures, better posturing, paralysis, barbiturates – these are discussed below.

### *4 Posture*

Head up (approx. 15°) and in the midline to facilitate venous drainage from the brain.

### *5 Paralyse*

Pancuronium 0.1 mg/kg p.r.n. Prevents muscle spasm and shivering that raise ICP. Seizure activity will be masked, hence some centres use continuous EEG monitoring, a loading dose of phenytoin and keep a vigil for autonomic signs of seizures that are not ablated by paralysis, i.e. rapid pupillary fluctuation, pulse and BP lability.

### *6 Control seizures aggressively*

Many centres give prophylactic phenytoin, especially if the child is receiving muscle relaxants because the signs of fitting may only be those of cardiovascular instability. Have a low threshold for using thiopentone 5 mg/kg over 5 min (may drop BP but responds to plasma expanders), followed by infusion at 1–3 mg/kg/h. High doses are needed for the first few hours until the fat stores are saturated.

### *7 Temperature control*

Core body temperature must be kept at 36.5–37.5°C. Higher temperatures increase brain metabolic requirements. Lower temperatures increase predisposition to severe sepsis. Cool the forehead with ice packs and use rectal paracetamol. If further cooling is required, use a cooling blanket or more ice packs, but paralyse the child to prevent shivering.

### *8 Mannitol*

0.25–0.5 g/kg/dose × 1 or 2, only if serum osmolality is < 330 mosm. Repeated doses may paradoxically increase brain water. Should be given with frusemide 1 mg/kg.

### *9 Fluid restriction*

This is secondary in importance to the goal of achieving adequate blood pressure, urine output, peripheral perfusion and by implication cerebral perfusion. However, if these goals have been achieved, restrict fluids to 0–30 ml/kg/day. Insertion of a central venous line will provide valuable information about the need for additional plasma expansion which is best achieved with small aliquots of albumin or whole blood. Regular assays of serum sodium and osmolarity of serum and urine are required in order to anticipate dilutional hyponatraemia and the syndrome of inappropriate ADH.

### *10 Gastric pH*

If < 5, give magnesium trisilicate 0.3–0.5 ml/kg/4 h via NGT. Alternatively, ranitidine 1 mg/kg/8 h slow IV or 3 mg/kg/12 h via NGT. There is some evidence that this may alter upper GI flora and in turn predispose to bacterial pneumonia.

### *11 Other drugs*

Steroids are of no benefit and may be harmful. High-dose barbiturate coma – controversial. Not in vogue at present.

### *12 Monitoring ICP*

Best done with intraventricular catheter.

## Further reading


Anon. (1987) Skull X-ray after head injury – the final word? *Lancet*, **i**, 667

Anon. (1988) When are cyclists going to wear helmets? *Lancet*, **i**, 159–160

[illegible] (19[illegible]) Delayed effects of head injury. *Br. Med. J.*, [illegible]

Langfitt, T. W. and Gennarelli, T. A. (1982) Can the outcome from head injury be improved? *J. Neurosurg.*, **56**, 19–25

Leonidas, J. C., Ting, W. and Binkiewicz, A. (1982) Mild head trauma in children: when is a Roentgenogram necessary. *Pediatr.*, **69**, 139–143

Thompson, R. S. *et al.* (1989) A case-control study of the effectiveness of bicycle safety helmets. *N. Engl. J. Med.*, **320**, 1363

# 8.8 (Near) drowning

Drowning is defined as death from submersion, within 24 h of the accident. Near drowning refers to victims who survive longer than 24 h. Here the terms will be used interchangeably. The differences between fresh- and salt-water drowning are clinically insignificant. The problems encountered commonly relate to the brain, occasionally the heart and lungs, and rarely electrolytes. There are numerous reports of normal survival after prolonged immersion; hence, prolonged effective first aid is crucial and it should be administered until the child is normothermic.

## PATHOPHYSIOLOGY

The main physiological consequence of near drowning is hypoxaemia, rather than ischaemia. The net result in the brain is cerebral oedema, and cellular increases in glucose uptake, glycolysis and lactate production.

## FACTORS AFFECTING OUTCOME

### *1 Physiological*

The diving seal reflex diverts blood away from tissues resistant to hypoxia (gut, skin, muscle) to those least tolerant of oxygen lack (brain, heart).

### *2 Hypothermia*

Decreases cerebral metabolism and therefore protects against the effects of hypoxia.

### *3 Duration of immersion*

Bears some relationship to outcome, but in any given individual the above factors may protect the brain. Continue first aid measures till arrival in hospital and normothermia.

### *4 First aid*

No other accident in children highlights the importance of a community knowledge of cardiopulmonary resuscitation (CPR) as well as drowning.

### *5 Post-immersion medical care*

Relates primarily to good neuro-intensive care.

## PREVENTION

Private swimming pools should be fenced.
Early swimming tuition.
Public awareness of risks of children playing unattended near water, however shallow.

## INTENSIVE CARE MANAGEMENT

Children, who on arrival in hospital are in deep coma, require CPR, have an arterial blood pH < 7.0, or a GCS of < 6 (see Table 8.4) are unlikely to have normal survival, although normothermia must be attained before neurological examination is valid. Neurological care is similar to that of a child with head injury (see Section 8.7). Intracranial pressure monitoring probably has no place in drowning.

### *1 Maintain cerebral perfusion pressure*

That is, maintain adequate BP and reduce ICP – see Section 8.7. This may involve:

**1.1 Restoration of circulating blood volume** A CVC line may help.

**1.2 Inotropic support of BP**

**1.3 Modest hyperventilation** To $P\text{CO}_2$ of 30–35 mmHg (4.0–4.6 kPa).

**1.4 Head up** 15° and keep head in midline.

**1.5 Normothermia** The dangers of hyper- or hypothermia are considerable.

### *2 Fluids*

Once circulating blood volume and cardiac output are restored, maintenance fluids should initially be < 30 ml/kg/day if the child is ventilated. Syndrome of inappropriate ADH is associated with cerebral hypoxia and IPPV.

### *3 Respiratory support*

Needed for cardiac, pulmonary and neurological reasons. Coma (GCS < 9) probably requires ETT for airway protection and ensuring mild hypocapnia. Any child unable to maintain $P\text{aO}_2$ > 90 mmHg (12 kPa) in 40% head box $O_2$ is likely to require ventilation.

### *4 Cardiac support*

A hypoxic myocardium suffers damage and may require dopamine or dobutamine (5–10 μg/kg/min).

### *5 Gastrointestinal dialysis*

Bloody diarrhoea suggests severe gut ischaemia. Give nil by mouth, and consider early TPN. As with all neurointensive care, consider antacids if gastric pH < 5.

### *6 Antibiotics*

No evidence that antibiotics are required. Indeed, antibiotics may select for resistant organisms.

### *7 Steroids*

Little rationale for their use. Not advised.

### *8 Monitoring*

Insertion of CVC and IA lines greatly facilitates management.

### *9 Rewarming*

Space blanket, electric blanket, warm IV fluids and humidified inspired gas are recommended. Occasionally use warm peritoneal lavage.

## PROGNOSIS

Those arriving at hospital awake have an excellent prognosis. Those with a GCS of 6 or more on arrival usually recover fully, provided that there is evidence of improvement within 6 h.

## Further reading

Bohn, D. J., Bigger, W. D., Smith, C. R. *et al.* (1986) Influence of hypothermia, barbiturate therapy and intracranial pressure monitoring on morbidity and mortality after near drowning. *Crit. Care Med.*, **14**, 529

Dean, J. M. and Kaufman, N. D. (1981) Prognostic indicators in pediatric near-drowning: The Glasgow Coma Scale. *Crit. Care. Med.*, **9**, 536–539

Orlowski, J. (1987) Drowning, near drowning and ice-water submersions. *Pediatr. Clin. N. Am.*, **34**, 75–92

Rogers, M. C. (1987) *Textbook of Pediatric Intensive Care*, Williams and Wilkins, Baltimore, pp. 721–739

# 8.9 The infant with a large head

A large head is usually considered in the context of the child's occipitofrontal circumference (OFC). It is best to take three measurements at a time to ensure that the tape measure has not inadvertently been malpositioned.

## AETIOLOGY

1. Normal variant.
2. Hydrocephalus.
3. Localized expanding lesions, e.g. subdural haematoma, intracerebral or arachnoid cyst.
4. Megalencephaly.

### *1 Normal variant*

This is a diagnosis made by repeated measurements of OFC over several months or years. The child is neurodevelopmentally normal and often has parents with large OFC. The child's OFC will usually have an initial accelerated rate of growth, but will settle into a growth pattern at a high level but parallel to the normal curve.

### *2 Hydrocephalus*

Excess CSF accumulation in the brain may be due to:

(a) increased production (rare);
(b) obstruction of the CSF pathway;
(c) diminished absorption through the arachnoid granulations into the veins.

Obstruction of CSF flow can be *non-communicating* where there is no communication between subarachnoid space and the ventricles, or *communicating* where the obstruction is beyond the basal cisterns.

Common causes of hydrocephalus are:

1. Spina bifida – associated with Arnold–Chiari malformation and aqueduct stenosis.
2. Sequelae of arachnoiditis – e.g. post-haemorrhagic hydrocephalus in premature infants, or post-purulent meningitis.
3. Stricture of the aqueduct – usually congenital.
4. Obstruction of CSF at any level by tumours, cysts, aneurysm of vein of Galen.

### *3 Subdural effusion/haematoma*

Many possible causes, including idiopathic/birth trauma; non-accidental injury; dehydration; haematological problems – leukaemia, haemophilia, scurvy.

**Axioms** (a) Seizures and a large head in an infant represent a subdural effusion till proven otherwise; (b) an unexplained subdural collection should prompt a search for other features of non-accidental injury.

### *4 Megalencephaly (rare)*

The ventricles are of normal size, but brain mass is increased. Mental retardation is common. Causes include the phakomatoses, storage diseases, metabolic diseases such as Tay–Sachs disease and Sotos syndrome, and commonly, no cause is found.

## CLINICAL FEATURES

### *1 History*

Acute rise in ICP – vomit, lethargy, convulsions.
Chronic rise in ICP – FTT, developmental delay, vomit.

Neonatal history – prematurity, IVH.
Developmental history.
Social/family environment.

### *2 Examination*

**2.1 Serial OFC** An isolated measurement is much less revealing than serial head growth. OFC of parents and siblings should also be plotted.

**2.2 Skull shape** Hydrocephalus causes frontal bossing with other features of 'setting sun' eyes, wide fontanelle, prominent scalp veins and high-pitched percussion note.
Prominent occiput – posterior fossa cyst.
Parietal bulge – porencephaly or subdural collection.
Small posterior fossa with 'occipital overhang' – aqueduct stenosis.

**2.3 Signs of raised ICP** Split sutures, bulging fontanelle, papilloedema.

**2.4 Skull transillumination** Requires a bright light in a very dark room. Diffuse transillumination is seen with uniform ventricular dilatation, hydranencephaly, bilateral subdural effusion. Asymmetrical translucency may indicate a subdural collection, or porencephaly. Posterior fossa transillumination suggests a Dandy–Walker cyst. Blood does not transilluminate.

**2.5 Fundi** Retinal haemorrhages suggest non-accidental injury or birth trauma.

**2.6 General examination** Signs of external trauma, focal or bilateral neurological signs, failure to thrive, developmental delay are all in keeping with subdural effusion.

## INVESTIGATION

Skull x-ray – split sutures, thinning of skull vault in hydrocephalus.
CT scan.
Ultrasound – safe, non-invasive, reliable way of brain imaging, if the anterior fontanelle is open. Posterior fossa lesions and subdural effusions are not well seen.

## MANAGEMENT

Not all children with rapidly growing heads require immediate investigation. An asymptomatic child can be followed until his OFC crosses percentile lines.
Hydrocephalus – VP shunt is the treatment of choice. Hydrocephalus occasionally resolves with ventricular taps or diuretics.

Tumours – excision, radiotherapy and/or chemotherapy.
Subdural effusion – if symptoms develop (lethargy, focal signs, fever suggesting empyema), a subdural tap is both diagnostic and therapeutic (see Section 4.3). It may need to be done as an emergency.

## 8.10 CSF shunt complications

Insertion of a ventriculoperitoneal (VP) shunt is the operation of choice in hydrocephalus. Occasionally, intracerebral cysts are drained with cystoperitoneal shunts. Ventriculo-atrial (VA) and ventriculopleural shunts are seldom used. In communicating hydrocephalus, lumboperitoneal shunts are occasionally inserted.

### COMPLICATIONS OF VP SHUNTS

#### *1 Obstruction*

The ventricular end becomes clogged with choroid plexus or cerebral tissue, or the lower end may obstruct when it displaces into an unsuitable position usually due to ongoing growth of the child.

#### *2 Infection*

May lead to septicaemia. Low-grade sepsis (usually *Staphylococcus epidermidis*) may erroneously be dismissed as 'contaminant'.

#### *3 Mechanical failure*

Usually fracture or separation of the tubing.

#### *4 VA shunts only*

Shunt nephritis, pulmonary hypertension.

### CLINICAL FEATURES

#### *1 Complete obstruction*

May cause acute or subacute onset headache, blurred vision, vomit, loss of coordination and declining conscious state. If the shunt 'pump' cannot be compressed or remains compressed, then one or more of the components may be occluded. Seizures alone do not indicate shunt dysfunction unless they are associated with the above neurological features (Hack *et al.*, 1990).

#### *2 Partial or intermittent obstruction*

Results in periodic headache, nausea, drowsiness, poor school performance. There is argument as to whether or not this is a real entity.

### *3 Shunt infection*

May present with unexplained fever, headache, nausea, malaise, splenomegaly or anaemia. Difficult to diagnose clinically.

## INVESTIGATION

### *1 Obstruction*

CT scan.

### *2 Fractured tubing*

X-ray the length of the tubing.

### *3 Infection*

Needle aspiration of the 'pump', C-reactive protein, haemoglobin, serial staphylococcal antibody titres.

## TREATMENT

All complications should be referred to a neurosurgeon.
Acute blockage is a surgical emergency.
Shunt infection usually requires replacement of shunt. Avoid casual use of antibiotics until diagnosis is bacteriologically confirmed.

## Further reading

Guertin, S. R. (1987) Cerebrospinal fluid shunts. *Pediatr. Clin. N. Am.*, **34**, 203–217

Hack, C. H., Enrile, B. G., Donat, J. F. and Kosnik, E. (1990) Seizures in relation to shunt dysfunction in children with meningomyelocele. *J. Pediatr.*, **116**, 57–60

Chapter 9

# Haematology and oncology

## 9.1 The new leukaemic child

### POINTS TO CONSIDER

1. Although the clinical picture and peripheral blood film may be highly suggestive of leukaemia, the only way to make an affirmative diagnosis is with bone marrow aspiration (BMA).
2. Treatment is seldom so imperative that one cannot wait until the next weekday to perform a BMA with surface markers and cytogenetics.
3. Any new leukaemic with high fever should be managed as a 'febrile neutropenic child' (see Section 9.2).
4. Leukaemic children should initially be managed in a regional oncology centre. There is no longer a place for the clinician who 'dabbles in a bit of oncology' to manage the induction phase of chemotherapy. However, oncology centres should increase the involvement of clinicians from smaller centres in the follow-up care of children.

### MANAGEMENT ON ADMISSION

#### *1 Insert IV line*

Take blood for: FBC, urea and electrolytes, Ca, $PO_4$, blood cultures (if appropriate), clotting screen, blood group and save some serum for cross-match, uric acid.

#### *2 Measure height and weight*

Calculate body surface area (see Section 3.7).

#### *3 Hydration*

4% dextrose/0.18% saline to run at 3 litres/$m^2$/day.

- *Do not add potassium to the infusion.*

#### *4 Allopurinol*

10 mg/kg/day oral in 2 or 3 doses.

## COMPLICATIONS IN THE FIRST TWO DAYS OF CHEMOTHERAPY

### *Tumour lysis syndrome*

In children with high white cell count (WCC >50 000/mm$^3$) or those with high bulk disease (e.g. lymphoma), rapid tumour lysis predisposes to uric acid nephropathy and hyperkalaemia. This is usually prevented by hydration and allopurinol for 12–24 h prior to chemotherapy. The duty house officer should be vigilant about:

Urea and electrolytes – need to be checked overnight.
$Ca^{2+}$ (it goes down), $PO_4^{2-}$ (it goes up).
No added $K^+$ to fluids.
Careful fluid balance.

If there is renal involvement (hypertension, palpable kidneys, renal failure), before commencing chemotherapy consider dialysis, deep x-ray therapy (DXRT), smaller induction doses, or more cautious hydration.

# 9.2 Management of the febrile neutropenic child

A neutropenic child can rapidly succumb to infection. Fever in such a child must be appraised and treated as a matter of urgency. The following is a modified version of the approach at Addenbrooke's Hospital, Cambridge. Each centre will have its own individual approach.

## DEFINITION OF NEUTROPENIA

Absolute neutrophil count (ANC) of <500/mm$^3$ (some centres use <1000/mm$^3$).

## DEFINITION OF FEVER

Pyrexia >39°C *or*
Pyrexia >38°C 2 h apart
(or unwell, hypotensive, neutropenic child even without pyrexia).

## INVESTIGATION

At least one set of blood cultures should be taken before commencing antibiotic treatment. Some other investigations are presented below, but they are to be tailored to the individual child.

FBC – to establish neutrophil count.
Blood culture – from peripheral vein *and* from any indwelling central line (Hickman, Broviac).
CXR.
MSU or SPA of bladder – microscopy and culture for cells, bacteria and *Candida*.
Serology for viruses (also occasionally for *Candida* and precipitins for *Aspergillus*).
Swab of: nose – ? *Aspergillus*;
throat – bacteria, viruses;
rectal – not perianal skin.
Stool culture.
Nasopharyngeal aspirate – viral immunofluorescence, if there is any evidence of lung disease.
LP – if indicated.
Culture any obvious site of infection.

If diarrhoea – faeces for bacterial culture, electron microscopy (EM) for viruses, ask specifically for *Clostridium difficile* cytotoxin (finding the organism alone does not implicate it in the illness).

If oral mucositis – swab in viral transport medium for *Herpes simplex*;
– swab in Stuart's medium for capnocytophagia (rare).

If persistent pneumonia – consider bronchial lavage for pneumocystis.

## THERAPY

Be guided by the microbiology department.
N.B. If the child has >500 neutrophils/mm$^3$ *and* is well *and* has no obvious focus of infection, treat as for any other child.

### *1 <500 neutrophils/mm$^3$*

Ceftazidime 30 mg/kg/8 h IV (or IM). Use 50 mg/kg/8 h if very sick.
Gentamicin 2.5 mg/kg/8 h IV.
Nystatin 100 000–500 000 u/6 h orally.

### *2 No response by 72 h*

**2.1 No clues** Cease ceftazidime, especially if there are ceftazidime-resistant Enterobacteriaceae in the child's upper respiratory flora.
Use – piperacillin 50 mg/kg/6 h (or ciprofloxacin 5–10 mg/kg/12 h. N.B. Reduce dose of theophylline). Use under microbiologist's guidance.

**2.2 Mucositis** Consider *H. simplex*. Use acyclovir 10 mg/kg/8 h IV over 1 h if swab positive (= high dose because of immunocompromise); consider capnocytophagia/anaerobes; add erythromycin and metronidazole.

**2.3 Diarrhoea *or* abdominal pain *or* abdominal distension** Perform a plain abdominal x-ray for evidence of neutropenic ileocaecitis. Consider other causes such as *C. difficile* enterotoxin, *C. septicum*, disturbance in Ca, Mg, K, $PO_4$ status.
Use – gentamicin 2.5 mg/kg/8 h; vancomycin 10–15 mg/kg/8–12 h (infuse over 30–60 min); metronidazole 7.5 mg/kg/8 h.

### 2.4 Pneumonia

*2.4.1 ?Pneumocystis* Cotrimoxazole (trimethoprim 1 mg/sulphamethoxazole 5 mg) at a dose of trimethoprim 5 mg/kg/6 h. Median intervals for return of normal clinical findings with treatment are: 4 days for fever, 7 days for respiratory rate, 8 days for $Pao_2$ and 9 days for CXR. If no improvement by expected time, consider open lung biopsy/steroids (N.B. Some use pentamidine).

*2.4.2 ?Aspergillus* Amphotericin B – test dose 1 mg in 20 ml 5% dextrose over 1 h, then 0.25 mg/kg/day (infuse over 6 h, protect from light). Increase by 0.25 mg/kg increments to a max. of 1 mg/kg/day. Reactions include: fevers, rashes, rigors which may require antihistamine/hydrocortisone/pethidine. Hypokalaemia is common and may require $K^+$ supplements.

5-Fluorocytosine (flucytosine): 50 mg/kg/8 h oral/IV over 30 min. Lower dose in renal impairment. Useful as an adjunct to amphotericin in *Cryptococcus*. Its benefit in *Aspergillus* is more questionable.

### *3 Granulocyte transfusions – rarely used*

May improve survival in Gram-negative sepsis. Occasionally used for localized infection, e.g. perianal abscess. Must be collected by experienced phaeresis unit and given daily for 4–7 days. Immunological reactions to the transfusion are common.

## 9.3 Varicella zoster in the immunosuppressed child

One-third of immunosuppressed children who develop varicella will have visceral dissemination most commonly involving the lung. Children off chemotherapy treatment for >6 months are at small risk of disseminated varicella, although preventative treatment after exposure should be offered to those within 1 year of ceasing treatment.

### PREVENTION

#### *1 Zoster immune globulin (ZIG)*

Give within 72 h of chickenpox exposure (see Section 6.1).

#### *2 Acyclovir*

Prophylaxis: as soon as possible after contact, as an alternative to ZIG.
Dose: 0–5 yr 200 mg q.d.s. orally for 21 days
6–10 yr 400 mg q.d.s.
>10 yr 800 mg q.d.s.
Treatment: as soon as varicella appears.
Dose: 500 mg/m$^2$/8 h IV over 1 h × 7 days.
Other treatments: Vidarabine, alpha-leucocyte interferon – probably more toxic and no longer used (*J. Pediatr.* (1982) **101**, 622).

## 9.4 The bleeding oncology patient

Haemostasis requires adequate numbers of functioning platelets, normal plasma clotting factors and vascular integrity. Any or all of these may be compromised in a child receiving treatment for cancer; however, thrombocytopenia is the most common abnormality.

### THROMBOCYTOPENIA

#### *1 Platelet count 10 000–30 000/mm$^3$*

May cause petechiae and mucocutaneous bleeding, but is not life threatening unless the child also seems unwell and febrile (i.e. ?septic, ?DIC).

#### *2 Platelet count < 10 000*

High risk of severe spontaneous internal haemorrhage.

### TREATMENT

#### *1 Platelet transfusion*

Usually given if platelet count <20 000/mm$^3$, although in practice each case is treated on its merits.
Dose: 6 u/m$^2$ or 0.2 u/kg will normally raise platelet count by approx. 75 000/mm$^3$. Administer over 30 min.
Side effects: fever, rigors, hypotension.
Treatment: slow down IV infusion;
antihistamines – chlorpheniramine 0.25 mg/kg IV;
hydrocortisone 2–4 mg/kg IV;
paracetamol.

### *2 Avoid agents that decrease platelet function*

These include aspirin, non-steroidal anti-inflammatory drugs, moxalactam, intralipid.

### *3 Avoid IM injections – or deep venepunctures*

### *4 Suppress menstruation*

Menstruation usually stops while patient is on chemotherapy, especially if ill enough to be thrombocytopenic. It is rare to have to use oestrogens for post-pubertal females.

*5 Epistaxis* (see Section 18.3)

## Further reading

Allegretta, G. J., Weisman, S. J. and Altman, A. J. (1985) Oncologic emergencies II. *Pediatr. Clin. N. Am.*, **32,** 614–616

# 9.5 The pale child/anaemia

A child may be pale without any underlying disorder. Pallor without anaemia is also recognized in acutely unwell children who may be suffering from infection or circulatory failure due to acute fluid or blood loss, congestive cardiac failure or septicaemia.

Long-standing pallor without anaemia may be normal or due to anxiety, eczema or, if the child is in poor health, one should consider chronic renal disease, rare inborn errors of metabolism or hypothyroidism.

Pallor may of course also be due to decreased haemoglobin (Hb) concentration. Children may tolerate very severe anaemia with very few or no symptoms and may only present because of an unrelated illness. Iron deficiency is by far the most common cause of anaemia in our community.

## DEFINITION OF ANAEMIA

Anaemia exists when the Hb and haematocrit fall below the normal range appropriate to the child's age (see Section 9.13).

## CLASSIFICATION OF ANAEMIA

(a) Decreased production of red blood cells (RBC).
(b) Increased destruction of RBC.
(c) Blood loss.

## (a) Decreased production of RBC

### *1 Deficiencies*

**1.1 Iron** Due to nutritional inadequacy, malabsorption or chronic blood loss.

**1.2 Folic acid** Nutritional inadequacy (goats' milk diet) or increased utilization in chronic haemolysis, phenytoin.

**1.3 Vitamin $B_{12}$** Intrinsic factor deficiency in congenital pernicious anaemia or poor absorption due to disease or resection of the terminal ileum. Vegans.

**1.4 Combined deficiencies** Malnutrition or malabsorption syndromes, e.g. coeliac disease.

### *2 Bone marrow defect*

**2.1 Infiltration** For example leukaemia, neuroblastoma, lipid storage disease.

**2.2 Aplastic anaemia** Congenital or drug induced. Selective aplasia of red cells may be due to congenital pure red cell aplasia (Blackfan–Diamond syndrome).

### *3 Chronic disease*

For example, chronic renal failure, chronic infection.

## (b) Increased destruction of RBC (haemolytic anaemia)

1. Neonatal ABO, Rh or minor blood group incompatibility.
2. Haemoglobinopathies – thalassaemia, sickle cell disease.
3. Disorders of RBC metabolism – hereditary spherocytosis (acholuric jaundice), G-6-PD and pyruvate kinase deficiency.
4. Immune haemolysis (Coombs' positive) – idiopathic, drugs, infection.
5. Others – haemolytic uraemic syndrome, DIC, hypersplenism, malaria.

## (c) Blood loss

1. GIT bleed – oesophagitis, cows' milk protein sensitivity, Meckel's diverticulum, oesophageal varices, hookworm infestation.
2. Haematuria – rarely causes anaemia.
3. Pulmonary – Goodpasture's syndrome, pulmonary haemosiderosis.
4. Too many blood tests.

# WHAT TO DO WITH THE ANAEMIC CHILD

(a) Take a history.
(b) Examine the child.
(c) Perform initial simple investigations.

*By obtaining a good history, examination, blood film and reticulocyte count one can virtually always reach a narrow differential diagnosis.*

## (a) History

### *1 All ages*

Jaundice, urine colour, medications, bleeding or bruising, racial origin and family history. Recent arrival from a tropical country might suggest malaria.

### *2 Neonatal period*

Prematurity – preterm and babies with intra-uterine growth retardation are prone to iron deficiency.
Jaundice – especially if required blood transfusion or exchange transfusion suggests neonatal haemolysis.
Haemorrhage – i.e. bruising or bleeding.

### *3 Infancy*

Diet – identify iron-containing foods in the diet (see Section 9.6); therefore, record what milk and solids the child takes, and at what age were they introduced?
Infection – recurrent/chronic infection or diarrhoea.

### *4 Childhood*

Diet.

## (b) Examination

Skin and mucous membranes – pallor, bruising, petechiae.
Conjunctivae – icterus, pallor.
Liver, spleen, lymph nodes – enlargement suggests reticulo-endothelial malignancy, connective tissue disease or haemolysis.
Growth failure – chronic systemic illness, malabsorption.

## (c) Possible initial investigations

Haemoglobin, haematocrit.
Peripheral blood film with total white cell and differential count.
Mean corpuscular volume, mean corpuscular haemoglobin (= red cell indices).
Reticulocyte count.
Urinalysis – haemoglobin, urobilinogen, bilirubin.
Serum bilirubin – conjugated and unconjugated.
Thick and thin blood film for malaria parasites – for recent travellers to the tropics (see Section 10.11).

Using the above results, refer to Figure 9.1 and then Tables 9.1 and 9.2 for further elucidation of the cause of the anaemia.

N.B. Some new automated blood cell analysers provide a measure of red blood cell volume distribution width (RDW) and a histogram of red blood cell volume distribution. RDW is a measure of the heterogeneity of distribution of red blood cell size which is the equivalent of anisocytosis in

**Table 9.1 Investigation of hypochromic microcytic anaemia***

| | *Fe deficiency* | *Thalassaemia* | *Chronic infection* |
|---|---|---|---|
| Serum iron | Dec. | N or inc. | N or Dec. |
| Transferrin | Inc. | Dec. | Dec. |
| Saturation | Dec. (<15%) | N or inc. | Dec. |
| Ferritin | Dec. | N or inc. | N |
| Red cell protoporphyrin | Inc. | Dec. | Inc. |
| Hb elecrophoresis | N | Abnormal | N |

* See Section 9.13 for normal values.
N, normal; Dec., decreased; Inc., increased.

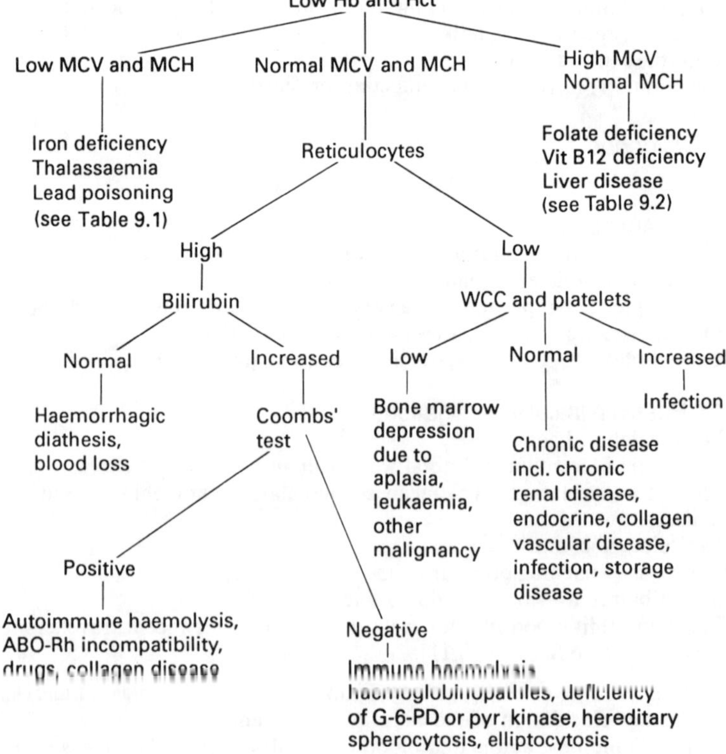


**Figure 9.1** Differentiation of causes of anaemia (Hb, haemoglobin; Hct, haematocrit; MCV, mean corpuscular volume; MCH, mean corpuscular haemoglobin; WCC, white cell count)

**Table 9.2 Investigation of macrocytic anaemia**

| | *$B_{12}$ deficiency* | *Folate deficiency* |
|---|---|---|
| Serum $B_{12}$ | Decreased | Normal |
| Serum folate | Normal or increased | Fluctuates with diet |
| Red cell folate | Decreased | Decreased |

analysis of the peripheral blood smear. Classification of anaemias by mean corpuscular volume (MCV) and RDW is a very sensitive way of reaching the correct classification of the anaemia (*Pediatr.* (1987) **80**, 251; *Am. J. Clin. Pathol.* (1983) **80**, 322–326).

# 9.6 Iron deficiency

This is usually a nutritional deficiency – the only nutritional deficiency disease seen commonly in the Western world.

Iron stores are acquired mainly in the 3rd trimester of pregnancy. The regulation of iron absorption is at gut mucosal level and is dependent on the amount and type of iron presented. Up to 20% of haem iron is absorbed, whereas less than 10% of inorganic iron is taken up. Cows' and human milk both contain 1.5 mg iron per 1000 ml. Up to 50% of human milk iron will be absorbed, in contrast with less than 10% for cows' milk.

Iron deficiency is rare before 4 months of age because of iron stores at birth and conservation of iron from physiological post-natal haemolysis. Those particularly at risk are ex-premature babies and babies fed on a predominantly cows' milk diet after 6 months with delayed introduction of mixed feeds.

## AETIOLOGY

### *1 Perinatal*

Prematurity, multiple pregnancy, placental bleeding, early clamping of cord.

### *2 Nutritional*

Prolonged cows' milk diet or late weaning from breast. Low iron content of foods, e.g. unfortified cereals.

### *3 Blood loss*

Oesophagitis, cows' milk sensitivity, Meckel's diverticulum, hookworm infestation, oesophageal varices.

### *4 Malabsorption*

Coeliac disease.

## CLINICAL FEATURES

Marked anaemia may be tolerated with few symptoms. Decompensation may occur with an intercurrent illness. Symptoms include pallor, lethargy, irritability, easy fatigability, pica, decreased learning capacity and frequent infections. Signs include pallor, tachycardia and cardiac failure.

## INVESTIGATIONS

Blood film and red cell indices reveal a microcytic hypochromic anaemia with poikilocytosis and target cells. Platelets are often raised with blood loss.
MCV is low (normal 80–96 $\mu m^3$), MCH is <20 pg (see Section 9.13).
Ferritin: <20 ng/ml.
Low serum iron and high total iron-binding capacity. The iron-binding protein (transferrin) is <15% saturated (Table 9.1).

## MANAGEMENT

### *1 Prevention*

Oral iron intake should be 1 mg/kg/day (max. 15 mg) after 4 months of age. This can be achieved by a diet rich in fortified cereals, green vegetables, haem iron (meat) and vitamin C to aid absorption. Breast feeding is the preferred milk or alternatively fortified formulae should be used until at least 6 months of age.

### *2 Treatment*

**2.1 Diet** See 'Prevention' (above).

**2.2 Elemental iron** 6 mg/kg/day in divided doses. Continue for 3 months (prophylaxis 1–2 mg/kg/day).

One mg elemental iron is present in 3 mg ferrous sulphate and 9 mg ferrous gluconate. The latter is better tolerated. Absorption is best if given between meals and with ascorbic acid.

Parenteral iron – gives frequent systemic and rare anaphylactic side effects. Use only for malabsorption, non-compliance or intolerance to oral iron.

Dose – calculated to raise Hb to 13 mg% is:

$$\text{Blood volume (80 ml/kg)} \times \frac{(13 - \text{Hb})}{100} \times 3.4 = \text{Dose in mg}$$

**2.3 Response to treatment** Reticulocytosis within 2–3 days.

**2.4 Slow blood transfusion** Indicated if in severe heart failure. Use packed cells and diuretics, or exchange transfusion.

# 9.7 Abnormal bleeding

The child with abnormal bleeding, bruising or petechial spots requires:

(a) a good history;
(b) careful examination;
(c) some simple investigations.

The tendency to abnormal bleeding can be considered as:

(i) thrombocytopenia or abnormal platelet function;
(ii) abnormality of clotting factors;
(iii) vasculitis or abnormality of blood vessels.

## (a) History

### *1 Onset*

Bleeding or petechiae in the neonatal period suggest the following: isoimmune thrombocytopenia, intra-uterine or post-natal infection (petechiae), vitamin K deficiency (GI bleed on days 2–5), haemophilia (post-circumcision), factor XIII deficiency (umbilical stump bleed), factor XI deficiency (post-circumcision).

### *2 Family history*

Ask at length about easy bleeding or bruising in siblings, parents, their relatives and antecedents. Commonly found inheritance characteristics are: factor VIII and factor IX deficiencies, Wiskott–Aldrich syndrome – sex-linked recessive; von Willebrand's disease and hereditary haemorrhagic telangiectasia – autosomal dominant. New mutations or poor expression of a gene may account for the absence of a typical family history.

### *3 Past history*

Ask about bleeding following surgery, trivial trauma, dental extractions, circumcision.

### *4 Site of bleeding*

The following are common associations:

haemarthrosis – haemophilia A or B;
epistaxis – von Willebrand's disease, abnormal platelet function, hereditary haemorrhagic telangiectasia;

petechiae – immune thrombocytopenic purpura, Henoch–Schönlein purpura (HSP), meningococcaemia;
gum bleed – haematological malignancy, scurvy (also periosteal and retro-orbital bleeding).

### *5 Diet*
Vitamin C intake.

### *6 Drugs*
All recently taken drugs should be suspected of having caused either decreased platelet function (e.g. aspirin, a cyclo-oxygenase inhibitor) or thrombocytopenia. The latter may be immune mediated (e.g. quinidine, which acts as a hapten) or related to decreased bone marrow production (sulphurs, phenylbutazone).

### *7 Associated disease*
Viral illness (rubella, infectious mononucleosis), leukaemia, SLE, liver disease/portal hypertension, giant haemangiomata.

## (b) Examination

### *1 Pallor*
Anaemia indicates an illness other than a simple coagulation disorder unless major bleeding has occurred.

### *2 Skin*
Petechiae – suggest thrombocytopenia, platelet dysfunction or vascular abnormality, not coagulation disorders which tend to cause ecchymoses. Henoch–Schönlein purpura causes a maculopapular erythematous rash that later becomes haemorrhagic in the centre, distributed predominantly on buttocks and lower limbs. Eczema is seen in Wiskott–Aldrich syndrome. Increased platelet consumption is seen in Kasabach–Merritt syndrome with cavernous haemangiomata on the trunk, extremities or abdominal viscera.

Bruising is seen with non-accidental injury and coagulation disorders. The presence of hyperelastic skin and joints, keloid or 'cigarette paper scars' suggests Ehlers–Danlos syndrome. Blue sclera or abnormal dentition occur in osteogenesis imperfecta.

### *3 Site of bleeding*
Joints: haemarthrosis in haemophilia A or B, arthritis in HSP.
GI haemorrhage: vitamin K deficiency in the neonate, portal hypertension in the older child. Hereditary haemorrhagic telangiectasia may demonstrate telangiectasis on nose, conjunctivae, ears, nasal mucosa, lips and tongue in older children.

### *4 Splenomegaly*

In isolation it suggests hypersplenism, but with hepatomegaly and lymphadenopathy, leukaemia and infectious mononucleosis must be excluded.

## (c) Screening investigations

### *1 Full blood count and film*

Isolated thrombocytopenia suggests idiopathic thrombocytopenic purpura (ITP) in an otherwise well child (see Subsection 9.8.1).

Thrombocytopenia with anaemia ± leucopenia or blasts = bone marrow aplasia or infiltration (leukaemia).

Petechiae with normal platelet count – vasculitis (HSP, meningococcaemia) or platelet dysfunction (see Subsection 9.8.2).

### *2 Prothrombin time* (PT) (see Figure 9.2)

Measures the integrity of the extrinsic and common pathways (factors II, V, VII, X).

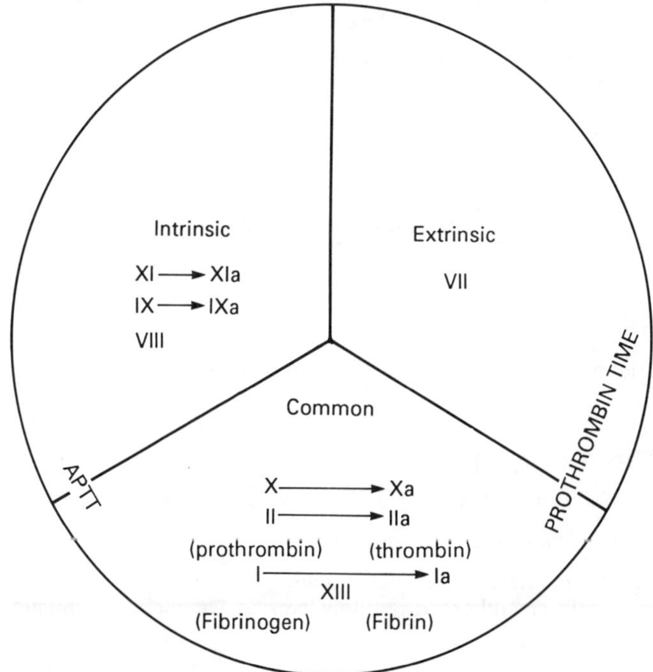


**Figure 9.2** Simplified coagulation cascade. Activated partial thromboplastin time (APTT) measures the integrity of intrinsic and common pathways; prothrombin time (PT) measures that of the extrinsic and common pathways

*3 Activated partial thromboplastin time* (APTT) (see Figure 9.2)
Measures the integrity of the intrinsic and common pathways.
Prolonged APTT (with normal PT) – deficiency of factors VIII or IX, or rarely factors XII or XI.
Prolongation of PT and APTT – disseminated intravascular coagulation.

*4 Bleeding time*
Prolongation occurs in thrombocytopenia or platelet dysfunction (von Willebrand's disease, uraemia, aspirin, etc.). The Ivy method uses a sphygmomanometer inflated to 40 mmHg and a no. 11 blade, with a piece of paper tape folded across the blade 3 mm from the tip, so that the depth of the puncture can be controlled. Three forearm punctures are each blotted with filter paper at 15 s intervals. The upper limit of normal for this method is 8 min. The template bleeding time is a modification of the Ivy method that has improved the sensitivity and reliability of the test. Reproducibility of the bleeding time depends on many variables including the experience of the person performing the test. It is too specialized for the inexperienced (Mielke, C. H. *et al.* (1969) *Blood,* **34**, 204). Ear lobe prick bleeding time (Duke method) is less sensitive than the Ivy method.

Armed with these tests it should be possible to slot the child into one of:

1. Thrombocytopenia or abnormal platelet function.
2. Abnormality of clotting factors.
3. Vasculitis or abnormality of blood vessels.

# 9.8 Platelet disorders

This group of bleeding disorders can be subdivided into conditions with low platelet numbers (thrombocytopenia) or diminished platelet function (rare).

## 9.8.1 Thrombocytopenia

### CAUSES OF THROMBOCYTOPENIA IN CHILDREN

*1 Disorders of increased destruction*

**1.1 Immune mediated** ITP, autoimmune disease, infectious mononucleosis, rubella and other viruses, drug induced, lymphoma, isoimmune (neonates).

**1.2 Non-immune** Consumptive coagulopathy – DIC, haemolytic uraemic syndrome.
Vascular – giant haemangioma, cyanotic heart disease.

### *2 Disorders of decreased production*

**2.1 Inherited** Wiskott–Aldrich syndrome, May–Hegglin anomaly, trisomy syndrome, Fanconi's anaemia, isovaleric acidaemia, Bernard–Soulier syndrome, thrombocytopenia absent radii (TAR) syndrome, megakaryocyte aplasia.

**2.2 Acquired**
Aplastic anaemia – idiopathic, drug induced, toxins, radiation, hepatitis.
Marrow replacement – leukaemia, neuroblastoma.
Megaloblastic anaemia – $B_{12}$/folate deficiency.

### *3 Disorders of platelet distribution*

Hypersplenism – portal hypertension, thalassaemia, malaria, storage disease.

## 9.8.2 Immune (idiopathic) thrombocytopenic purpura (ITP)

- *A well child with isolated thrombocytopenia is likely to have ITP.*
- *An unwell child is likely to have leukaemia.*

ITP is not a rare problem for the paediatrician, with an incidence of 4–10 cases per 100000 children per year. Both the acute and chronic forms have an immunological basis, with the chronic variety probably being an autoimmune disease. The lifespan of platelets (normally about 9 days) may be reduced to hours as they are coated with antibody, sequestrated in and destroyed by the spleen. Overall mortality is 0.3% of cases. Peak age incidence is 2–6 years. The major laboratory feature is thrombocytopenia in the presence of a bone marrow with normal or increased megakaryocyte production.

### CLINICAL FEATURES

Typically, a previously healthy child develops bruising, petechiae and perhaps epistaxis, 1–3 weeks following a viral infection. Physical examination shows petechiae and ecchymoses but no pallor, hepato splenomegaly, or lymphadenopathy.

### INVESTIGATION AND DIFFERENTIAL DIAGNOSIS

### *1 Full blood count*

Shows thrombocytopenia, normal haemoglobin, WCC and film. There are no pathognomonic features of ITP and the diagnosis rests on excluding the causes of secondary thrombocytopenia.

### *2 Bone marrow aspiration (BMA) examination*

Usually done to document adequacy of megakaryocytes, and exclude aplasia and bone marrow infiltration, especially leukaemia. If a child is well with no abnormal physical features, it is permissible to withhold BMA and watch serial blood counts for recovery of platelet count. BMA is always indicated in thrombocytopenia if the child is unwell or if therapeutic intervention is to be commenced.

### *3 Drugs*

All should be regarded as aetiological suspects and ceased.

### *4 Paired viral antibody sera and EBV serology*

May reveal infectious mononucleosis or unsuspected rubella.

### *5 Short stature or congenital anomalies*

Suggest an inherited thrombocytopenia.

### *6 Eczema and/or a history of repeated infection in boys*

Possible Wiskott–Aldrich syndrome.

### *7 A toxic unwell child*

? Leukaemia, haemolytic uraemic syndrome, DIC. Check blood film, renal function and clotting profile.

### *8 Chronic ITP*

May be confused with the rare conditions of hereditary thrombocytopenia and pure megakaryocyte aplasia which can be excluded by a family history and bone marrow examination.

## NATURAL HISTORY

### *1 Acute ITP*

Self-limiting (by definition) within 6 months (by convention). Eighty-five per cent of children with ITP are in this group of whom 90% will have resolved by 3 months. The group typically consists of younger children of equal sex ratio who often have preceding infection and a short history of petechiae (days).

### *2 Chronic ITP*

Ten per cent of children with ITP will be thrombocytopenic for >6 months. They tend to be older children, female and have a long history (weeks) of petechiae usually without preceding infection. Platelet count is usually between 30 000 and 120 000/mm$^3$. Chronicity by no means precludes spontaneous remission.

### *3 Recurrent ITP*

About 5% of children with ITP have intermittent disease.

## MORBIDITY

Spectacular nose-bleeds can occasionally occur. Petechiae are painless. Soft-tissue and intra-articular bleeds do not occur. Menorrhagia can be a problem in adolescents.

## MORTALITY

Intracranial haemorrhage is the only potentially fatal complication.

## MANAGEMENT

### *1 Acute ITP*

**1.1 Hospitalization** Admit all new cases. Intracranial haemorrhage, although rare, usually occurs in the first few days, but it has been known up to a year after diagnosis. Keeping the child in hospital longer than 2–3 days is hard to defend.

**1.2 Minimize risks** Avoid aspirin-like drugs and vigorous contact sports. Excessive physical restrictions on a child, however, are unreasonable and impractical.

**1.3 Intracranial haemorrhage** Urgent neurosurgical treatment along with:

(a) IV gamma globulin 400 mg/kg;
(b) IV methylprednisolone 15–30 mg/kg;
(c) platelet transfusion;
(d) consider emergency splenectomy.

**1.4 Steroids** There is insufficient evidence to recommend their routine use. Although steroids probably accelerate the recovery of the platelet count, stabilize capillaries and do no harm, they have no proven effect on preventing intracranial haemorrhage. If used, recommended dose of prednisolone is 1–2 mg/kg/day for 10–28 days. Alternatively, high-dose IV methylprednisolone has been advocated at 30 mg/kg/day over 30 min for 3 days (*J. Pediatr.* (1988) **113**, 563–566).

**1.5 IV gamma globulin (IVGG)** Causes a prompt rise in platelet count, although its influence on morbidity is unknown. A death has occurred during therapy, it is expensive (£15–20/g) and adverse reactions and viral contamination are known. The beneficial effects are transient and there is no evidence that it 'cures' the disease. Dose: 400 mg/kg/day for 5 days. It is unjustified to spend several hundred pounds on treating a common mild self-limiting illness. It should only be used for an acute haemostatic emergency.

### *2 Chronic ITP*

The risks associated with *not* actively treating this group are negligible. Fatalities are rare. The major morbidity encountered includes bruising, epistaxis, menorrhagia and operative bleeding. All treatments should be assessed with the essentially benign nature of the illness in mind. Optimum treatment is only to minimize risks (see 'Acute ITP' – above).

**2.1 Minimize risks** See above. This is the mainstay of treatment.

**2.2 Steroids** High-dose long-term therapy is contraindicated. It may be used on a short-term basis for bleeding (e.g. complicating a viral infection), trauma or surgical procedures. Dose – prednisolone 2 mg/kg/day for 3 days or methylprednisolone 15 mg/kg/day for 3 days (*Arch. Dis. Child.* (1984) **59**, 777–779). These courses may also induce short-term remissions.

**2.3 IVGG** There is no evidence that IVGG 'cures' chronic ITP. About 75% will show a rapid but transient response. It is thought to work through transient reticulo-endothelial blockade due to a decrease in Fc receptor affinity for platelet-associated IgG, and competition for Fc receptors by the increased serum IgG. Most children with chronic ITP require no treatment. It can be of use in the young child with annoying, recurrent, cutaneous or mucosal bleeding in whom splenectomy and long-term steroids are inappropriate. Other indications for use are as described above for steroids. Dose: 400 mg/kg/day × 5 days.

**2.4 Splenectomy** Results in an elevated platelet count. Should be reserved for life-threatening disease because the risk of overwhelming sepsis (and fatal malaria in future travels) makes it a procedure with a mortality far in excess of the condition it is supposed to treat.

**2.5 Other treatments** The following have had mixed success: azothiaprine, cyclophosphamide, vinca alkaloids, plasmaphaeresis, plasma infusion, danazol, exchange transfusion, cyclosporin, anti-Rh(D) immunoglobulin.

## Further reading

**Buchanan**, G. R. (1987) The non treatment of childhood idiopathic thrombocytopenic purpura. *Eur. J. Pediatr.*, **146**, 107–112

Chessels, J. (1989) Chronic idiopathic thrombocytopenic purpura: primum non nocere. *Arch. Dis. Child.*, **64**, 1326–1328

Lilleyman, J. S. (1986) Changing perspectives in idiopathic thrombocytopenia purpura. In *Recent Advances in Paediatrics* (ed. Meadow, R.), Churchill Livingstone, Edinburgh, pp. 239–258

### *Secondary thrombocytopenia*

Many disorders other than ITP can cause thrombocytopenia – see 'Causes of thrombocytopenia in children' – above. In particular, one should always consider leukaemia or other neoplastic bone marrow infiltration, acquired bone aplasia, especially drug-induced aplasia, DIC, hypersplenism (portal hypertension, thalassaemia, malaria) and auto-immune disorders.

### 9.8.3 Disorders of platelet function

These disorders are suspected on the grounds of a prolonged bleeding time with normal platelet numbers, PT and APTT. Aspirin can interfere with platelet function for 7 days. Von Willebrand's disease is often unsuspected (N.B. APTT may also be prolonged). All other disorders in this group are rare. They include Glanzmann's disease and platelet storage pool disorders.

## 9.9 Coagulation disorders

Haemostasis is initiated by vascular constriction and platelet adhesion and aggregation; however, for permanent haemostasis in large vessels, the addition of fibrin to the 'haemostatic plug' is essential. Fibrin formation is the end product of a 'coagulation cascade' of what are mostly pre-enzyme–enzyme transformations, except for factors VIII and V which are cofactors for the enzyme generated in the preceding stage (factors IXa and Xa, respectively). The cascade has intrinsic, extrinsic and common pathways. All must be functioning well for normal haemostasis.

#### COAGULATION PATHWAY

See Figure 9.2.

#### INHIBITORS OF COAGULATION

Protein C – inactivates factors VIII and V and may inactivate plasminogen.
Protein S – regulates protein C.
Antithrombin III – regulates thrombin.

## FIBRINOLYSIS

The physiological removal of fibrin (fibrinolysis) occurs when it binds to tissue plasminogen activator (TPA) and plasminogen, resulting in the formation of plasmin and various fibrin degradation products (FDP) – see Figure 9.3.

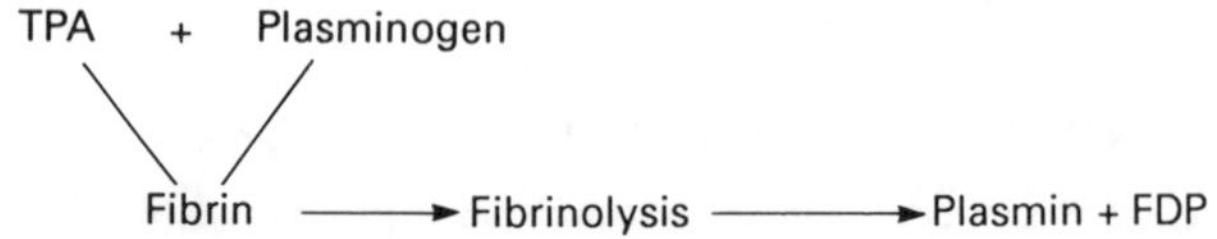


**Figure 9.3** Simplified fibrinolytic pathway (TPA, tissue plasminogen activator; FDP, fibrin degradation products)

Fibrinolytic activity is assessed by:

1. Estimation of plasma activator activity or euglobulin lysis.
2. Fibrin degradation products.

## CLOTTING FACTOR DEFICIENCIES

### *1 Inherited*

Factor VIII – haemophilia A, von Willebrand's syndrome (also platelet function abnormality).
Factor IX – haemophilia B (Christmas disease).
Others – factors XI, XIII.

### *2 Acquired*

Vitamin K deficiency – liver disease, dysbiotic gut flora, malabsorption.
Consumption coagulopathy (DIC).

# 9.10 Haemophilia A (factor VIII deficiency)

Both haemophilia A and haemophilia B are inherited in an X-linked recessive fashion and they are clinically similar, although B tends to be a milder disorder. Only haemophilia A will be discussed in detail. Tragically, in the decade preceding 1986 many haemophiliacs were exposed to the human immunodeficiency virus (HIV). Each year more of these individuals develop HIV-related disease.

## INCIDENCE

4–10 per 10 000 live births.

## CLINICAL FEATURES

Degree of factor VIII (F VIII) deficiency roughly correlates with severity of clinical manifestation (Table 9.3).

**Table 9.3 Factor VIII level correlated with clinical severity**

| *Blood level of F VIII* (% of normal) | *Clinical picture* |
|---|---|
| 50–100 | Nil |
| 25–50 | Excessive bleeding after major trauma |
| 5–25 | Severe bleeding after minor trauma or surgery |
| 1–5 | Occ. haemarthroses, and spontaneous bleeding |
| <1 | Frequent haemarthroses, deep tissue bleeds, intracranial haemorrhage |

## TYPICAL FEATURES

Neonatal period – post-circumcision bleeding.
Infancy – bleeding into muscles and soft tissues.
Toddlers – haemarthroses and bleed into soft tissues.

## MAJOR MORBIDITY

AIDS
Intracranial bleeding – the cause of death in 7% of haemophiliacs.
Arthropathy – acute painful haemarthroses, chronic synovial hypertrophy and destruction of articular surfaces.
Forearm bleed – Volkmann's ischaemic contracture.
Retroperitoneal bleed – paralytic ileus, compression of femoral nerve under inguinal ligament.

## PREVENTION

Avoid contact sports.
Avoid IM injections and aspirin-like drugs.
Regular dental care to minimize need for extractions.

## INVESTIGATION

APTT – prolonged when F VIII levels are <40% of normal.
PT, platelet count, bleeding time – normal.
Assay for F VIII antibodies.
HIV antibodies in those who received F VIII before heat-treated F VIII became available.

## MANAGEMENT OF ACUTE BLEEDING EPISODE

### *1 Factor VIII*

**1.1 Dose** If a child has low levels of intrinsic F VIII (<5%), then treat as follows:

| | |
|---|---|
| Haemarthrosis/soft tissue bleed: | 20 u/kg |
| Major bleeds (psoas haematoma): | 30 u/kg |
| Head injury: | 50 u/kg |

*or*

$$\text{Units of F VIII required} = \frac{\text{Weight (kg)} \times \text{Desired \% rise in factor VIII}}{1.5}$$

1 u of F VIII is the amount found in 1 ml of normal plasma.
1 u F VIII/kg gives an increase in total body F VIII of 2% of normal.

**1.2 Preparations of factor VIII** Lyophilized F VIII is prepared from pooled plasma. It carries a relatively high risk of hepatitis.
Cryoprecipitate is a plasma fraction obtained by slow thawing of frozen plasma and dissolving it in 10–20 ml of plasma supernatant. It contains about 20 times the normal plasma F VIII concentration.
Fresh frozen plasma has about 1 u F VIII/ml. Its use is limited by volume considerations. Give 15–20 ml/kg, then 10 ml/kg/12 h. F VIII levels will only rise to 10–20% of normal.

### *2 Desmopressin (DDAVP)*

It is a synthetic agent free of side effects such as AIDS and hepatitis, acting to increase F VIII release from the vascular lining. It is the treatment of choice in mild–moderate haemophilia (intrinsic F VIII level of 8–20%), low-level carriers and von Willebrand's disease, i.e. wherever it is judged that a three-fold increase in F VIII will be sufficient to stop the bleeding.
Dose: 0.03 μg/kg IV over 1 h/12–24 h IV. By day 2 or 3 there is usually a suboptimal response (tachyphylaxis). Some give it intranasally, but the response is less predictable.

### *3 Restore normal function/prevent deformity*

Immobilize limb for 24–48 h for pain control. Then use graded exercise and mobilization with aid of physiotherapy.

### *4 Analgesia*

Prompt and liberal F VIII administration and immobilization.
Simple (non-aspirin) analgesia – paracetamol.
Rectal proladone may be needed – least addictive opiate. Other opiates are contraindicated.

### *5 Inhibition of fibrinolysis*

Useful in persistent mouth, nose and surgical bleeding and dental extraction. Contraindicated in renal tract bleeding.
Prophylaxis: oral tranexamic acid (Cyclokapron) 20–30 mg/kg/8 h, for 7–10 days (decrease dose in renal impairment).
Treatment: 15 mg/kg/12 h by slow IV until bleeding stops, then manage as for prophylaxis.

### *6 Facilitate normal emotional/social development*

Home treatment programmes encourage self-reliance and independence from the hospital.

## SPECIAL CIRCUMSTANCES

### *1 Suspected intracranial haemorrhage*

*Do not* do a lumbar puncture.
*Do* give F VIII 50 u/kg push dose.
*Do* a CT scan.

### *2 Elective surgery*

Preoperative test for F VIII antibodies and half-life (normal 8–12 h). Replacement therapy:

100% replacement (i.e. 50 u/kg/day) for 3 days;
50% replacement for 3 days;
25% replacement for 7 days.

For bone and joint surgery – as above, plus antifibrinolytic agents.
Intracranial surgery – 100% normal for 21 days.
Dental extraction – antifibrinolytic therapy for 1 day preoperatively and 10 days postoperatively. Give intraoperative F VIII to 50% normal once.

### *3 Haemophilia with F VIII antibodies*

Incidence: seen in about 10% of haemophiliacs under the age of 20 years.

Low antibody levels: use standard treatments more frequently or prothrombin complex concentrates – same dose as for F VIII.

High antibody levels: prothrombin complex concentrates. Alternatives are heterologous F VIII, plasmaphaeresis, immunosuppressants, regular twice weekly F VIII (anamnestic response), factor VIII inhibitor bypassing activity (FIBA).

#### *4 Mouth/gum bleed*

Use standard dose of F VIII and antifibrinolytic therapy (as above). Some also recommend penicillin orally.

### *Von Willebrand's disease*

DDAVP (see above) is the treatment of choice, often given with antifibrinolytic agents. Uncommonly, one also gives cryoprecipitate. *T*½ of von Willebrand's factor is 4 h. Factor VIII levels increase for 48–72 h after the infusion.

### *Christmas disease (factor IX deficiency)*

Treated with fresh frozen plasma or prothrombin concentrate (Prothrombinex: factors II, IX, X).

$$\text{Units of F IX required} = \frac{\text{Weight (kg)} \times \text{Desired \% rise in factor IX}}{1.2}$$

### Further reading

Nathan, D. G. and Oski, F. A. (1987) *Hematology of Infancy and Childhood,* W. B. Saunders, Philadelphia

## 9.11 Vascular defects

1. Anaphylactoid purpura.
2. Infection – meningococcaemia.
3. Deficiencies – vitamin C.
4. Miscellaneous.

### 9.11.1 Anaphylactoid purpura (Henoch–Schönlein purpura – HSP)

This is an illness of uncertain aetiology, which results from vasculitis of small blood vessels. It mainly affects children aged 2–8 years. There are no diagnostic tests; the diagnosis is a clinical one.

#### CLINICAL PICTURE

May follow upper respiratory tract infection (URTI) or streptococcal pharyngitis.

### *1 Rash (in 100% of cases)*

Usually on lower extremities and buttocks. Initially it is an erythematous maculopapular eruption, eventually becoming petechial. Rarely one sees erythema multiforme or nodosum or angioneurotic oedema.

### *2 Arthritis (66% of cases)*

A serous effusion with leucocytosis, involving large joints especially knees and ankles.

### *3 Gastrointestinal involvement (66% of cases)*

Colicky severe abdominal pain, occasionally accompanied by haematemesis or rectal bleeding. Unnecessary laparotomy may be performed if one does not inspect the legs for a rash. Rarely, HSP causes intussusception or perforation.

### *4 Renal (25%)*

Usually focal mesangial proliferative glomerulonephritis with microhaematuria and proteinuria. Two per cent of children get severe nephritis, some of whom may go on to develop chronic renal failure.

### *5 CNS*

Hypertensive encephalopathy is renal in origin. Seizures, pareses and coma are due to CNS vasculitis.

### *6 Rarely*

Rheumatoid-like nodules, cardiac involvement, testicular swelling and pain.

## INVESTIGATIONS

Platelet count – to exclude thrombocytopenia.
Urine – microscopy, protein.
Urea and electrolytes.
If the diagnosis is seriously in doubt, the following tests may rarely (if ever) be performed. Biopsy of newly affected skin will usually show perivascular deposition of IgA. Serum IgA may be elevated, $C_3$ is normal.

## DIFFERENTIAL DIAGNOSIS

### *1 Rash*

Haemorrhagic diathesis is excluded by normal platelet count and clotting profile. Septicaemic children are much sicker, but if in doubt take blood cultures anyway.

### *2 GIT*

Appendicitis, intussusception.

*3 Other vasculitis*
Polyarteritis nodosa, SLE (usually have high ESR).

*4 Renal*
SLE, acute post-streptococcal nephritis give rash and nephritis.

### TREATMENT

*1 Steroids*
May help GIT and CNS manifestations, but they are of no use in renal disease.

*2 Analgesia*

*3 Long-term follow-up*
For all those with ongoing haematuria, proteinuria or urinary sediment.

### PROGNOSIS

Very good outlook if there is no associated renal disease. Illness lasts up to 6 weeks. Twenty-five per cent have renal involvement; 25 per cent of those may have persistent urinary sediment for years. These should have long-term follow-up of their urinalysis, blood pressure and renal function.

### *Meningococcaemia*

This is a vasculitis with septicaemia and endotoxaemia (see Section 10.1).

## 9.11.2 Miscellaneous abnormalities of blood vessels

Vascular wall or supporting tissue defects causing bleeding are recognized in:

Vitamin C deficiency.
Hereditary haemorrhagic telangiectasia.
Polyarteritis nodosa.
Uraemia.
Ehlers–Danlos syndrome.
Cushing's syndrome.
Cutis laxa.

## 9.11.3 Vitamin C (ascorbic acid) deficiency/scurvy

Vitamin C is essential for the normal formation of collagen, including that of bone, cartilage, teeth and the intercellular substance of capillaries. Scurvy causes spontaneous haemorrhages and defective ossification.

## AETIOLOGY

Breast milk has adequate amounts of vitamin C unless the mother has subclinical avitaminosis C. Most proprietary infant milk formulae have adequate vitamin C content. Cows' milk and all boiled, dried or evaporated milks are deficient in vitamin C.

## CLINICAL FEATURES

It most commonly presents in children aged 6–24 months. After a period of vague symptoms such as irritability and loss of appetite, bruising, petechiae, subperiosteal and gingival bleeding may appear as may retro-orbital bleeding with proptosis, periorbital ecchymosis (black eye). An affected child is usually pale, miserable, lies immobile with legs in a 'frog position', and resents handling because of painful subperiosteal bleeding.

## INVESTIGATION

X-ray of the wrist – dense lines (of Fraenkel) at the metaphysis of radius and ulna, and 'eggshell'-like epiphyses.

## DIFFERENTIAL DIAGNOSIS

Pseudoparesis of scurvy may be confused with polio or other neuropathy and pyogenic bone or joint disease. The other features of scurvy rapidly clarify the diagnosis. A peripheral blood examination will exclude leukaemia.

## TREATMENT

Vitamin C: 100–200 mg/day orally.

## PREVENTION

Breast-fed babies whose mothers have a diet that includes 100 mg/day of ascorbic acid need no supplements. Formula-fed babies need 35 mg/day. Children or adults need 50 mg/day.

# Further reading

Nathan, D. G and Oski, F. A. (1987) *Haematology of Infancy and Childhood*, W. B. Saunders, Philadelphia

# 9.12 Transfusion of blood and platelets

Volume of blood required (ml) =

1. For packed cells: desired rise in Hb (g/100 ml) × Wt (kg) × 3.
2. For whole blood: above result × 2.
3. Alternative method (N.B. Circulating blood volume = 80 ml/kg).

Volume of packed cells needed to raise haematocrit (Hct) =

$$\frac{\text{Circulating blood vol.} \times (\text{Desired Hct} - \text{Present Hct})}{\text{Hct of packed RBCs}}$$

Most packed RBCs have Hct of 60–70%.

## PLATELET TRANSFUSION

4–6 u/m$^2$ (or 0.2 u/kg) should raise platelet count by 50 000–75 000/mm$^3$. In practice, number of units administered is often regulated by availability as determined by the blood bank.
Infuse over 30 min.

# 9.13 Normal haematological data

## RED BLOOD CELLS

Mean ± 2 SD (95% range).

| *Age* | *Hb* (g/100 ml) | *Reticulo-cytes* (%) | *MCV* (μm$^3$) | *MCH* (pg) | *MCHC* (g%) |
|---|---|---|---|---|---|
| Birth | 16.5 ± 3.0 | 3.2 | 106 (mean) | 36 (mean) | 32 |
| 2 wk | 15.0 ± 3.0 | 0.3–1.5 | 102 (mean) | 32 (mean) | 32 |
| 3 mo | 11.0 ± 1.5 | 0.5–1.5 | 95 (mean) | 29 ± 5 | 33 ± 2 |
| 1 yr | 12.0 ± 1.0 | 0.5–1.5 | 78 ± 8 | 27 ± 4 | 33 ± 2 |
| 3–13 yr | 13.0 ± 1.5 | 0.5–1.5 | 80 ± 9 | 29 ± 3 | 33 ± 2 |

## PACKED CELL VOLUME/HAEMATOCRIT

An approximate estimation of PCV(%) is Hb (mg/100 ml) × 3.

## PLATELETS

At any age: 150–450 × $10^9$/litre.

## HAEMATINICS

| | |
|---|---|
| Serum iron | 9–27 µmol/litre (0.5–1.5 mg/litre) |
| TIBC | 45–72 µmol/litre (2.5–4.0 mg/litre) |
| % Saturation | 16–33% |
| Ferritin | 10–300 µg/litre |
| Serum folate | >1.8 µg/litre (>4 nmol/litre) |
| Red cell folate | >120 µg/litre (270 nmol/litre) |
| Serum vitamin $B_{12}$ | 160–925 ng/litre |

## COAGULATION VALUES

Prothrombin time (Quick): 10–15 s.
Partial thromboplastin time (PTT): <1 mo 25–60 s; >1 mo 25–45 s.
Ivy bleeding time: 2–8 min (varies greatly with method used).
Fibrinogen: 1.5–4.0 g/litre. It is an acute phase reactant.
Fibrin degradation products: <10 µg/ml.

## HAEMOGLOBIN ELECTROPHORESIS

Foetal haemoglobin:

at birth – 60–95%
at 3 mo – 15–30%
at 6 mo – 2–4%
at 9 mo – <2%

Haemoglobin $A_2$:
after 4 months of age: 1.0–4.0%.

Chapter 10

# Infection and antibiotics

## 10.1 Meningococcaemia

Meningococcal septicaemia ranges clinically from a fulminating lethal illness to low-grade infection. Early recognition and treatment is vital. A DHSS circular (3 February 1988) recommends giving parenteral penicillin to patients with suspected meningococcaemia before transferring them to hospital. Cases may occur sporadically or in epidemics.

### PATHOLOGY

The organism resides in the nasopharynx from where it may invade the body, causing septicaemia, endotoxaemia and vasculitis, with subsequent disseminated intravascular coagulation (DIC). Haemorrhage and necrosis may occur in any organ system. There is bleeding and plasma leak into the skin and subcutaneous tissues. Adrenal haemorrhage is seen, causing shock (Waterhouse–Freidrichsen syndrome). Rash is due to a local Schwartzmann reaction, circulating immune complexes, or DIC. There are several different antigen groups, group B being responsible for most infections in the UK and Europe. Group C is less common and groups A, Y and W135 together comprise <10%.

### CLINICAL

#### *1 Fulminating septicaemia*

Very sudden onset. Aggressive behaviour, rapidly deteriorating consciousness, fever, shock, cardiac and renal failure, DIC. The rash may initially be a pink macular one, which very rapidly becomes petechial, purpuric or occasionally ecchymotic (*Lancet* (1988) I, 1166–1167).

#### *2 Meningitis*

#### *3 Chronic meningococcaemia*

Rare in children. Fluctuating anorexia, weight loss, rigors, arthralgia, arthritis are seen.

## DIAGNOSIS

### *1 Blood culture*

May take a week to grow. If prior antibiotics have been given, diagnosis may still be confirmed by countercurrent immunoelectrophoresis or latex agglutination of urine, serum or CSF (of doubtful value for group B).

### *2 LP*

Only if the child is clinically stable.

## TREATMENT

### *1 Antibiotics*

IV benzyl penicillin 60 mg (100 000 u)/kg/4 h. It is wise also to use chloramphenicol 40 mg/kg loading dose, then 25 mg/kg/6 h to be ceased once the diagnosis is confirmed, because *Haemophilus* septicaemia may occasionally give a similar picture. Continue treatment for 1 week. Penicillin and chloramphenicol resistance is recognized outside the UK (*Lancet* (1988) **i**, 54 and 702). Ceftazidime, cefotaxime (*Pediatr. Inf. Dis.* (1986) **5**, 402–407 and 408–415) and ceftriaxone (*Eur. J. Clin. Microbiol.* (1983) **2**, 509–515) have been used successfully.

### *2 Cardiorespiratory support*

In severe disease there is rapid clinical decline. Vascular leak is common but usually vastly underestimated, which is one of several reasons for severe shock. Some or all of the following may be needed:

Admission to intensive care.
Insert several large-bore IV cannulae including a central venous line.
Give 20 ml/kg/IV bolus of colloid. Repeat as necessary to restore circulating blood volume. Much more may be needed later.
Restrict maintenance fluids to 50–60 ml/kg/day and top up with 10–20 ml/kg aliquots of colloid as necessary to maintain BP, CVP and urine output.
Dopamine or dobutamine infusion 5–10 μg/kg/min.
Paralysis and ventilation are often needed.
Hydrocortisone 10 mg/kg bolus and 2.5 mg/kg/6 h is controversial, but should be given if in shock.
DIC is managed with fresh frozen plasma and platelets.
$Ca^{2+}$ – Significant inotropic support may be obtained from Ca gluconate 10% 0.5 ml/kg (max. 20 ml) slow IV push, plus infusion of 0.2–0.5 ml/kg/h. This is only the writer's personal observation, although there are published data that those who are severely ill often have low ionized calcium (*J. Pediatr.* (1989) **114**, 990–991 and associated articles).

### 3 Renal failure
Peritoneal dialysis or haemofiltration may be needed.

### 4 Close monitoring
Hb, renal function, $Na^+$, $K^+$, $Ca^{2+}$, $Mg^{2+}$, albumin, PT, APTT, platelets.

### 5 Prophylaxis
Rifampicin: adults 600 mg b.d.; children >1 month 10 mg/kg/12 h; children <1 month 5 mg/kg/12 h – for 2 days. 1 h before or 2 h after meals.

It should be offered to:

household contacts;
the patient;
day-care nursery contacts;
medical staff (when there has been mucous membrane contact);
close school contacts (not the whole class).

Other effective agents include ceftriaxone (*Lancet* (1988) **i**, 1240–1242) and ciprofloxacin 750 mg, single dose oral (*Pediatr. Inf. Dis. Newsletter* (1989) **15**, 1).

### 6 Notify
The regional medical officer for environmental health.

### 7 Unproven treatments
Plasmaphaeresis (worth trying – *Pediatr. Inf. Dis. J.* (1989) **8**, 399–400), leucopheresis, exchange transfusion (*N. Engl. J. Med.* (1979) **300**, 1277; *Br. Med. J.* (1984) 439–441).

### 8 Vaccination
Given to schools where there have been more than 1 case of non-group B meningococcus. Available for epidemics of groups A, C, W135, Y.
Field trials of a vaccine against group B are under way.

## PROGNOSIS

Bad prognostic factors include, absence of meningitis, widespread peripheral purpura, shock, absence of leucocytosis, fever >40°C, disseminated intravascular coagulation, and cardiac or renal failure.

## Further reading

Jones, D. M. (1989) Control of meningococcal disease. *Br. Med. J.*, **298**, 542–543
Raman, G. V. (1988) Meningococcal septicaemia and meningitis: a rising tide. *Br. Med. J.*, **296**, 1141–1142
Smith, H. (1986) Chemoprophylaxis of meningitis. *Arch. Dis. Child.*, **61**, 4–5

## 10.2 Some morbilliform (measles-like) eruptions

*1 Viral*
Measles.
Rubella.
Echovirus 16.
Roseola infantum.
Erythema infectiosum (fifth disease).
Infectious mononucleosis.
Pityriasis rosea.

*2 Others*
Drug eruptions – commonly amoxycillin, ampicillin, but any drug should be suspected.
Bacteria – streptococci, scarlet fever.
Reactive erythemas – erythema multiforme, papular urticaria.

## 10.3 Measles (rubeola)

A highly contagious disease caused by RNA paramyxovirus.

### SPREAD

Droplet.

### INCUBATION PERIOD

10–11 days.

### CLINICAL FEATURES (see Figure 10.1)

Day 1 – Fever, malaise.
Day 2 – Coryza, conjunctivitis, cough.
Days 2–3 – Koplik's spots – over the buccal and labial mucosa. Initially bright red with a central blue-white speck, later becoming like grains of salt on a red background. Often persist until days 2–3 of the rash.

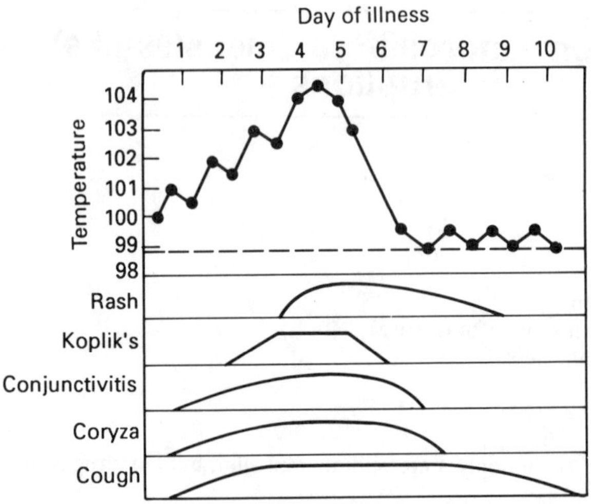


**Figure 10.1** Clinical course of typical measles (From Krugman, S. *et al.* (1985) *Infectious Diseases of Children,* CV Mosby, St. Louis, Missouri, with permission)

Day 4 – Rash – erythematous maculopapular. First appears behind the ears, then spreads downwards to involve trunk, arms and finally reaching the feet by day 7 when it starts to fade in order of appearance.
Other manifestations: lymphadenopathy, giant cell pneumonia.

## COMPLICATIONS

1. Otitis media ± mastoiditis.
2. Pneumonia – viral or secondary bacterial. Suspect it if child develops respiratory distress. Bacterial pathogens are streptococci, *Staphylococcus, Haemophilus influenzae.*
3. Croup.
4. Acute encephalitis – in 0.1% of cases. Usually within 1 week of the appearance of the rash. Usually CSF shows pleocytosis and mildly raised protein. 60% recover, 15% die, 25% show long-term CNS damage.
5. Subacute sclerosing panencephalitis (SSPE) – in 1 per 100 000 cases: Occurs months–years after measles.
   Clinical features: myoclonic jerks, dementia, death within 6 months.
   EEG: paroxysmal spikes at regular intervals, depressed activity between spikes.
   CSF – high CSF globulin, predominantly IgG. High measles antibody titre.
6. Pregnancy – the virus does not appear to be teratogenic.

## PREVENTION

Universal measles/mumps/rubella vaccination at 12–18 months. Measles immunization given within 3 days of contact may be protective in susceptible individuals.
Immunocompromised children exposed to measles should have gamma globulin (see Section 6.1).

## MANAGEMENT

Supportive – antibiotics should not be used routinely.
Conjunctivitis can usually be managed with simple eye toilet.
Paracetamol for fever.
Otitis media – amoxycillin or cotrimoxazole.
Pneumonia – see Section 7.14.
Encephalitis – good neurointensive care. Prevent overhydration and control seizures (see Section 8.2).

## INFECTIVITY

It can be spread from 2 days before until the fifth day after the appearance of the rash, after which the child can go back to school.

# 10.4 Rubella – acquired post-natally

The typical features are a mild or absent prodrome, a 3-day rash and lymph node (post-auricular) enlargement. The prognosis is excellent. It is a potent teratogen in the first trimester of pregnancy. Universal MMR vaccination aims at eradicating it from our community.

## INCUBATION PERIOD

14–21 days.

## CLINICAL FEATURES (see Figure 10.2)

Day 1 – malaise, mild coryza and conjunctivitis are the first complaints.
Day 4 – rash consists of discrete, pink/red macules which occasionally coalesce on the trunk but not on limbs, and fade after 3 days.
Lymphadenopathy – from day 1 onwards. Usually generalized, but suboccipital, post-auricular and cervical nodes are most prominent, ± splenomegaly.

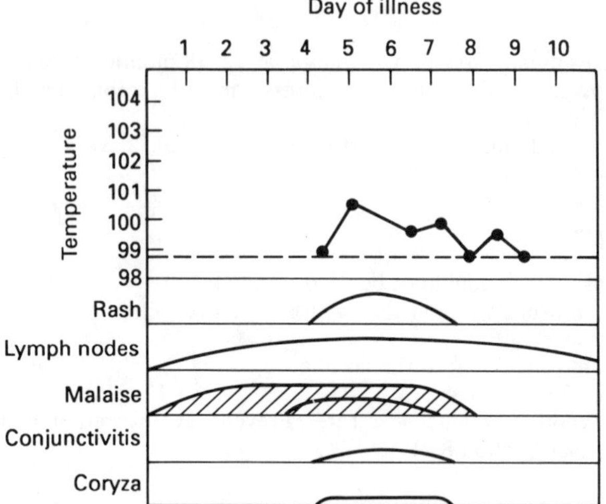


**Figure 10.2** Clinical course of typical rubella (From Krugman, S. *et al.* (1985) *Infectious Diseases of Children,* CV Mosby, St. Louis, Missouri, with permission)

## COMPLICATIONS–UNCOMMON

1. Arthritis – large or small joints, usually in older children or adults. Occurs as the rash is fading.
2. Encephalitis – rare.
3. Purpura – thrombocytopenic or non-thrombocytopenic.

## PREVENTION

MMR vaccine at 12–18 months is to be strongly encouraged. It may be given later at any age in those not immunized.

## TREATMENT

Symptomatic.

## INFECTIVITY

It can be spread from the later part of the incubation period to the end of the 3rd day of the rash (neonates with congenital rubella may excrete the virus for much longer).

## EXPOSURE TO RUBELLA IN PREGNANCY

Rubella vaccination in pregnancy is contraindicated but is nevertheless probably harmless (see Section 6.1).

MMR immunization prior to child-bearing age should be the rule. For a mother in 1st trimester of pregnancy who is exposed to suspected rubella:

1. Test maternal serum for rubella antibodies (result within 24 h). If antibody is present, there is no risk of infection.
2. If antibody is not detected, give 20 ml IM gamma globulin.
3. 4 weeks later – repeat antibody titre or specific IgM. A 4-fold increase in antibody titre indicates infection and termination of pregnancy must be considered.

N.B. Infants born with rubella embryopathy should be isolated because they shed virus for weeks–months.

# 10.5 Varicella – chickenpox

The varicella–herpes zoster virus causes both chickenpox and shingles. Only chickenpox will be discussed.

## INCUBATION PERIOD

10–21 days (usually 15).

## CLINICAL FEATURES (see Figure 10.3)

The disease begins with fever and malaise. The rash starts off as pruritic small macules, but within 6–8 h they become papules and then vesicles

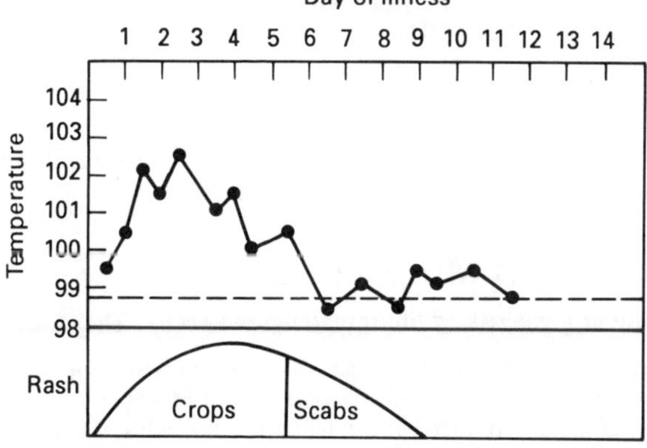


**Figure 10.3** Clinical course of typical chickenpox (From Krugman, S. *et al.* (1985) *Infectious Diseases of Children,* CV Mosby, St. Louis, Missouri, with permission)

surrounded by an erythematous area. Crusting begins almost immediately. Lesions appear in crops involving most of the body. Mucous membranes may also be involved. Lesions are seen in all stages of metamorphosis. The rash resolves completely over 3 weeks.

## COMPLICATIONS

1. Impetigo.
2. Encephalitis – 1:1000 cases. It may occur as an isolated cerebellar ataxia, usually as the rash is resolving, in which case the prognosis is excellent without any treatment. Cerebral encephalitis has a more guarded prognosis, but may respond to acyclovir.
3. Pneumonia – occurs 1–5 days after onset of rash. Gives typical nodular CXR appearance. Common in immunocompromised children.

## PREVENTION

None is recommended for the normal child who has been exposed. For the leukaemic child within 1 year (some say 6 months) of completing treatment, or any other immunocompromised child, zoster immune globulin or acyclovir is recommended (see Section 6.1).

## MANAGEMENT

Most children will only require symptomatic treatment with topical antipruritic lotion (Calamine, Caladryl). Caladryl (1% diphenhydramine) should not be given with oral diphenhydramine (Benadryl) because of the risk of toxic encephalopathy (Schunk, D. and Svendsen, D. (1988) *Am. J. Dis. Child.*, **142,** 1020–1021).

Paracetamol is commonly given, although there is some evidence that it does not alleviate symptoms and may prolong the illness (Doran, T. F. *et al.* (1989) *J. Pediatr.*, **114**, 1045–1048).

## TERATOGENICITY

A congenital varicella syndrome has been described, but it is rare. It has occurred with maternal infection as late as 28 weeks' gestation.

## NEONATES IN CONTACT WITH VARICELLA

Some neonates are at great risk of life threatening varicella. They are:

1. Neonates born 6 days or less after onset of maternal chickenpox or whose mothers develop it from delivery to 1 month of age.
2. Neonates who come in contact with chickenpox but whose mothers have no history of previous varicella (i.e. no passive immunity) – see Section 6.1.

# 10.6 Mumps

Caused by RNA myxovirus. Transmission is by droplet spread or direct contact with virus-carrying droplets, or fomites. It is easily the most common cause of parotitis in children. Immunity is lifelong.

## INCUBATION PERIOD

16–18 days.

## CLINICAL FEATURES

Thirty-five per cent have subclinical infection. The remainder mostly have unilateral (25%) or bilateral parotitis, often with sublingual and submandibular involvement. Typically, a child complains of ear-ache, and the following day the parotid begins to swell. This will usually 'obliterate' the concavity which lies just posterior to the mandible and inferior to the ear lobe (antero-inferior to the mastoid) and will persist for 6–10 days.

## COMPLICATIONS

1. Meningoencephalitis – including sensorineural deafness.
2. Pancreatitis.
3. Orchitis – sterility is exceedingly rare in children with mumps.

## INVESTIGATIONS

In practice, no tests are needed. The virus may be isolated from saliva, urine and CSF (if indicated). Mumps serology may be of use. Raised pancreatic amylase is an unreliable test.

## MANAGEMENT

Symptomatic.

## INFECTIVITY

From several days before parotitis until subsidence of the swelling (average 7–10 days).

## DIFFERENTIAL DIAGNOSIS OF PAROTID SWELLING

Infections such as *Staphylococcus aureus* and viruses (para-influenza, Coxsackie), drugs, metabolic (diabetes), parotid tumour, obstruction of Stensen's duct.

# 10.7 Roseola infantum (exanthem subitum)

This is a common benign infectious disease of infancy. The aetiology is probably human herpesvirus 6 (HHV-6; see *Lancet* (1988) **i**, 1065). The typical clinical course is described in Figure 10.4. The rash appears as the fever recedes. The lesions are discrete rose-pink macules or maculopapules, and characteristically first appear on the trunk and spread to reach face and extremities. The rash resolves over 1–2 days. There are virtually no complications apart from simple febrile convulsions.

Incubation period is 5–15 days, and period of infectivity is not known.

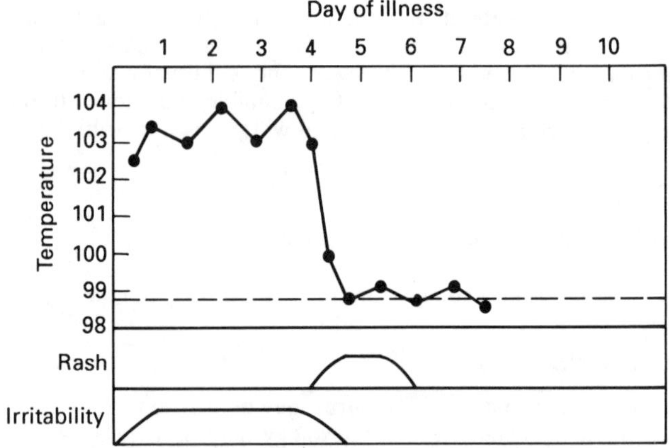


**Figure 10.4** Clinical course of typical roseola infantum (From Krugman, S. *et al.* (1985) *Infectious Diseases of Children,* CV Mosby, St. Louis, Missouri, with permission)

# 10.8 Erythema infectiosum (fifth disease)

It has been called fifth disease because it is the fifth of six childhood exanthems (Shapiro, 1965). In 1984 it was first associated with human parvovirus B19 which is now accepted as its primary cause.

## INCUBATION PERIOD

13–18 days (Joseph, P. R. (1986) *Lancet,* **ii**, 1390–1391).

## CLINICAL FEATURES

About 50% have a 1–4-day mild febrile prodrome. The rash is a bright, erythematous, macular facial one, giving a slapped cheek appearance. It may be associated with circumoral pallor and fine desquamation. By day 2 the rash typically has spread to involve proximal arms and legs (extensor surfaces), and then spreads to the flexor surfaces and trunk. Recent reports indicate that palms and soles may be involved. The facial rash usually disappears first, but the body rash may evanesce over days–weeks.

## INVESTIGATIONS (of academic interest only)

Parvovirus IgM remains elevated for at least 3 months.

## TERATOGENICITY

There has been some evidence to suggest that maternal B19 infection may be associated with foetal death and congenital hydrops. If this is indeed the case, then the risks are exceedingly small. Serological antibody testing is not widely available for those in contact with B19; however, many people in the community have antibodies, and for those who do not, the teratogenic risk is either non-existent or exceedingly small.

# Further reading

## *Erythema infectiosum*

Anderson, L. J. (1987) Role of human parvovirus B19 in human disease. *Pediatr. Inf. Dis.,* **6**, 711–718

Anon. (1988) Fifth disease, pregnancy outcome – implications for management. *Pediatr. Alert,* **13**, 46–49

Shapiro, L. (1965) The numbered diseases: first through sixth. *J. Am. Med. Ass.,* **194**, 680

## *Exanthem subitum*

Yoshiyama, H., Suzuki, E., Yoshida, T., Kajii, T. and Yamamoto, N. (1990) Role of human herpesvirus 6 in infants with exanthem subitum. *Pediatr. Inf. Dis. J.,* **9**, 71–74

## *Measles, rubella, mumps, varicella, roseola*

Krugman, S. L., Katz, S., Gershon, A. A. and Wilfert, C. M. (1985) *Infectious Diseases of Children,* CV Mosby, St. Louis, Missouri

# 10.9 Periorbital and orbital cellulitis

Periorbital (preseptal) cellulitis is a bacterial infection confined to the area anterior to the orbital septum – a fascial layer that separates the orbit from the eyelids. True orbital cellulitis is posterior to the septum. The anatomical proximity of the sinuses, as well as the relationship between the venous drainage of the nose, paranasal sinuses and orbit, provide routes for the spread of infection.

## CLINICAL FEATURES

### *1 Periorbital cellulitis*

It causes erythema, oedema and induration of the eyelids.
Conjunctival injection and oedema may be present.

### *2 Orbital cellulitis*

It causes pain on eye movement. Limitation of extraocular muscle movements or proptosis are serious signs that may indicate an abscess.

## PREDISPOSITIONS

### *Periorbital cellulitis*

Skin trauma/infection, URTI, otitis media and uncommonly sinusitis.

### *2 Orbital cellulitis*

Clinical or radiographic evidence of sinusitis is implicated in >75% of cases.

## AETIOLOGY

*Haemophilus influenzae* (more common in <5 yr), staphylococci, *Streptococcus pneumoniae* and other streptococci cause between 75% and 95% of cases.

## COMPLICATIONS

Periorbital cellulitis is associated with meningitis in 2% of cases.
Orbital cellulitis is a far more serious illness, having as its complications, meningitis, brain abscess, cavernous sinus thrombosis, orbital and periosteal abscess, optic atrophy and blindness.

## INVESTIGATION

1. If there is a suspicion of orbital cellulitis, an ophthalmologist should examine for orbital involvement. If this is confirmed, an ENT surgeon should be involved with a view to drainage of an affected sinus.
2. Blood culture.
3. Conjunctival swab – of limited help.
4. One can do a needle aspiration of the spreading cellulitic edge by injecting 0.5 ml saline and attempting to aspirate a drop.
5. If there are signs of orbital cellulitis, perform a CT or x-ray of sinuses.
6. Consider LP if there is a suspicion of meningitis.

## TREATMENT

### *1 Periorbital cellulitis*

Cefuroxime 35 mg/kg/8 h IV (alternatives are chloramphenicol 40 mg/kg/ loading dose, then 25 mg/kg/6 h, or cefotaxime). If the organism is identified, treat according to sensitivities. If no organism is isolated, change to augmentin 10–15 mg/kg/8 h once the child is improving, for a total of 7 days' treatment.

### *2 Orbital cellulitis*

Antral washout of infected sinus.

Antibiotic treatment as above. Alternatives include a third-generation cephalosporin or chloramphenicol, +/– flucloxacillin. Continue treatment for 10–14 days.

## Further reading

Anon. (1986) Orbital cellulitis. *Lancet,* **ii**, 497

Israele, V. and Nelson, J. D. (1987) Periorbital and orbital cellulitis. *Pediatr. Inf. Dis.,* **6**, 404–410.

# 10.10 Some antimicrobial agents

## COMMENTS

### *1 Cephalosporins*

None works against MRSA. The first-generation cephalosporins are very active against *S. aureus* and penicillin-sensitive streptococci. The third-generation cephalosporins have weak anaerobic cover, but are very active against most Gram-negative enteric infection and *H. influenzae.*

**Table 10.1 Spectrum of activity of some old and new antibiotics**

| | *SA* | *MRSA* | *S. faec.* | *E. coli* | *H. inf.* | *Kleb./ Serra./ Entero.* | *Ps. aer.* | *Anaer.* |
|---|---|---|---|---|---|---|---|---|
| Cefazolin | ++ | – | – | + | + | + | – | + |
| Cefoxitin | + | – | – | ++ | ++ | + | – | ++ |
| Cefotaxime | + | – | – | +++ | +++ | ++ | + | + |
| Ceftriaxone | + | – | – | +++ | +++ | ++ | + | + |
| Ceftazidime | + | – | – | +++ | +++ | ++ | ++ | + |
| Aztreonam | – | – | – | +++ | +++ | ++ | ++ | – |
| Piperacillin / Azlocillin | – | – | + | – | ++ | + | ++ | + |
| Amox./clav. | ++ | – | + | ++ | ++ | + | – | + |
| Tic./clav. | + | – | + | ++ | ++ | + | ++ | ++ |
| Imipenem | ++ | + | + | ++ | ++ | ++ | ++ | ++ |
| Quinolones | ++ | + | + | ++ | ++ | ++ | ++ | ++ |

*Key to symbols and abbreviations*
+++ = active against 98% of strains. – = inactive against 98% of strains. +, ++ = intermediate activity. SA = *Staphylococcus aureus*. MRSA = methicillin-resistant *S. aureus*. S. faec. = *Streptococcus faecalis* (Enterococci). H. inf. = *Haemophilus influenzae*. Kleb./Serra./Entero. = *Klebsiella, Serratia,* Enterobacteriaceae. Ps. aer. = *Pseudomonas aeruginosa*. Anaer. = anaerobes. Amox./clav. = amoxycillin/clavulanic acid. Tic./clav. = ticarcillin/clavulanic acid.

**1.1 First generation** These include: cephalothin (Keflin), cefalozin (Ancef), cephalexin (Keflex, Ceforal), cephapirin.

They are active against *S. aureus*, including penicillinase-producing strains. It is best to become familiar with an oral (cephalexin 10–15 mg/kg/6 h) and a parenteral (cefazolin 10–35 mg/kg/8 h) drug, rather than trying to know them all.

**1.2 Second generation** These include: cefamandole, cefoxitin (Mefoxin), cefuroxime (Zinacef), cefaclor (Ceclor). These have better activity against *H. influenzae*, including some β-lactamase-producing strains while retaining good activity against *S. aureus* and *Pneumococcus*. Cefuroxime (30–40 mg/kg/8 h IV, IM – use double dose in meningitis) is the only one with good CSF penetration through inflamed meninges, although it is no longer recommended for meningitis. Cefaclor (10–15 mg/kg/8 h) is orally [illegible]

**1.3 Third generation** Cefotaxime (Claforan), ceftriaxone (Rocephin), ceftazidime (Fortaz), cefoperazone (Cefobid), latamoxef (Moxalactam). These have broad-spectrum activity against Gram-negative enteric bacteria, including many that are resistant to aminoglycosides or earlier cephalosporins. They are also highly active against *H. influenzae* and

*Neisseria*, but have less activity against Gram-positive cocci than the first-generation drugs. They demonstrate good CSF penetration in all ages, but lack activity against enterococci and *Listeria*, which cause meningitis in neonates; hence in this group ampicillin should also be used.

Ceftriaxone (100 mg/kg/day IM, IV, single daily dose) has a longer half-life than cefotaxime (50 mg/kg/6 h IV) and both have been very successful in treating meningitis. Ceftazidime has considerable anti-pseudomonal activity. Latamoxef (Moxalactam) does not cover strepto-cocci (including *Pneumococcus*), but has good anaerobic activity. It should probably not be used in children.

### 2 Monobactams

Aztreonam was the first to be licensed. It has minimal cross-hypersensitivity with penicillins and cephalosporins. It is of little use against Gram-positive or anaerobic organisms, but has excellent activity against most Gram-negative aerobic infection. It should be used with an aminoglycoside in pseudomonal infection.

### 3 Carbapenems

Imipenem – the first thienamycin antibiotic – is a potent broad-spectrum β-lactam antibiotic. It is effective against a wide range of Gram-positive, Gram-negative and anaerobic infections. It comes with cilastatin (1:1 ratio) which prevents renal breakdown of the imipenem by dihydropepti-dase I. Resistance in *Ps. aeruginosa* has been observed (they produce imipenemase). Its activity against Gram negatives may be diminished by concurrent use of other β-lactams. It is resistant to β-lactamase, but also induces it. It is not ideal for MRSA or enterococci.

Monobactams and carbapenems can be given to those with suspected penicillin allergy (Holgate, S. T. (1988) Penicillin allergy: how to diagnose and when to treat. *Br. Med. J.*, **296**, 1213–1214), although alternatives should be sought in one who has had an anaphylactic response.

### 4 Clavulanic acid

A potent inactivator of many β-lactamase enzymes. It is combined with amoxycillin (Augmentin) and ticarcillin (Timentin).

Augmentin is active against β-lactamase-producing *H. influenzae* as well as staphylococci, streptococci, *Branhamella catarrhalis*, anaerobes. Most β-lactamase-producing strains of *E. coli*, *Proteus* and *Klebsiella* spp. will be susceptible to concentrations of the combination present in urine (Donowitz and Mandell, 1988). It has no antipseudomonal activity. It is used in children (excessively) for upper respiratory and ear infection; however, it should probably be reserved for use as a second-line drug in relapsed streptococcal throats (*J. Pediatr.* (1988) **113**, 400–403), frequent otitis media, or urinary tract infection. Timentin for parenteral use provides very broad-spectrum cover. For *Pseudomonas* infection it should be used with an aminoglycoside.

### 5 Quinolones

Nalidixic acid was the forerunner of this group. Ciprofloxacin is the most widely used drug in this category, and may be given enterally and parenterally. It provides broad-spectrum cover in particular against Gram-negative aerobes. *In vivo* activity may well be better than *in vitro*. It results in increased levels of theophylline and caffeine, and may precipitate theophylline seizures. Chloramphenicol and rifampicin inhibit its action. The quinolones have limited use in growing children because of possible adverse effects on the cartilage growth plate (see discussion, *J. Pediatr.* (1989) **115**, 1022–1024).

### 6 Chloramphenicol

This much and unfairly maligned drug is active against most Gram-positive organisms and Gram-negative bacilli (not *Ps. aeruginosa*), anaerobes, *Mycoplasma* and *Rickettsia*. The emergence of ampicillin-resistant *H. influenzae* and the increased recognition of *Bacteroides fragilis* as a human pathogen have increased its clinical utility. Recent emergence in some countries of resistant *H. influenzae* is resulting in a swing to third-generation cephalosporins in the treatment of meningitis, but in most communities it is still the drug of choice. Against *H. influenzae* it is bactericidal at low concentrations and bacteristatic against most other organisms. Other clinical uses are cerebral abscess, rickettsial infection, acute epiglottitis, osteomyelitis, salmonellosis (including typhoid), orbital cellulitis and intraocular infection.

Idiosyncratic aplastic anaemia occurs in 1:40 000 patients treated with the drug. Dose-related, reversible bone marrow suppression occurs with plasma levels >25 μg/ml.

It is available in capsules (chloramphenicol base), suspension (palmitate ester) and parenteral (succinate ester) forms. The oral preparations are well absorbed and give higher active drug levels than parenteral administration, such that in meningitis, once the child is conscious and not vomiting, it is advisable to switch to an oral preparation (under inpatient supervision).

Chloramphenicol use in neonates is dangerous unless levels are closely monitored becuase they reach toxic levels more readily and unpredictably, resulting in cardiovascular collapse (grey baby syndrome).

## Further reading

Donowitz, G. R. and Mandell, G. L. (1988) Beta lactam antibiotics I and II. *New Engl. J. Med.*, **318**, 419–426 and 490–499

Finch, R. (1988) Anti infectives. *Br. Med. J.*, **296**, 261–264

Jacobs, R. F. (1986) Imipenem-cilastatin: the first thienamycin antibiotic. *Pediatr. Inf. Dis.*, **5**, 444–448

Laferriere, C. I. and Marks, M. I. (1982) Chloramphenicol: properties and clinical use. *Pediatr. Inf. Dis.*, **1**, 257–264

Martinez, J. L. *et al.* (1987) Resistance to β lactam/clavulanate. *Lancet*, **ii**, 1473

Neu, H. C. (1987) Clinical use of the quinolones. *Lancet*, **ii**, 1319–1322

# 10.11 Malaria – treatment and prophylaxis

While malaria is certainly not commonly encountered in paediatric practice, the treatment of cerebral malaria is a medical emergency and may be encountered in those returning from foreign parts. Questions regarding prophylaxis are common.

Sensible advice in the UK is available from:

British National Formulary 1988, pp. 224–227.
Birmingham: Dept of Communicable and Tropical Diseases, E. Birmingham Hospital, Bordesley Green Road B9 5ST (tel. 021-7724311).
Glasgow: Communicable Disease Unit, Ruchill Hospital, Glasgow G20 9NB (tel. 041-9467120).
Liverpool: Liverpool School of Tropical Medicine, Pembroke Place, Liverpool L3 5QA (tel. 051-7089393).
London: Ross Institute of Tropical Hygiene, London School of Hygiene and Tropical Medicine, Keppel Street, London WC1E 7HT (tel. 071-636 8636).
PHLS Malaria Reference Library. Recorded message 071-636 7921 or personal enquiry 071-636 3924 (0930–1030 and 1400–1500).

Alternatively, one may peruse the following guidelines.

**Axioms** (a) All those who develop fever within 12 months of returning from an endemic zone should have malaria excluded with a blood slide. (b) When a person within 2 months of returning displays any signs of falciparum malaria, such as coma, convulsions, clouded conscious state, jaundice, then investigation and treatment for severe malaria is a medical emergency.

## MANAGEMENT OF SEVERE *PLASMODIUM FALCIPARUM* MALARIA

This is 'mainstream' advice. For advice regarding resistance patterns in specific regions, check with the above institutions.

Severe falciparum malaria may cause coma, haemolysis, hypoglycaemia, lactic acidosis, pulmonary oedema, acute renal failure. Anyone recently returned from a malaria endemic area, who has a febrile illness with diminished conscious state, must be assumed to have falciparum malaria.

### *1 Assume chloroquine resistance*

### *2 Investigations*

Record weight, thick and thin blood film, LP to exclude meningitis and consider other causes of coma, urea and electrolytes, blood glucose.

When peripheral blood parasitaemia is high (5–50%), admit to an intensive care unit.

### 3 Quinine dihydrochloride salt

Amp. 300 mg/ml, 10 mg of salt = 8.3 mg of quinine base. Give 20 mg/kg of salt IV over 4 h (or IM), then 10 mg/kg over 4 h 8 hourly for 5 days. Change to oral quinine sulphate 10 mg/kg/8 h as soon as conscious state improves. N.B. Steroids are not indicated; heparin is dangerous.

### 4 Watch for

Hypoglycaemia, renal failure, pulmonary oedema, DIC.

### 5 Restrict fluids

Less than half maintenance. Ideally, fluid input should be tailored to central venous pressure measurements, as the balance between over- and under-hydration may be a delicate one.

### 6 On day 5

Give one dose of oral Fansidar: <1 yr, one-half tab.; 1–4 yr, 1 tab.; 4–8 yr, 1.5 tab.; 8–12 yr, 2 tab.; 12–14 yr, 2.5 tab.; >14 yr, 3 tab.

### 7 Exchange transfusion

? Useful in those with major complications and parasite count >10%.

## TREATMENT OF VIVAX, OVALE, MALARIAE OR SENSITIVE FALCIPARUM MALARIA

### 1 Chloroquine (150 mg base tablet)

5 mg/kg/8 h on day 1, and once a day on days 2 and 3.

### 2 Eradication of the exo-erythrocytic phase

(i.e. within the liver where it is not killed off by chloroquine). Only required for vivax and ovale and only given when the patient has left the malaria zone. Primaquine 0.25 mg/kg on days 4–17. Contraindicated in those with G-6-PD deficiency.

## MALARIA PROPHYLAXIS

*P. falciparum* demonstrates great ingenuity in its ability to develop resistance to chemoprophylaxis.

### 1 General advice

Seek advice on local resistance patterns from one of the aforementioned institutions. Instruct travellers that malaria can develop as early as 8 days after exposure and that delaying treatment of a suspected infection can have serious consequences.

### *2 Personal protection – this is as important as chemoprophylaxis*

Malaria transmission occurs primarily between dusk and dawn:

1. After dusk, wear long-sleeved shirt, trousers, and long nightwear.
2. Use mosquito nets.
3. Use personal insect repellent on all exposed surfaces after dusk. The most effective repellents contain *N,N*-diethyltoluamide (DEET). The higher the concentration, the longer lasting the effect. It should not be used to cover the whole body, but only the exposed surfaces.
4. Pyrethrum-containing insect spray – use indoors after dusk and before going to sleep.

### *3 Chemoprophylaxis*

It provides relative not absolute protection. Should be started 1–2 weeks prior to departure.

**3.1 Areas with no chloroquine resistance** Chloroquine base 5 mg/kg orally once a week.

**3.2 Medium–high level resistance** Chloroquine 5 mg/kg once a week *and* one of:

Proguanil daily, <2 yr, 50 mg; 2–6 yr, 100 mg; 7–10 yr, 150 mg; >10 yr, 200 mg *or*
Maloprim (pyrimethamine 12.5 mg, dapsone 100 mg) weekly, oral. <15 kg, one-quarter tab.; 15–30 kg, one-half tab.; 30–50 kg, three-quarter tab. *or*
Fansidar (pyrimethamine 25 mg, sulphadoxine 500 mg) weekly, oral. 2–11 mo, one-eighth tab.; 1–3 yr, one-quarter tab.; 4–8 yr, one-half tab.; 9–14 yr, three-quarter tab.

**3.3 Side effects** Proguanil – mouth ulcers, mild abdominal discomfort, mild vomiting.
Fansidar – severe Stevens–Johnson syndrome. Avoid using it for prophylaxis.
Maloprim – agranulocytosis, when used twice weekly. If only taken once weekly, risk is very slight (1:10 000 prescriptions).

### *4 Breast fed infants*

Individual prophylaxis is required; negligible amounts of anti-malarial drugs found in breast milk.

### *5 Pregnant women*

Advised to avoid visiting malaria-endemic countries; however, if they do, the benefits of prophylaxis far outweigh the risks of taking anti-malarial drugs.

### 6 Treatment while overseas

In areas without ready access to health workers, all travellers should carry one treatment course for severe malaria (oral quinine and fansidar) and mild malaria (chloroquine) as well as their regular prophylaxis.

## Further reading


Anon. (1988) Recommendations for the prevention of malaria in travellers. *M.M.W.R.*, **37**, 277–284

Anon. (1990) Exchange transfusion in falciparum malaria. *Lancet,* **335**, 324–325

Bradley, D. J. and Howard, P. A. P. (1989) Prophylaxis against malaria for travellers from the United Kingdom. Report of a meeting convened by the Malaria Reference Laboratory and the Ross Institute. *Br. Med. J.*, **299**, 1087–1089

Cook, G. C. (1988) Prevention and treatment of malaria. *Lancet,* **i**, 32–37

Howard, P. A. P., Bradley, D. J., Blaze, M. and Hurn, M. (1988) Malaria in Britain 1976–86. *Br. Med. J.*, **296**, 245–248

Phillips, R. E. (1988) Malaria treatment and prophylaxis. *Prescribers' J.*, **28**, 72–77

Winstanley, P. (1986) Malaria prophylaxis – benefit vs. risk. *Adverse Drug Reaction Bull.*, **117**, 436–439


# 10.12 Diseases notifiable* under the Public Health (Control of Disease) Act 1984†

Acute encephalitis
Acute poliomyelitis
Anthrax
Cholera
Diphtheria
Dysentery (amoebic or bacillary)
Food poisoning
Leprosy
Leptospirosis
Malaria
Measles
Meningitis
Meningococcal septicaemia (without meningitis)
Mumps
Ophthalmia neonatorum
Paratyphoid fever
Plague
Rabies
Relapsing fever
Scarlet fever
Smallpox
Tetanus
Tuberculosis
Typhoid fever
Typhus fever
Viral haemorrhagic fever
Viral hepatitis
Whooping cough
Yellow fever

*Notification of disease can be done through most microbiology departments. Alternatively, one can report diseases directly to the regional Medical Officer for Environmental Health.

†Source: Galbraith, N. S. (1988) Changes in notifiable infectious diseases. *Br. Med. J.*, **297**, 1291

Chapter 11

# Orthopaedics and rheumatology

## 11.1 The child with a limp

In a young child it is often difficult to identify the site and source of pain in a limb. Causes range from a stone in the shoe or plantar papilloma to a cerebral tumour. Irritable hip is the most common cause of presentation to hospital with limp and joint pain. If there is fever and local bony tenderness, admission is required for investigation of septic arthritis or osteomyelitis. An erythematous or purpuric rash predominantly on lower extremities suggests Henoch–Schönlein purpura (HSP) (see Section 9.11). Neurological findings in the legs should prompt a search for a spinal lesion. A young child may simply refuse to walk rather than limp.

### CAUSES OF LIMP (see Table 11.1)

### HISTORY

Ask about:

#### *1 Trauma*

Trauma is frequently mistakenly blamed, when other causes should be considered. Uncommonly, innocuous injuries result in fractures through pathological bone.

#### *2 Pain*

Some limps are painless. Try to identify possible source of pain, but bear in mind that children often do not localize pain accurately. Low back pain may be referred to buttock and lateral thigh. Hip pain often refers to groin and inner thigh or knee. Constant pain suggests tumour or bone infection, whereas pain related to joint movement is often soft-tissue injury or arthropathy.

#### *3 Age* (see Table 11.1)

**Table 11.1 Causes of limp according to age**

| *Age* | *Common* | *Uncommon* |
|---|---|---|
| All ages | Trauma<br>Osteomyelitis<br>Septic arthritis<br>JCA, HSP<br>Cancer–leukaemia, bone sarcoma, osteoma<br>Neuroblastoma | Discitis<br>Spinal infection<br>Other rheumatic diseases, e.g. SLE, Rh. fever, dermatomyositis, IBD, Kawasaki, psoriatic arthritis, reactive arthritis (salmonella, shigella, yersinia).<br>Other infections: hepatitis, influenza, EBV, rubella, brucella |
| 1–2 yr | Cerebral palsy<br>CDH<br>Spiral fracture tibia<br>Haemophilia | Hemiatrophy<br>Coxa vara<br>Sickle cell disease |
| 2–5 yr | Mild spastic hemiplegia<br>Synovitis | Tuberculosis<br>Muscular dystrophies |
| 5–10 yr | 'Irritable hip'<br>Legg–Calvé–Perthes' disease<br>Kohler's disease | |
| 10–15 yr | Osgood–Schlatter's<br>SUFE | Hysteria |

JCA, juvenile chronic arthritis; CDH, congenital dislocation of the hip; IBD, inflammatory bowel disease; HSP, Henoch–Schönlein purpura; SLE, systemic lupus erythematosus; EBV, Epstein–Barr virus; SUFE, slipped upper femoral epiphysis.

### *4 General well-being*

Toxaemia – suggests infection, connective tissue disease, leukaemia.
Bleeding, bruising – leukaemia, HSP.
Chronic diarrhoea – reactive arthritis, inflammatory bowel disease.

### *5 Family or past history*

Arthritis – ?Juvenile chronic arthritis (JCA), ?Rheumatic fever.
F/H – TB, *Brucella*, haemophilia.
Diet – ?Vitamin C deficiency.

## EXAMINATION

Assess for fever and state of well-being.

### *1 Inspect and palpate*

Have the child clad only in underwear. Ask the child to walk unassisted to and fro several times.
Muscle wasting – a soft flat gluteal suggests a hip lesion.
All of limb including interdigital spaces should be checked.

Hop on affected leg – if successful, excludes major disease.
Groin skin folds – increased in shortening or congenital dislocation of hip.
Rash – erythematous or petechial – HSP, leukaemia;
– butterfly malar rash – SLE
Palpate the whole limb, feeling for localized heat that might suggest bone or joint sepsis, or swelling and tenderness suggesting fracture.

### *2 Joints*

'True arthritis' is defined as a red, hot, swollen, tender joint with restricted range of movements. Check for wasted muscles around joints. Compare opposite joints. Crepitus and pain with compression of patella over the femoral condyle suggest chondromalacia patellae. Jerking of patella on flexion/extension suggests subluxation.

### *3 Leg lengths*

True and apparent shortening, seen in congenital dislocation of the hips (CDH), slipped upper femoral epiphysis (SUFE), spinal or neurological problems. External rotation in SUFE.

### *4 Complete neurological examination*

Examine for spasticity and hyperreflexia that suggests cerebral palsy. Examine lower back for cutaneous evidence of spinal dysraphism. Cavus foot and clawed toes suggest Charcot–Marie–Tooth disease.

### *5 Eyes*

Uveitis. Best assessed by an ophthalmologist.

### *6 Cardiovascular*

Rheumatic fever, Kawasaki syndrome.

### *7 Reticulo-endothelial system*

Hepatosplenomegaly and lymphadenopathy are features of JCA, SLE, Kawasaki disease, some malignancies and brucella.

### *8 Gait*

Assess the 'stance' phase when foot is in contact with floor, and the 'swing' phase when foot is off the floor.

**8.1 Antalgic gait** Short stance phase, not wishing to weight-bear for long on a painful limb.

**8.2 Trendelenburg gait** If gluteus medius (hip abductor) is weak, the opposite side of the pelvis dips down during stance phase. It is recognized in CDH. If it is bilateral, a waddling gait is seen.

**8.3 Spastic gait** The child tends to walk on tiptoes, on the affected leg. The diplegic child will cross legs when trying to walk (scissoring).

## INVESTIGATIONS

Some of the following may be appropriate:

Blood culture, FBC, ESR.
Bone x-ray – helpful in trauma and suspected Perthes' disease. Septic arthritis will often only show soft-tissue swelling. X-ray changes of osteomyelitis usually take at least 10 days to appear.
Clotting screen – prolonged partial thromboplastin time in haemophilia, normal in HSP.
Rheumatoid factor, antinuclear antibodies.
Antistreptolysin-O titre and ECG in suspected rheumatic fever.
Bone scan.
Joint aspiration for suspected bone and joint sepsis, and inflammatory joint disease (see Table 11.2).
(Antineutrophil cytoplasm antibodies of research interest in vasculitis.)

**Table 11.2 Synovial fluid (After Ansell, B. M. (1980) *Rheumatic Disorders of Childhood*, Butterworths, London)**

*Non-inflammatory*
Clear/light yellow (straw coloured)
WBC: $<1.0 \times 10^9$/litre ($<1000/mm^3$)
Protein: 1 g/litre
Sugar: within 1 mmol/litre of serum

*Inflamed synovial fluid*
Turbid
WBC – septic $>100 \times 10^9$/litre ($>100\,000/mm^3$): >75% polymorphs
– inflammatory (JCA) $30–100 \times 10^9$/litre: >50% polymorphs
– viral $5–20 \times 10^9$/litre mononuclear
– traumatic $<2 \times 10^9$/litre

Glucose – septic: >2.8 mmol/litre (50 mg/100 ml) below serum
– inflammatory (JCA): 1–2.8 mmol/litre below serum
Protein – 20–40 g/litre

WBC, white blood cell; JCA, juvenile chronic arthritis.

# 11.2 Irritable hip – transient synovitis

This is the commonest hip disease of childhood, occurring between ages 2 and 10 years. It is a result of a synovitis of uncertain origin, often preceded by a viral illness or trauma. Pain may be in the hip or referred to the knee, or not present at all. There are no obvious signs of inflammation. Range of hip movements is limited, especially at the extremes of movement, by pain or muscle spasm.

Resolution occurs spontaneously over 2 days–4 weeks. Treatment is with rest and simple analgesia. Uncommonly, traction is needed for pain relief.

## INVESTIGATIONS

X-ray is normal (and will help to exclude Perthes' disease). Moderate elevation of temperature and ESR are not uncommon. Bone scan (usually not necessary) shows mild diffuse uptake over the entire joint.

## DIFFERENTIAL DIAGNOSIS

### *1 Early septic arthritis*

May be difficult to differentiate the two. Septic hip is usually 'frozen' or at least more restricted in range of movement, whereas an irritable hip can usually be moved with care. Irritable hip tends to not cause severe fever or toxaemia. When in doubt, aspiration of hip and adjacent femur may uncommonly be needed.

### *2 Perthes' disease*

Chung (1986) claims that about 10% of children with 'irritable hip' eventually develop Perthes' disease. Even if this is overstated, nevertheless, the point is well taken. The differentiation is made radiologically (see Section 11.4).

### *3 Slipped upper femoral epiphysis (SUFE)*

Tends to occur in overweight teenagers. Typical signs are shortening and external rotation of the limb (see Section 11.6).

### *4 Rheumatic fever*

Typically causes migratory polyarthralgia, but the hip joint may be the first joint affected. B haemolytic streptococcal infection precedes joint pain by 2–3 weeks. Examination usually reveals other major/minor manifestations (see Section 11.9).

### *5 Others* (see Table 11.1)

Always consider juvenile chronic arthritis and leukaemia.

## Further reading

Chung, S. M. K. (1986) Diseases of the developing hip joint. *Pediatr. Clin. N. Am.*, **33**, 1457–1473

## 11.3 Osteochondritis juvenilis

These are conditions which involve the epiphyses of growing bones. They are usually self-limited illnesses. Perthes' disease of the femoral head, and Osgood–Schlatter's disease of the tibial tuberosity are the most noteworthy. Other affected bones are:

Tarsal navicular (Koehler's disease).
Head of metatarsal (Freiberg).
Patella (Larsen–Johansson).
Vertebral (Scheuerman) – needs physiotherapy and orthopaedic brace to prevent long-term kyphosis.
Capitellum of radius (Panness).
Carpal scaphoid (Kienboeck).

## 11.4 Perthes' disease

This is an osteochondritis of the femoral head, resulting in avascular necrosis, and oedema of adjacent tissues. It occurs primarily in children aged between 4 and 8 years, with a boy to girl ratio of 5:1.

### CLINICAL FEATURES

The child presents with stiffness and occasionally pain in groin, hip or referred to knee, often commencing several weeks or months before presentation. The child has an antalgic gait with limited range of hip movement, especially decreased abduction in flexion. Muscle wasting is common as is constitutional delay of growth (with delayed bone age).

### INVESTIGATIONS

#### *1 X-ray*

One must request AP and 'frog leg' lateral views. The earliest change is subtle widening of cartilage space. Later, one sees increased density and decreased size of femoral head with distorted shape from areas of bone absorption, collapse and repair.

#### *2 Bone scan*

Initial decrease and later increased uptake in capital femoral epiphysis.

### TREATMENT

Treatment is by orthopaedic surgeons and aims at minimizing distortion of the femoral head, containing it in the acetabulum. Therapeutic options are rest, braces, casts or femoral osteotomy.

## 11.5 Osgood–Schlatter's disease

An osteochondritis or chronic stress fracture of tibial tuberosity, usually seen in early adolescent boys. It causes ache, swelling and tenderness of tibial tuberosity. The x-ray shows an enlarged, fragmented tibial tuberosity. It resolves completely over months, with symptomatic treatment. Severe pain is alleviated by a plaster cylinder for a month.

## 11.6 Slipped upper femoral epiphysis (SUFE)

The epiphyseal plate between femoral head and neck is disrupted and the femoral head slips posteriorly and medially. The peak age incidence is 10–15 years, with a boy to girl ratio of 3:1, with 20% being bilateral. The major complication with or without treatment is avascular necrosis. The aetiology is unknown.

### CLINICAL FEATURES

The child is usually obese, with relatively small external genitalia and delayed puberty, although it is recognized in tall thin adolescents. The slip may be acute and mimic fractured neck of femur, i.e. the child cannot walk, the leg lies in external rotation, or chronic which gives an insidious ache in the hip over months. The child has an antalgic gait and mild fixed external rotation of the leg. It is often passed off as a 'sprained hip'.

### MANAGEMENT

X-ray – a lateral or 'frog lateral' view is essential.
Treatment usually involves pinning the femoral head.

## Further reading

Ansell, B. M. (1980) *Rheumatic Disorders in Childhood*, Butterworths, London
Chung, S. M. K. (1986) Diseases of the developing hip joint. *Pediatr. Clin. N. Am.*, **33**, 1457–1473
Jones, P. G. and Woodward, A. A. (1986) *Clinical Paediatric Surgery*, Blackwell Scientific Publications, Melbourne

# 11.7 Bone and joint sepsis

Osteomyelitis (OM) and septic arthritis (SA) still have a significant morbidity. Early diagnosis and treatment are crucial. The use of surgery is an important adjunct to antibiotic treatment in some cases. They are often initially clinically indistinguishable from one another. SA usually gives a 'frozen' joint. The two will be considered together.

## PATHOPHYSIOLOGY

Both are usually secondary to bacteraemia. There are no phagocytes in the end-artery loops beneath the epiphyseal plate of bones, hence this is where bone infection is likely to develop. Infection tracks to the subperiosteal space, strips periosteum from bone along with blood supply to the underlying cortex, resulting in formation of sequestrum. In SA, lysosomal enzymes released in pus attack the mucopolysaccharide component of articular cartilage even after the offending microorganisms have been killed.

## AETIOLOGY

### *1 Neonates*

Group B streptococcus, *Staphylococcus aureus*, Enterobacteriaceae.
Rarely – *Gonococcus, Salmonella, Haemophilus influenzae* b, *Pseudomonas, Candida.*

### *2 Infants and children*

*S. aureus* is the most common pathogen.
Less commonly – *H. influenzae* b, *Pneumococcus, E. coli.* Salmonella OM is well described in children with sickle cell disease, and occasionally in those without. *Pseudomonas* is recognized following penetrating injuries to the foot.

## CLINICAL FEATURES

### *1 Osteomyelitis*

Bone pain and tenderness, often with overlying red, hot, swollen skin. ?Effusion of adjacent joint, but some movement is usually possible. Fever, signs of toxaemia.

### *2 Septic arthritis*

Red, hot, swollen, tender, 'frozen' (minimal mobility) joint. Fever, toxaemia.

### *3 Neonates*

Usually have few typical signs. It can be extraordinarily difficult to suspect bone or joint sepsis in an unwell neonate because of the paucity of signs.

## MANAGEMENT

### *1 Initial investigation*

Blood culture × 2.
White cell count, ESR – both are usually but not invariably raised.
Diagnostic arthrocentesis in suspected SA – culture, WCC, glucose, protein.
X-ray – will usually show normal bone in early OM.

### *2 Orthopaedic treatment*

In SA, formal arthrotomy and drainage under GA or repeated needle aspiration are usually recommended. In suspected OM, opinion is divided between immediate needle aspiration at point of maximal tenderness on admission, or observation for 48 h to assess response to treatment, given that early OM without abscess responds very well to medical treatment alone. Orthopaedic intervention is vital in all cases that do not show significant improvement within 48 h.

### *3 Initial medical treatment*

Treatment must not be delayed in children with suspected bone/joint infection.

**3.1 Neonate** Flucloxacillin 50 mg/kg/6 h (give it 12 hourly in first 2 weeks of life, 8 hourly in third week of life) *and* gentamicin 2.5 mg/kg/8 h (given 12 hourly if aged <2 weeks).

**3.2 Infants and children** Initial therapy should cover *S. aureus, H. influenzae* and *Pneumococcus.* Cefuroxime 35–50 mg/kg/8 h IV is good treatment.

### *4 Further investigation*

Bone x-ray is of little help in the first 10 days of OM.
Bone scan is useful.

### *5 Oral antibiotics*

If the child has prompt resolution of systemic and local signs, change to an appropriate oral antibiotic according to sensitivities. Penicillin V, amoxycillin, flucloxacillin and chloramphenicol have all shown good penetration into bone and synovial fluid. Use 1.5–2 × the normal recommended dose except in the case of chloramphenicol where dose adequacy can be assessed by drug levels. If no organism is identified, broad-spectrum oral antibiotic cover can be obtained with augmentin or cefuroxime axetil. Assess adequacy of oral treatment by measuring serum bacterial titre of the patient's serum against the offending organism, on blood taken 1–2 h after the dose. The titre should be at least one-eighth (1/32 for streptococci). Inadequate titres imply the need for a higher dose, or the addition of probenecid (for penicillins or cephalosporins), or poor compliance.

### *6 Duration of treatment*

If good response is maintained, treat SA for a total of 2 weeks and OM for 3 weeks (usually completed in hospital). OM complicated by abscess or sequestrum formation may require a longer course of therapy. Some clinicians regard ESR as a reliable marker of treatment response.

### *7 Other measures*

Immobilization of bone or joint during the period of acute pain and swelling. Remobilization with physiotherapy may be needed once swelling subsides.

## Further reading

McCracken, G. H. and Nelson, J. D. (1983) *Antimicrobial Therapy for Newborns*, Grune and Stratton, New York, pp. 172–177

Syrogiannopoulos, G. A. and Nelson, J. D. (1988) Duration of antimicrobial therapy for acute suppurative osteoarticular infections. *Lancet,* **i**, 37–40

Tetzlaff, T. R., McCracken, G. H. and Nelson, J. D. (1978) Oral antibiotic therapy for skeletal infections of children II. Therapy of osteomyelitis and suppurative arthritis. *J. Pediatr.*, **92**, 485–490

Wolfson, J. S. and Swartz, M. N. (1985) Serum bactericidal activity as a monitor of antibiotic therapy. *N. Engl. J. Med.,* **312**, 968–975

# 11.8 Rheumatic disease

Rheumatic or collagen vascular disease in childhood includes many illnesses, each involving many disciplines. Some are listed in Table 11.3. Only a few will be described here.

Some possible initial investigations of a suspected rheumatic disease are listed in Table 11.4.

**Table 11.3 Rheumatic diseases of childhood (After Abelson, W. H. and Smith, R. G. (1987) *Residents' Handbook of Pediatrics*: The Hospital for Sick Children, Toronto, Canada. BC Decker, Toronto)**

| | *Monoarticular* | *Polyarticular* |
|---|---|---|
| Juvenile chronic arthritis (see Section 11.9) | + | + |
| Spondyloarthropathies: | | |
| Ankylosing spondylitis | + | + |
| Inflammatory bowel disease arthritis | + | + |
| Reactive arthritis: | | |
| Reiter's syndrome | + | + |
| Post-gastrointestinal dialysis infection (*Yersinia, Salmonella, Shigella, Campylobacter*) | + | + |
| Psoriatic arthritis | + | + |
| Systemic lupus erythematosus | | + |
| Dermatomyositis | | + |
| Scleroderma | | + |
| Mixed connective tissue disease | | + |
| Vasculitis syndromes: | | |
| Henoch–Schönlein purpura (see Subsection 9.11.1) | | + |
| Kawasaki disease | | + |
| Polyarteritis nodosa | | + |
| Behçet's syndrome | | + |
| Rheumatic fever | | + |

**Table 11.4 Initial investigation of suspected rheumatic disease**

*1. Blood*

FBC and differential white cell count
ESR
AST (formerly SGOT), alkaline phosphatase
Immunoglobulins
ANA
Rheumatoid factor
C3, C4 (in suspected SLE)
ASOT
Urea, creatinine

*2. Urine*

Microscopy
Urinalysis

*3. Others*

Consider: ECG, x-ray of any affected joints, joint aspiration, ophthalmological referral

FBC, full blood count; ESR, erythrocyte sedimentation rate; AST, aspartate aminotransferase; SGOT, serum glutamic oxaloacetic transaminase; ANA, antinuclear antibodies; SLE, systemic lupus erythematosus; ASOT, antistreptolysin-O titre; ECG, electrocardiogram.

# 11.9 Juvenile chronic arthritis (JCA, juvenile rheumatoid arthritis)

## CLINICAL FEATURES

There are many subgroups, only one of which resembles adult rheumatoid arthritis – see Table 11.5. Most children can be slotted into a subgroup on the basis of number of joints involved, severity, or laboratory tests.

Systemic onset JCA is characterized by high intermittent fevers, rheumatoid rash, hepatosplenomegaly, anaemia, lymphadenopathy, serositis. The systemic manifestations are dramatic but rarely life threatening.

Polyarticular rheumatoid factor positive (RF+) JCA is associated with severe destructive arthritis and bad prognosis.

Young children (mainly girls) with pauciarticular disease need quarterly slit-lamp examinations. Uveitis can be insidious and can begin as late as 10 years after the arthritis. If not treated it will cause permanent scarring. Those most at risk have antinuclear antibodies positive (ANA+).

## INVESTIGATION

RF, ANA, HLA type – see Table 11.5.

Acute phase reactants – ESR, C-reactive protein. Although generally regarded as helpful, there is surprisingly poor correlation between ESR and clinical activity (Giannini, E. H. and Brewer, E. J. (1987) Poor correlation between ESR and clinical activity in JRA. *Clin. Rheumatol.*, **6,** 197–201). Only 50% of those with JCA have raised ESR. It must not be used to confirm or eliminate possible disease, it is not a determinant of long-term outcome, and it is inferior to clinical examination as a measure of response to treatment (*Lancet* (1989) **ii**, 1531–1532).

## MANAGEMENT

### Aims

(a) Normalize life at home and at school.
(b) Prevent contractures and deformity.
(c) Well-integrated multidisciplinary approach involving physiotherapist, occupational therapist, social worker, schoolteacher, orthopaedic surgeon.

#### *1 Rest*

Only when disease is active. Irreversible damage can arise from prolonged bed rest.

#### *2 Maintain posture, range of movement and muscle strength*

Requires good physiotherapy and occupational therapy. Splints are

**Table 11.5 Juvenile chronic arthritis**

| *Mode of onset* | *Per cent of patients* | *Sex* | *Clinical findings* | *Lab. findings/prognosis* |
|---|---|---|---|---|
| Systemic | 20 | F:M 1.5:1 | Fever, rash, lymphadenopathy, hepatosplenomegaly, pleurisy, pericarditis<br>Any joints may be involved | 25% severe arthritis<br>RF–, ANA– |
| Polyarticular RF– | 25 | Mostly F | Acute or insidious onset. Small and large joints | 10% severe arthritis<br>25% remission<br>25% ANA+ |
| Polyarticular RF+ | 5 | Mostly F | Any joints. Severe destructive arthritis<br>Resembles adult rheumatoid arthritis | RF+ in 100%<br>ANA+ in 75%<br>HLA–DR4 associated<br>50% severe disability |
| Pauciarticular<br>Early childhood onset<br>(type I) | 35 | Mostly F | Hips and sacroiliac joints spared.<br>Anterior uveitis in 50% which can be chronic and cause permanent damage | RF–, ANA+ in 70%<br>Assoc. with HLA–DRW 8, 6 and 5.<br><20% have severe arthritis<br>Need 3 monthly ophthalmology |
| Pauciarticular<br>Late childhood onset<br>(HLA–B27+)<br>(type II) | 15 | F:M<br>1:9<br>Mostly male | Tendinitis, heel pain, sacroiliac joint and lumbar spine<br>No iritis<br>May have positive F/H for spondyloarthropathies | 75% HLA B27+<br>ANA–, RF–<br>May develop adult spondyloarthropathy |

RF±, rheumatoid factor positive or negative; ANA±, antinuclear antibodies positive or negative; HLA, human leucocyte antigen; F/H, family history.

Polyarticular implies 5 or more joints within the first 6 months. Pauciarticular implies less than 5 joints within the first 6 months. Systemic onset implies a systemic illness characterized by fever, rash, hepatosplenomegaly, lymphadenopathy, anaemia, serositis.

widely used. Exercise is the most valuable form of physiotherapy. May require resisted exercise, exercise aids, hydrotherapy, etc. Heat (e.g. warm bath) may prevent morning joint stiffness and facilitate morning exercise.

### *3 Drugs*

**3.1 Aspirin** Still very much the first drug of choice. Initial dose: 20–30 mg/kg/6 h oral with food to bring disease under control (>25 kg, 2.4–3.6 g/day).

*3.1.1 Side effects* Tinnitus, over-breathing, vomit, drowsiness.

*3.1.2 Serum level* If side effects occur or high dose is needed for more than a week. Take blood midway between doses. Maintain level at 1.0–2.0 mmol/litre (× 13.8 = mg/100 ml), in which case hepatotoxicity will be most unlikely.

*3.1.3 Subsequent doses* Try to reduce to 30 mg/kg/12 h.
Benorylate (aspirin – paracetamol ester) 100 mg/kg/12 h will often maintain an ambulant child in a satisfactory state (Ansell, 1980).

**3.2 Non-steroidal anti-inflammatory agents**

*3.2.1 Naproxen* 5–10 mg/kg/12 h (max. 1.0 g/day) has similar analgesic properties to aspirin but does not lower fever.

*3.2.2 Tolmetin* 5–10 mg/kg/8 h (max. 2.0 g/day) compares favourably with aspirin. Has little effect on fever.

*3.2.3 Indomethacin* 1.5–3.0 mg/kg/day (max. 200 mg/day) in 2 or 3 divided doses. Available as suspension. 1 mg/kg at night is useful for avoiding morning stiffness when used as an adjunct to full salicylate dosage by day.

**3.3 Steroids** Used topically for iridocyclitis. Only used systemically for serious acute disease.

**3.4 Second-line drugs** Chloroquine, gold, penicillamine, methotrexate, azathioprine, cyclophosphamide, chlorambucil. It is rarely necessary to consider these drugs. They should be used under the close guidance of a rheumatology clinic. Their use is well reviewed by Rosenberg (1989).

## Further reading

Ansell, B. M. (1980) *Rheumatic Disorders in Childhood*, Butterworths, London
Miller, M. L. (1986) Pediatric rheumatology. *Pediatr. Clin. N. Am.*, **33**, 1015–1263
Rosenberg, A. M. (1989) Advanced drug therapy for juvenile rheumatoid arthritis. *J. Pediatr.*, **114**, 171–178
Schaller, J. G. (1986) Arthritis in children. *Pediatr. Clin. N. Am.*, **33**, 1565–1580

# 11.10 Rheumatic fever

The dramatic decline in rheumatic fever (RhF) over the past four decades probably owes as much to socioeconomic factors as to the use of antibiotics. RhF is probably the result of an abnormal host immune response to certain antigens of group A beta haemolytic streptococci (GABHS). The most significant effect is endocarditis which may recur with subsequent GABHS infections. Lifelong penicillin prophylaxis is recommended. Recent experience in the USA suggests that we may be witnessing a recrudescence of this disease.

## CLINICAL FEATURES

The diagnosis is a clinical one. If there are 2 major or 1 major and 2 minor of the revised Jones criteria (Table 11.6), *plus* evidence of preceding streptococcal infection (ASOT or other antistreptococcal titres such as anti-DNase B, *or* positive throat culture for GABHS), then the diagnosis is made. N.B. Failure to meet the criteria does not exclude rheumatic fever.

**Table 11.6 Acute rheumatic fever – revised Jones criteria**

| *Major* | *Minor* |
|---|---|
| Carditis | Previous rheumatic fever |
| Polyarthritis | Arthralgia |
| Chorea | Fever |
| Erythema marginatum | Raised ESR (false −ve in CCF) |
| Subcutaneous nodules | Raised CRP |
| | ECG: prolonged PR or QT interval |

*Notes*
Polyarthritis – flitting; initially may mimic septic arthritis.
Erythema marginatum – a large red rash with a clear edge which spreads at 2–4 mm/12 h (Ansell, 1980).
Nodules – on elbows, knees and knuckles after about 6 weeks of illness.
Carditis – may be a pancarditis. Characteristic features include a soft apical pansystolic murmur ± mid-diastolic (Carey Coombs) murmur in mitral area, pericardial friction rub, prolonged PR interval on ECG (>0.18 s), heart failure.

ESR, erythrocyte sedimentation rate; CCF, congestive cardiac failure; CRP, C-reactive protein; PR, pulse rate

## INVESTIGATIONS

ESR, CRP, CXR, ECG, ASOT or anti-DNase B.

## INITIAL MANAGEMENT

### *1 Rest*

Especially if there is carditis. Gradual ambulation after 2 weeks.

### *2 Penicillin*

Will not attenuate an existing case, but most would nevertheless give a 10-day treatment course.

### *3 Aspirin*

For fever, arthritis and perhaps mild carditis, although not in severe carditis or heart failure: 20–25 mg/kg/6 h for 4–6 weeks, then gradually reduce. Optimum serum level 20–25 mg/100 ml (1.5–2.0 mmol/litre).

### *4 Prednisolone*

No objective evidence of any benefit; however, Ansell (1980) and many others recommend giving 1–2 mg/kg/day for 4–6 weeks in those with serious carditis.

## PROPHYLAXIS (SECONDARY PREVENTION) FOR THOSE WITH OR WITHOUT CARDITIS

Penicillin V 125–250 mg twice daily *or* benzathine penicillin 1.2 million u/month IM (every 3 weeks, *J. Pediatr.* (1986) **108**, 299). Second attacks are most common in the first 12 months, but most would agree that treatment should be lifelong in those who have had cardiac involvement and at least till mid-twenties for those who have not.

Alternative prophylaxis: sulphadiazine 0.5 g/day for those < 30 kg; 1.0 g/day if >30 kg, *or* erythromycin 250 mg/12 h oral.

## BACTERIAL ENDOCARDITIS PROPHYLAXIS

Children with valvular heart disease require *additional* short-term antibiotic prophylaxis for some dental and surgical procedures (see Section 15.2).

## PREVENTION OF ACUTE RHEUMATIC FEVER (PRIMARY PREVENTION)

There is evidence that some group A streptococci are becoming more 'rheumatogenic'. Prevention relies on vigilance in treating group A streptococcal pharyngitis (see Section 7.1).

# Further reading

Ansell, B. M. (1980) *Rheumatic Disorders in Childhood*, Butterworths, London

Bissenden, J. G. (1988) Transatlantic warning bells sound on rheumatic fever. *Br. Med. J.*, **296**, 1215

Dajani, A. S., Bisno, A. L., Chung, K. J. *et al.* (1989) Prevention of rheumatic fever: a statement for health professionals by the Committee on Rheumatic Fever, Endocarditis and Kawasaki Disease, of the Council on Cardiovascular Disease in the Young, the American Heart Association. *Pediatr. Inf. Dis. J.*, **8**, 263–266

Stollerman, G. H. and Markowitz, M. *et al.* (1985) Report of the *ad hoc* committee to revise Jones criteria (modified), of the Council on Rheumatic Fever and Congenital Heart Disease of the American Heart Assoc. *Circulation,* **32**, 664–668

# 11.11 Kawasaki syndrome (KS)

KS or mucocutaneous lymph node syndrome is an acute multisystem disease of childhood, with vasculitic features. Twenty per cent of patients have cardiovascular involvement, but overall mortality is <1%. Clinical and epidemiological factors suggest an infectious aetiology, possibly due to a human retrovirus. The use of intravenous gamma globulin in the acute phase of the illness has dramatically reduced the coronary artery abnormalities. Pathological features of fatal cases of KS are indistinguishable from infantile polyarteritis nodosa. Eighty per cent of cases are in children <4 years and the syndrome is unusual after 8 years. Japanese and Koreans are at highest risk.

## CLINICAL FEATURES

Diagnostic criteria and associated features are found in Tables 11.7 and 11.8. Additional clinical features are described below.

**Table 11.7 Diagnostic criteria for Kawasaki syndrome**

1. Fever of 5 or more days' duration, unresponsive to antibiotics
2. Bilateral conjunctival injection
3. Oropharyngeal changes* such as strawberry tongue, injected lips, dry fissured lips, injected pharynx
4. Changes* in extremities such as reddening of palms and soles, induration/oedema of hands and/or feet, desquamation of digits
5. Rash – polymorphous, non-vesicular
6. Cervical lymphadenopathy – usually unilateral

* One sign is sufficient.

Note: Patients should meet 5 out of the 6 criteria *and* have other diseases excluded.

**Table 11.8 Associated features of Kawasaki syndrome**

| *Clinical* | *Laboratory* |
|---|---|
| Urethritis | Raised ESR, CRP, alpha-1 antitrypsin |
| Arthritis/arthralgia | Thrombocytosis after day 10 |
| Carditis (myo- or peri-) | Sterile pyuria |
| Aseptic meningitis | Negative ASOT |
| Diarrhoea | |
| Gall bladder hydrops | |
| Obstructive jaundice | |
| Pneumonitis | |

ESR, erythrocyte sedimentation rate; CRP, C-reactive proteins; ASOT, antistreptolysin-O titre.

### *1 Fever*

This is spiking, remittent and prolonged (usually 1–2 weeks) but resolves within 3 days of commencing high-dose aspirin.

### *2 Eye changes*

**2.1 Conjunctival injection** Unique in that it involves bulbar rather than palpebral conjunctivae. It is non-exudative and appears within 1 week of onset of fever. It usually lasts 1–2 weeks and resolves without treatment.

**2.2 Anterior uveitis** Occurs in 80% of children with KS and requires no treatment. A slit-lamp examination early in the illness may help to differentiate those with KS from other febrile children with fever, rash and conjunctivitis.

### *3 Oral changes*

Ulceration of mouth is so rare as to suggest an alternative diagnosis such as herpes simplex or Stevens–Johnson syndrome.

### *4 Skin*

**4.1 Rash** Usually appears within 5 days of onset of fever and may be erythematous, morbilliform, urticarial, scarlatiniform or erythema multiforme. Desquamation, especially on the digits, is usually noted between days 10 and 20. A perineal rash beginning 3–4 days after the onset of the illness and desquamating by days 6–7 has been described (Urbach, A. H. *et al.* (1988) *Am. J. Dis. Child.*, **142**, 1174–1176).

**4.2 Woody induration** of palms and soles is unique.

**4.3** Occasionally, **Raynaud's phenomenon** and rarely **severe gangrene** of fingers and toes occur.

### 5 Cervical lymphadenopathy

Seen in 50% of cases, whereas the other criteria are seen in >90%. A firm unilateral node or clump of nodes measuring >1.5 cm diameter is required.

### 6 CNS

Virtually all cases seem very irritable ± meningeal signs, but only rarely do they have seizures or hemiparesis.

### 7 Abdomen

Hydropic gall bladder may be palpable. Hepatomegaly may be due to cardiac failure.

### 8 Cardiovascular

**8.1 Carditis** Tachycardia may be a response to fever or an early sign of heart failure or myocarditis. Distant heart sounds, pansystolic murmur (mitral regurgitation), friction rub are all features of carditis.

**8.2 Aneurysms** A regular search should be made for aneurysms in all major arteries including axillae, femoral, scalp, intracranial (bruits). Coronary aneurysms are detected on ultrasound at a mean of 10 days after the onset of fever.

## MANAGEMENT

### 1 Clinical examination of the heart

At least twice daily during acute period. Frequency of echocardiography is determined by clinical signs; however, in general it should be carried out at the time of diagnosis, several days later, 3 weeks into the illness, and at 8 weeks.

### 2 Aspirin

20–25 mg/kg/6 h to reduce inflammation and hasten defervescence of fever. By day 14 after onset of illness, if the child is afebrile, reduce dose to 3–5 mg/kg/day to inhibit platelet aggregation, but if fever is high continue on high-dose regimen.

If there is echocardiographic evidence of coronary artery abnormalities, continue low-dose therapy for at least a year and thereafter until coronary vasculature returns to normal. Some would also add dipyridamole 1–1.5 mg/kg/8 h.

### 3 IV gamma globulin

400 mg/kg/day × 4 days. Must be given at presentation, preferably within the first 10 days of the illness. It helps prevent coronary artery disease and has therefore recently received the endorsement of the American Academy of Pediatrics (*Pediatrics* (1988) **82**, 122). The mechanism is

unknown. It may block immunological activation or inflammatory response directed to vascular surfaces, saturate Fc receptors on platelets or reticulo-endothelial cells, lead to immunomodulation, or provide a specific antibody against an as yet unidentified causal agent.

### *4 Fibrinolytic therapy*

For acute coronary thrombosis, prompt treatment with streptokinase, urokinase or tissue plasminogen activator should be initiated at a tertiary care centre.

## DIFFERENTIAL DIAGNOSIS

Viral exanthems, scarlet fever, staphylococcal scalded skin syndrome, toxic shock, Stevens–Johnson syndrome, drug reaction, juvenile chronic arthritis.

## MORTALITY

Twenty per cent of patients with KS develop coronary artery abnormalities (mainly aneurysms). Case fatality rate is <1% (was 3% in early 1970s). Most fatalities are at 2–12 weeks after onset of illness, usually from coronary aneurysm thrombosis.

## Further reading

Hicks, R. V. and Melish, M. (1986) Kawasaki syndrome. *Pediatr. Clin. N. Am.*, **33,** 1151–1175

Newburger, J. W., Takahashi, M. and Burns, J. C. (1986) The treatment of Kawasaki syndrome with intravenous gamma globulin. *N. Engl. J. Med.*, **315**, 314–317

Rowley, A. H., Gonzalez-Crussi, F. and Shulman, S. T. (1988) Kawasaki syndrome. *Rev. Inf. Dis.*, **10**, 1–15

Rowley, A. H. and Shulman, S. T. (1988) What is the status of intravenous gamma-globulin for Kawasaki syndrome? *Pediatr. Inf. Dis. J.*, **7**, 463–466

Shulman, S. T. *et al.* (1989) Management of Kawasaki syndrome: a consensus statement prepared by North American participants of the Third International Kawasaki Disease Symposium, Tokyo, Japan, December 1988. *Pediatr. Inf. Dis. J.*, **8**, 663–665

Smith, L. B., Newburger, J. W. and Burns, J. C. (1989) Kawasaki syndrome and the eye. *Pediatr. Inf. Dis. J.*, **8**, 116–118

Chapter 12

# Gastroenterology

## 12.1 Food refusal: 'My child won't eat a thing'

The overwhelming majority of children who, according to their parents, 'do not eat a thing' are in fact normal healthy children, with normal appetites and normal growth. Despite this, in innumerable homes there is a daily battle. On one side, parents advance with any number of tricks and devices to encourage 'just one more spoonful', and on the other side, 'a little tyrant holds the fort, either refusing to surrender or else capitulating on his own terms. Two of his most powerful weapons of defence are vomiting and dawdling' (Brenneman, H. (1932) Psychological aspects of nutrition in childhood. *J. Pediatr.*, **1**, 145; cited in Illingworth, 1975). In this daily battle, the child will always win.

A neonate who goes off his food is likely to have an organic illness such as infection (UTI, otitis media, meningitis), CNS damage (e.g. kernicterus if the baby is severely jaundiced), organ failure (renal, cardiac, hepatic, etc.) or an inborn error of metabolism.

If an older infant or child goes off his food, plot the child's weight, height and head circumference on a centile chart along with previous recorded measurements. If the growth velocity is normal (i.e. follows an acceptable growth line), then the absolute weight is of little consequence. Therefore, if a child is on the 10th centile for weight and has always been so, then he has appropriate growth and it is inappropriate to expect him to be on the 50th centile (49% of children are below the 50th centile).

### THE CHILD WITH INADEQUATE WEIGHT GAIN

The child who moves away from his expected weight centile on the growth chart has failure to thrive (see Section 19.4). Typically, weight falls away from the expected growth curve before linear or head growth.

### THE CHILD WITH NORMAL WEIGHT GAIN

Such children 'won't eat' for three major reasons:

### 1 The child eats an amount appropriate to his growth

It is the parents' perception of the child's intake that is a problem. Children of small build (? familial or related to low birthweight) may have a smaller than average food requirement. The author finds it helpful to offer the example of a car with a small engine using less petrol than one with a large engine. Parents should be told that in all children the rate of weight gain falls off as the child gets older and food intake may seem to decrease. Demonstrating this on the growth chart is useful.

### 2 Between-meal snacks

The child has an adequate intake much of which is snacks consumed in between meals; hence at meal times food consumption is low.

### 3 Food forcing

Feeding the child 'by force' or repeatedly entreating the child to eat more. Often bribes or punishments are offered as added 'inducements'. Infants and children rapidly learn that parents can easily be manipulated through food. It becomes a battleground and the child invariably wins, further aggravating the parents, and thus a vicious circle is set up.

## MANAGEMENT

As with all behaviour problems, avoid appearing to criticize the parents for their management.

Explain to parents that the child has demonstrated good growth. Show them the growth charts and explain their significance. Tell them that however little the child is taking, he is obviously taking enough on which to thrive. Commend the parents on how they have demonstrably done a good job in difficult circumstances.

Advice should be given regarding offering sensible, balanced meals, and letting the child determine his own intake. It may be of use to eliminate 'junk food' from the house. The parents' obligation is to offer the child a balanced diet, not to make him consume it. There are little eaters and big eaters. Efforts to make little eaters eat more often leads to the opposite of the desired effect.

Lastly, parents should emerge from the consultation reassured that there is no underlying illness in their child. This can only be done by spending time listening to the parents' concerns and being seen to have carried out a thorough examination.

## Further reading

Illingworth, R. S. (1975) *The Normal Child*, Churchill Livingstone, Edinburgh

# 12.2 Neonatal vomiting

This is a problem with a multitude of possible causes. Vomiting in the first one or two days of life should make one think more of congenital causes, e.g. oesophageal or duodenal atresia. Beyond that period, infection, other causes of intestinal obstruction as well as renal or metabolic diseases, must be considered.

## AETIOLOGY

### *1 Non-organic causes*

Posseting.
Problems with mother–child interaction, overfeeding, incorrect feeding technique.

### *2 Organic causes (not in order of frequency)*

Infection – septicaemia, UTI, meningitis, omphalitis.
GIT – reflux, oesophageal atresia (rarely causes vomit), pyloric stenosis, duodenal atresia, volvulus, Hirschsprung's disease, meconium ileus.
CNS – subdural haematoma, cerebral anoxia.
Renal – UTI, chronic renal disease, renal tubular acidosis.
Metabolic – congenital adrenal hyperplasia, inborn errors of carbohydrate, amino acid and organic acids metabolism (e.g. phenylketonuria, galactosaemia).

## CLINICAL FEATURES

Polyhydramnios during pregnancy – suggests high intestinal obstruction.
Bile-stained vomitus (bile is green, not yellow) – suggests GIT obstruction distal to the ampulla of Vater.
Drowsy, poor sucking – suggests infection or metabolic disorder.
Projectile vomiting – a non-specific symptom, although typically associated with pyloric stenosis.
Failure to pass meconium within 24 h of birth – suggests Hirschsprung's disease or other intestinal obstruction.
Failure to regain birth weight – a non-specific warning sign.
Palpable abdominal mass – meconium ileus, large kidneys, palpable bladder (urethral valves).
Bulging fontanelle – raised ICP, meningitis.

## SPECIFIC CONDITIONS

### *1 Posseting*

Small-volume regurgitation of milk in a healthy happy child with no weight loss.

### *2 Infection*

Few hard clinical clues to sepsis in a neonate. Vomiting may indicate the need for LP, blood culture, SPA urine and close examination of umbilical stump.

### *3 GIT obstruction*

**3.1 Oesophageal atresia** Polyhydramnios is a harbinger of oesophageal atresia. It is usually associated with distal tracheo-oesophageal fistula (TOF). Vomiting (an uncommon feature) and respiratory distress typically commence after the first feed. Attempting to pass a soft 8–10 Fr. catheter (radio-opaque) into the stomach will usually encounter resistance at 10 cm from the lips (T3–T5). The atresia should be confirmed radiologically either by injecting air through the catheter, giving an air contrast outline of the blind-ending pouch, or by inserting 0.5 ml of bronchography contrast medium (e.g. Dionosil, Glaxo) under fluoroscopic control. Treatment is to cease all feeds, have a suction tube in the pouch, and early surgery once any respiratory distress has been stabilized.

**3.2 Duodenal atresia** In 90% of cases, obstruction is distal to the ampulla, hence vomiting is usually bile stained and commences within the first 2 days of life. Abdomen is undistended. 'Double bubble' appearance on abdominal x-ray. May be associated with Down's syndrome and imperforate anus.

**3.3 Large bowel obstruction** Causes abdominal distension and vomiting which later becomes bile stained.

**3.4 Hirschsprung's disease (congenital megacolon, aganglionosis coli)** Usually causes partial bowel obstruction, although it can present with complete obstruction (in neonates) or enterocolitis. Commonly the child will not have passed meconium in the first 24 h of life. Later features are: failure to thrive, vomit, abdominal distension (megacolon), constipation, foul-smelling liquid stools (spurious diarrhoea). Rectal examination may reveal a tight empty rectum, and will often result in the explosive release of foul-smelling liquefied meconium or faeces and air. Barium enema may not be diagnostic, but will exclude other pathology. If barium is still present after 24 h, then it suggests Hirschsprung's disease. Rectal biopsy demonstrates absent ganglion cells in the myenteric plexus. Surgical treatment is often done in stages which include: colostomy, excision of the aganglionic segment, and anastomosis to the anal canal.

**3.5 Meconium ileus** Results in abdominal distension from birth, in addition to bile-stained vomiting ± peritonitis. Abdominal x-ray shows distended bowel often with 'ground glass' appearance and intra-abdominal calcification. A gastrografin or 'Hypaque and Muco-myst' enema will be diagnostic and often therapeutic. Cystic fibrosis must be excluded in all cases.

**3.6 Others** Pyloric stenosis (see Section 12.5), volvulus (see Section 12.3), gastro-oesophageal reflux (GOR) (see Section 12.4).

## 12.3 Vomiting in infancy

### AETIOLOGY

*1 Non-organic causes*
'Wind', posseting.
Milk supply – too fast, too slow, too much, incorrectly made up. Maternal anxiety.

*2 Organic causes*
GIT – gastro-oesophageal reflux, pyloric stenosis, volvulus, gastroenteritis, coeliac disease, appendicitis, strangulated inguinal hernia, intussusception, cows' milk protein allergy.
Infection – UTI, otitis media, tonsillitis, meningitis, others.
CNS – meningitis, hydrocephalus, subdural effusions, tumours.
Respiratory – asthma/bronchiolitis, whooping cough.
Metabolic – inborn errors of metabolism.
Drugs – theophylline, erythromycin.

### CLINICAL FEATURES

Non-bile-stained vomit and good weight gain in a child who is contented and well suggest posseting or mild GOR. Projectile vomit is a typical but not invariable feature of pyloric stenosis. A pyloric tumour will often be palpated (see Section 12.5). Bile-stained vomit (green), failure to thrive, abdominal distension, bulging fontanelle or spreading cranial sutures all suggest a pathological cause.

### SOME SPECIFIC CONDITIONS

*1 Non-organic vomiting*
Many infants posset milk. 'Wind' is a vague term applied to babies purported to have swallowed air. This may be due to sucking for too long on an empty breast or on a teat with too small a hole, or to an over-abundance of breast milk. Although most parents are scrupulous about 'winding' their baby after a feed, it is curious how in many developing countries the practice is unknown without apparent harmful effect. Many medical and paramedical workers will recommend a bewildering succession of different powdered milk formulae for the baby

who cries or vomits: 'The differences between the dried milks are so trivial that it is never necessary to change from one to the other' (Illingworth, 1988), except in the unusual situations of cows' milk allergy or lactose intolerance.

### *2 Malrotation and volvulus*

Malrotation may occur with Ladd's bands and an unstable narrow mesenteric isthmus, thus predisposing the neonate to a volvulus. The volvulus may be intermittent which results in recurrent vomiting usually becoming bile stained. Strangulated volvulus is associated with bile-stained vomit, abdominal distension and occasionally rectal blood loss – it is a surgical emergency.

**2.1 Diagnosis** Abdominal x-ray demonstrates multiple fluid levels or relatively gasless abdomen. Barium meal and small bowel follow through will define the ligament of Treitz and the caecum.

**2.2 Treatment**

*2.2.1 Resuscitation* Correct fluid, electrolyte and acid-base abnormalities.

*2.2.2 Nasogastric tube* On free drainage or suction.

*2.2.3 Surgery* Immediately, even if resuscitation is incomplete. If the ileocaecal valve is preserved, the neonate can survive with only 25 cm of remaining gut.

### *3 Others*

Gastro-oesophageal reflux (see Section 12.4), pyloric stenosis (see Section 12.5).

## Further reading

Harries, J. T. (1975) *Essentials of Paediatric Gastroenterology*, Churchill Livingstone, Edinburgh

Illingworth, R. S. (1988) *Common Symptoms of Disease in Children*, Blackwell Scientific Publications, Oxford

# 12.4 Gastro-oesophageal reflux (GOR)

A common problem that is only sometimes associated with hiatus hernia. In the first 6 months of life, frequent posseting may be a normal phenomenon. By convention, a diagnosis of reflux implies an excess of this normal posseting or the development of complications such as aspiration, weight loss, GI bleeding.

## CLINICAL FEATURES

A bewildering array of problems may be caused by reflux, including: chronic vomiting/regurgitation, haematemesis, occult faecal blood loss, iron deficiency (microcytic) anaemia, anorexia, chronic wheeze and cough either due to or independent of recurrent aspiration, poor weight gain, cyanosis, reflex central apnoea/bradycardia, chest pain, dysphagia, oesophagitis (often seen in those with surprisingly little vomiting), oesophageal strictures. It is more common in the mentally handicapped.

## INVESTIGATION

The diagnosis is often made clinically rather than with many investigations.

### *1 Tests for reflux*

**1.1 Barium meal** Excludes strictures and gastric outlet obstruction and defines anatomy (hiatus hernia), but has many false positives and false negatives for reflux.

**1.2 Oesophageal pH monitor** Documents and quantitates reflux in doubtful cases, and establishes relation to sleep, feeding, apnoea, etc.

**1.3 Oesophageal manometry** Lower oesophageal sphincter pressure of $<10$ mmHg has a high correlation with incompetent sphincter mechanism, but is rarely necessary except as a research tool.

### *2 Tests for aspiration*

**2.1 Gastro-oesophageal scintography (milk scintiscan)** Demonstrates pulmonary aspiration. A negative test does not exclude it.

**2.2 Bronchoscopic lavage and aspirate** For lipid-laden macrophages.

### *3 Tests for oesophagitis*

**3.1 Blood loss** Microcytic anaemia on FBC or testing of faeces for occult blood loss suggest oesophagitis.

**3.2 Endoscopy and oesophageal biopsy.**

## TREATMENT

### *1 Thicken feeds* (see Table 12.1)

This traditional treatment has been shown to be efficacious or ineffective in different controlled trials. Baby rice and cornflour increase caloric density of feeds. They are not 'medicines', and may therefore diminish the

**Table 12.1 Thickeners of infant feeds**

| *Thickener* | *Dose* | *Content* |
|---|---|---|
| Cornflour | 1 teaspoon/100 ml feed | 145 kJ (35 kcal)/tablespoon |
| Baby rice | 1 tablespoon dry rice/30 ml formula | |
| Infant Gaviscon | < 2 months: ½ sachet/feed<br>> 2 months: ½–1 sachet/feed<br>Liquid Gaviscon: 1 ml/30 ml of milk | Sugar-free alginic acid and antacids. 4 mmol $Na^+$/sachet |
| Carobel | 1 scoop/200 ml feed | 79% hemicellulose |

medication mentality of a parent. Carobel is convenient. Gaviscon may best suit breast-fed babies and has antacid properties which may combat oesophagitis. Early introduction of solids is desirable.

### 2 Positioning

Some doubts have been cast on the time-honoured method of sitting the child up as straight as possible or in the semi-recumbent position 60° from the horizontal, and it has been suggested that these postures may aggravate reflux (Orenstein and Whitington, 1983). While he is asleep, lying the child prone with head elevation of 20–30° is probably best. However, the child may slide down the bed while asleep unless suspended in a harness, and it is not an easy posture to maintain while awake. The best posture for an awake child is not clear, although sitting fully upright puts pressure on the abdomen and is probably best avoided.

### 3 Time

The natural history is one of gradual improvement usually within the first year of life, probably due to sphincter maturation, assumption of upright posture and a diet primarily of solids rather than liquids.

### 4 Drugs

**4.1 Metoclopramide** Of controversial value (Machida, H. M. *et al.* (1988) *J. Pediatr.*, **112**, 483–487; Tolia, V. *et al.* (1989) *J. Pediatr.*, **115**, 141–145). There is a significant incidence of dystonic reactions in infants and it therefore should be avoided. If its use is considered necessary, use only for short periods under close supervision. Dose 0.125 mg/kg/6 h oral, half an hour before feeding.

**4.2 Domperidone** Also controversial. Avoid using unless all the above fail. Dose 0.03–0.06 mg/kg/6 h oral.

**4.3 $H_2$ receptor antagonists** For oesophagitis.

*5 Fundoplication*
If all else fails.

## Further reading

Orenstein, S. R. and Orenstein, D. M. (1988) Gastroesophageal reflux and respiratory disease in children. *J. Pediatr.*, 847–858

Orenstein, S. R. and Whitington, P. F. (1983) Positioning for prevention of infant gastro-oesophageal reflux. *J. Pediatr.*, **103**, 534–537

Ulshen, M. H. (1987) Treatment of gastro-esophageal relux: is nothing sacred? *J. Pediatr.*, **110**, 254–255

# 12.5 (Hypertrophic) pyloric stenosis

This is an important surgical condition of infancy because it is common, there is a significant morbidity and the operative treatment is readily available and simple. The onset is usually between the 2nd and 6th weeks of life (later in prems). Males are affected 5 times more commonly than females. There is an increased incidence within families (polygenic inheritance).

## CLINICAL FEATURES

The typical presentation is with forceful or projectile vomiting, after which the baby may still be hungry. Later features are weight loss, dehydration, constipation, persistent jaundice. Vomitus may contain altered blood.

The diagnosis is often made clinically by feeding the child (in mother's arms) while gently 'massaging' midway between umbilicus and xiphisternum just to the right of the midline. Palpating over 15 min usually reveals a pea–olive sized pyloric tumour. It is often felt most easily immediately after the baby vomits. This can be further facilitated by inserting a no. 10 Fr. nasogastric tube and leaving it on suction while the child's abdomen is being palpated. Peristaltic waves may be seen crossing the abdomen from left to right. Once the tumour is felt, no further diagnostic investigations are indicated.

## DIAGNOSTIC INVESTIGATIONS

These are often unnecessary if patience and clinical acumen are used (McNicholl, B. (1988) *Lancet,* **ii**, 222). Abdominal ultrasound is gradually replacing barium meal as the investigation of choice, although either in experienced hands is acceptable and reliable.

## DIFFERENTIAL DIAGNOSIS

Gastro-oesophageal reflux.
Infections – especially UTI.
Congenital adrenal hyperplasia – especially if $Na^+$ is low and $K^+$ is high.

## LABORATORY INVESTIGATIONS

Biochemical findings – metabolic alkalosis, hypokalaemia, hypochloraemia.

## TREATMENT

### *1 Nil by mouth*

Also nasogastric tube on free drainage.

### *2 Dehydration and alkalosis*

Rehydrate over 24 h using 0.45% saline plus 15–20 mmol KCl/500 ml at 150–200 ml/kg/day. Alkalosis will then self-correct. If the child is shocked or >10% dehydrated, first restore circulating blood volume with 10–20 ml/kg 0.9% saline rapidly.

### *3 Surgery – pyloromyotomy*

Postoperatively one may commence refeeding as soon as the baby seems well (usually within 4 h of returning from theatre). There is no known benefit to gradual reintroduction of feeds, although this is widely practised.

## Further reading

Harries, J. T. (1975) *Essentials of Paediatric Gastroenterology*, Churchill Livingstone, Edinburgh

Zeidan, B., Wyatt, B., Mackersie, A. and Brereton, R. J. (1988) Recent results of treatment of infantile hypertrophic pyloric stenosis. *Arch. Dis. Child.,* **63**, 1060–1064

# 12.6 Acute diarrhoea and dehydration

Most acute diarrhoea is caused by self-limiting infection (usually viral). Dehydration is the most important problem. The differential diagnosis must be considered in every case and includes infections such as pneumonia, otitis media, UTI, meningitis, and surgical problems such as appendicitis, intussusception and pyloric stenosis. The most important message that must be imparted to parents is that the child must drink more fluid than usual, more often than usual. For the vast majority of Western children, the choice of fluid is less important than the volume consumed. Antibiotics and antidiarrhoeal agents are usually unnecessary, may be harmful, and in general should be discouraged.

## AETIOLOGY

### *1 Virus*

Rotavirus (the most common pathogen), Norwalk agent, enteric adenovirus, small round virus, coronavirus, calcivirus.

### *2 Bacteria*

*Campylobacter jejuni, Escherichia coli* (enterotoxogenic, enteropathogenic, entero-invasive, entero-adherent), *Salmonella* spp., *Shigella* spp., *Yersinia, Clostridium difficile, Aeromonas* spp.

### *3 Parasites*

*Cryptosporidium, Entamoeba histolytica, Giardia lamblia.*

## SOME USEFUL QUESTIONS TO POSE

Ask about fluid intake, frequency and description of stool, urine output, vomiting.

Fever, blood, abdominal pain – suggest bacterial diarrhoea.

Weight loss, prolonged or bloody diarrhoea – suggest amoeba, *Giardia* (blood unlikely) or chronic inflammatory bowel disease.

Seafood ingestion – may alert the laboratory to using the culture medium for *Vibrio*, or suggest other causes of food poisoning.

An outbreak within a family or group – suggests food poisoning. An incubation period of <6 h is consistent with *Staphylococcus* or *Bacillus cereus*; 12–18 h suggests *Clostridium perfringens, B. cereus.* Neurological symptoms suggest shigella encephalopathy, simple febrile convulsions,

electrolyte disturbance. If diarrhoea is accompanied by nicotinic or muscarinic signs, ask about pesticide exposure (see Section 5.11).
Associated respiratory tract symptoms – suggest viral diarrhoea.
Other questions – recent travel, antibiotic use, other illnesses.

## CLINICAL SIGNS OF DEHYDRATION

### *1 Mild (subclinical): <5% bodyweight loss*

Thirsty and alert.

### *2 Moderate: 5–10% bodyweight loss*

Restless, lethargic but irritable, tachycardia, diminished skin turgor, depressed fontanelle, dry mucous membranes, absent tears, decreased urine output. N.B. Wet nappies may be due to urine or watery stools.

### *3 Severe: >10% bodyweight loss*

Drowsy, limp, cold, hypotensive, obvious sunken eyes, poor skin turgor, anuria, acidotic (Kussmaul) breathing.

Beware of underestimating dehydration in obese infants, and overestimating it in malnourished infants. It is possible that the above time-honoured assessment of dehydration may overestimate % bodyweight loss (Mackenzie, Barnes and Shann, 1989).

## MANAGEMENT

Continue breast feeding, encourage oral fluids in smaller amounts than usual but given more frequently, cease antibiotics, and be wary of commencing new ones (see below).

### *1 Treat at home if:*

Family coping, vomiting not interfering with fluid intake, no signs of dehydration.

### *2 Consider admission if:*

Diagnosis in doubt, child under 3 months, excessive vomiting, coexisting chronic diseases (e.g. diabetes, chronic renal or cyanotic heart disease, malnutrition).

### *3 Admit if:*

Clinically dehydrated, family not coping, poor oral intake.

## INVESTIGATIONS

### *1 Urea, creatinine, electrolytes and acid-base status*

Not routinely needed. Indicated for those with any of the following:

clinical dehydration, especially if requiring intravenous fluids;
changes in conscious state;
convulsions;
consider in any child under 3 months;
bloody diarrhoea – raised creatinine might suggest haemolytic uraemic syndrome (HUS).

If serum $Na^+$ is >150 mmol/litre, check for hypocalcaemia and hyperglycaemia.

### 2 Stool culture and rotavirus latex agglutination

Not routinely indicated. Consider if suspected epidemic, suspected food poisoning, blood in stool, institutionalized child, positive Wright's stain for faecal leucocytes, chronic diarrhoea. N.B. Positive stool culture does not necessarily imply pathogenesis nor a need for antibiotic therapy.

### 3 Microscopy

Gross blood and mucus indicates colitis.
Faecal leucocytosis (see Section 12.9 for staining) is often seen in *Campylobacter*, shigella, salmonella, typhoid fever, *Clostridium difficile*, ulcerative colitis and Crohn's disease.

Parasites are best found in a fresh specimen with saline and Lugol's solution staining.

### 4 Full blood count and film

Indicated in bloody diarrhoea to assess anaemia, but more importantly, thrombocytopenia or evidence of haemolysis on the film implicates HUS.

## FLUIDS

### 1 Mild dehydration

**1.1 Breast-fed infants** Should continue breast feeding *and* receive extra clear fluids.

**1.2 Bottle-fed infants** Can continue receiving normal formula *plus* additional clear fluids (see Section 12.7). There is little evidence to support the time-honoured management of starving the hungry child, giving only clear fluids for at least 24 h and only then reintroducing feeds. However, if this regimen is followed, regrading of feeds is unnecessary. It should only be considered if symptoms return with the reintroduction of feeds.

**1.3 Older children** Can continue normal feeding in addition to having supplementary clear fluids.

The type of fluid offered to well-nourished children is relatively unimportant so long as there are not excessive concentrations of salt or sugar.

Vomiting is not a contraindication to oral fluids. It is usually transient and may be overcome by giving small amounts frequently.

### *2 Moderate dehydration*

Administer a proprietary oral rehydration solution for 24 h (see Section 12.7), giving at least 200 ml/kg/day (1 Dioralyte sachet/kg/day). Then resume normal feeds. Older children may continue normal diet if they so desire with added oral fluids.

### *3 Severe dehydration*

**3.1 Restore circulation** Normal saline (or Hartmann's solution) 10–20 ml/kg rapidly. Repeat × 1 if necessary.

**3.2 Subsequent volume replacement** Use one-half to one-fifth normal saline with 2.5–4% dextrose. Add 10 mmol KCl to each 500 ml of fluid once urine output is re-established. For hyper- or hyponatraemia, see below.

Volume replacement = Deficit + Maintenance + Ongoing losses

For example, a 15 kg child who is 10% dehydrated:

| | *Total* |
|---|---|
| *Deficit* = | |
| 15 kg × 10% = 1500 ml | 1500 ml |
| *Maintenance* = | |
| 100 ml/kg for 1st 10 kg | |
| 50 ml/kg for each kg between 11 and 20 kg | |
| 25 ml/kg for each kg beyond 20 kg | |
| i.e. 10 × 100 ml/kg = 1000 ml | |
| + 5 × 50 ml/kg = 250 ml | |
| = 1250 ml | 1250 ml |
| *Ongoing losses* | |
| Estimated ongoing losses depend on: degree of ongoing diarrhoea – say 250 ml/day | 250 ml |
| *Total* = | 3000 ml |

*Therefore*, administer 3000 ml over the first 24 h.

## DRUGS

Antibiotics, antidiarrhoeals and anti-emetics are generally not recommended for children with diarrhoea. They have harmful side effects and deflect attention away from the importance of oral rehydration.

### *1 Antibiotics*

These may worsen viral diarrhoea and often prolong the carrier state of *Salmonella* (*J. Pediatr.* (1973) **83**, 646–650). Seldom will they favourably alter the course of the illness. Some exceptions are the early use of antibiotics in travellers' diarrhoea (cotrimoxazole), metronidazole for *Giardia* and *Amoeba*, cotrimoxazole (10 mg/kg/day of trimethoprim) or ampicillin (50–100 mg/kg/day) or nalidixic acid for *Shigella*. Erythromycin may be of use against *Campylobacter jejuni* if commenced early.

### *2 Antidiarrhoeals*

Deaths have been reported with diphenoxalate, loperamide and aspirin. Kaolin and pectin are unlikely to work (*Am. J. Med.* (1987) **78**, 81).

### *3 Anti-emetics*

Metoclopramide and prochlorperazine. Dystonic reactions are relatively common in young dehydrated children. Vomiting is usually transient and may be improved by giving small amounts of fluids more frequently. Hence, drugs should not be used for this indication.

## SPECIAL CIRCUMSTANCES

### *1 Lactose intolerance, sucrose intolerance*

Lactase deficiency causes watery frothy acidic stools, excessive flatus, excoriated buttocks, and reappearance of diarrhoea with introduction of lactose-containing milk. It is diagnosed by adding 1 Clinitest tablet (Ames) to 5 drops of faecal fluid and 10 drops of water. A blue or blue/green colour is negative (<0.5% reducing sugars). Green, green/brown, yellow or orange indicates the presence of significant (0.5% or more) reducing sugar. The intolerance may be self-limiting or may require 2–4 weeks of a lactose-free milk (Delact, Digestelac, Lactaid, soy-based milks). Less frequently, sucrose intolerance occurs. Sucrose is not a reducing sugar and must be hydrolysed by boiling faecal fluid with a 1 N HCl for 30 s to be detected by Clinitest.

### *2 Hypernatraemic dehydration – serum Na > 150 mmol/litre*

Usually a result of diarrhoea with inappropriately high solute load given as replacement fluid. Shock is a late manifestation. Skin turgor is of a doughy consistency rather than demonstrating the tenting usually seen in severe dehydration. Hyperglycaemia and hypocalcaemia may be seen.

Restore circulation with 20 ml/kg normal saline quickly if the child is very unwell or shocked. Correct remainder of dehydration over 48 h with half normal saline (4% dextrose, 0.18% saline if hypoglycaemic) + 20 mmol/litre of KCl + 10 ml/litre of 10% Ca gluconate. Total fluid input should be 70–100 ml/kg/day for infants. Serum sodium must not drop by more than 10 mmol/litre/day. Rapid infusion of low sodium solution is dangerous.

### 3 Hyponatraemic dehydration – Serum $Na^+$ <125 mmol/litre

*Sodium deficit* =
$[(135 - Na^+) \times Wt \times 0.6] + (TBWD \times Na^+)$
TBWD = total body water deficit (litres). Calculate as above.
$Na^+$ = current serum sodium.
Wt = current weight.
135 mmol/litre = desired serum sodium.
0.6 = correction factor; sodium distributes in the TBW which is 60% of weight.

For example, a 10 kg child with $Na^+$ 125, who is 10% dehydrated:
TBWD = 10% × 10 kg = 1 litre.
Maintenance fluids = 100 ml/kg/day × 10 kg = 1 litre.
Therefore, total fluids over 24 h = 2 litres.

*Sodium deficit is:*
$[(135 - 125) \times 10 \times 0.6]$ = 60
+ 1 × 125 = 125

185 mmol

*Sodium maintenance is:*
3 mmol/kg/day = 3 × 10 kg = 30 mmol

*Total sodium to be given over 24 h* = 215 mmol
This is to be given in 2 litres of fluid = 107 mEq $Na^+$/litre = three-quarters normal saline.

*In practice* – one can avoid messy calculations by giving 0.45% NaCl + 2.5% dextrose + 10 mmol KCl/500 ml as the replacement fluid over 24 h and letting the kidneys do the fine tuning, assuming that renal function is adequate. 'The most stupid kidneys are cleverer than the smartest resident.'

### 4 Antibiotic-associated diarrhoea

Often caused by *Clostridium difficile*. The initial management is to cease all antibiotics. The diagnosis can be confirmed by finding *C. difficile* toxin in the stool. Usually the only treatment needed is to cease all antibiotics; but if the diarrhoea persists, or is relapsing, one may try metronidazole or vancomycin. Bacitracin, cholestyramine and *Lactobacillus* have their advocates (*Lancet*, 1987, **ii**, 1519).

## Further reading

Anon. (1986) Oral rehydration therapy for treatment of diarrhoea in the home. WHO/CDD/SER/86.9

Anon. (1988) Preventing traveller's diarrhoea. *Lancet*, **ii**, 144

Brown, K. H. *et al.* (1988) Effect of continued oral feeding on clinical and nutritional outcomes of acute diarrhoea in children. *J. Pediatr.*, **112**, 191–200.

Gorbach, S. L. (1987) Bacterial diarrhoea and its treatment. *Lancet*, **ii**, 1378–1382
Mackenzie, A., Barnes, G. and Shann, F. (1989) Clinical signs of dehydration in children. *Lancet*, **ii**, 605–607
Santosham, M., Daum, R. S., Dillman, L. *et al.* (1982) Oral rehydration therapy of infantile diarrhoea. A controlled study of well nourished children hospitalized in the United States and Panama. *N. Engl. J. Med.*, **306**, 1070–1074
Wharton, B. A., Pugh, R. E., Taitz, L. S. *et al.* (1988) Dietary management of gastroenteritis in Britain. *Br. Med. J.*, **296**, 450–452

# 12.7 Oral rehydration

Commonly used fluids include carbonated soft drinks, fruit-flavoured squash (cordial) diluted roughly 1:5, and fruit juices; they are all hyperosmolar (approx. 800 mosm/litre) and mostly low in electrolytes.

### *1 For mild (i.e. subclinical) dehydration*

In the presence of mild to moderate diarrhoea, electrolyte depletion will be insignificant. Hydration can be maintained by liberal use of the following readily available solutions of sugar and water (without added salt). Fruit juice or soft drink should be diluted by 1 part:3 parts water (i.e. quarter-strength). Fruit squash (cordial) should be made up to only one-third its normal diluted strength. Table sugar: 1 heaped teaspoon to 200 ml water. Alternatively, give proprietary oral rehydration solutions at 200 ml/kg/day. See Table 12.2.

**Table 12.2 Solutions for oral rehydration**

| *Powder* (volume water per sachet) | *Concentration of solution* (mmol/litre) | | | | | |
|---|---|---|---|---|---|---|
| | Na | Cl | K | Base | Glucose | Osmolarity (mosm/litre) |
| Dioralyte (200 ml) | 35 | 37 | 20 | 18 (bicarb.) | 200 | 310 |
| WHO/UNICEF solution (1000 ml) | 90 | 80 | 20 | 10 (citrate) | 110 | 310 |
| Fruit juices* | <2.5 | | 25–50 | | | 600–800 |
| Carbonated drinks | <2 | | <2 | | | 600–800 |
| Fruit squash* (diluted roughly 1:5) | <5 | | <2 | | | 600–800 |

* Heath, P. J., Walker, S. and Park, G. R. (1986) *Lancet*, **ii**, 1397.

Home-made sugar–salt solutions ('a pinch of this and 2 pinches of that') are unnecessary for this group, show unacceptable variability in composition and may be dangerous.

### *2 Moderate dehydration (5–7%)*

Sugar–salt solutions have the potential to facilitate absorption of water and electrolytes even though many of the small bowel enterocytes have been damaged. Sachets of the powder are readily available (at pharmacists), cheap, and when added to the correct volume of water, provide optimum, safe treatment for the child with mild–moderate fluid losses.

## 12.8 Gastrointestinal bleeding

Gastrointestinal blood loss is best investigated bearing in mind the age of the patient and the amount and colour of the haemorrhage.

### AETIOLOGY

| | *Haematemesis* | *Melena/rectal bleeding* |
|---|---|---|
| ***Infants*** | | |
| | Swallowed blood | Infectious colitis |
| | Pyloric stenosis | Cows' milk allergy colitis |
| | Reflux oesophagitis | Intussusception |
| | Peptic ulcer | Volvulus |
| | | Tubular duplications |
| | | Anal fissure |
| | | Meckel's diverticulum |
| | | Swallowed blood |
| | | Duplications |
| ***Older children*** | | |
| | Mallory–Weiss tear | Meckel's diverticulum |
| | Peptic ulcer | Polyps |
| | Oesophageal varices | Oesophageal varices |
| | Stress ulcers | Peptic ulcer |
| | (Burns, head injuries, steroids) | Inflammatory bowel disease |

### ANORECTAL BLEEDING

Bright blood, usually on the surface of the stools, tend to arise from the large bowel. Dark denatured blood usually comes from higher up the GIT.

### *1 Anal fissure*

Diagnosed by parting the buttocks and exposing fissures in the anal mucosa. It is an innocent condition that may be associated with painful defaecation for several days despite the astonishing rapidity of fissural healing. Treatment for constipation may be useful as may topical application of lignocaine 2% gel.

### *2 Intussusception*

A painful condition with colicky spasms lasting 2 or 3 min during which the infant screams, draws up his knees and clenches his fists, relaxing as the spasm eases. Spasms occur at intervals of 15–20 min. Vomiting occurs in the first hour or two of the spasms, but may not recur once the stomach is empty. Rectal bleeding (resembling redcurrant jelly) is by no means always observed, nor always found on rectal examination. The child is usually between 2 months and 2 years, and may have had a recent upper respiratory infection, gastroenteritis, or Henoch–Schönlein purpura.

On examination, the child looks pale, clammy and exhausted (probably the most reliable physical sign). A sausage-shaped mass may be palpable in the right hypochondrium. Diagnosis is by barium enema or ultrasound. Treatment is by rehydration and conventionally hydrostatic reduction (90 cm (3 ft) of barium for 3 min × 3 attempts = 75% success), with close collaboration between surgeon and radiologist, or surgical reduction. Increasingly, pneumatic reduction is being used. Barium reduction is contraindicated if there is gut perforation, and should be done with circumspection if the symptoms have been present for more than 24 h.

### *3 Ulcerative colitis*

Frequent loose stools and weight loss are common presenting features. Diagnosis is by barium enema and sigmoidoscopy (see Section 12.11).

### *4 Massive GI bleed*

Only two conditions commonly present in this fashion.

**4.1 Meckel's diverticulum** This is present in 2% of the population, situated 60 cm (2 ft) proximal to the ileocaecal junction, with symptoms usually (not invariably) manifesting in the first 2 years of life. It is a persistence of a segment of vitello-intestinal duct which retains its communication with the ileum, and may contain ectopic pancreatic or gastric mucosal tissue or both. The commonest complication is the painless passage per rectum of a large volume of melena or bright blood.

Diagnosis is with a $^{99m}$Tc scan. A negative test does not exclude the condition because there may be insufficient ectopic gastric mucosa to take up the technetium. Once diagnosed, a laparotomy is required. If the scan is negative, it is generally permissible to wait for a second haemorrhage before proceeding to laparotomy.

**4.2 Portal hypertension** This uncommon problem is caused by many conditions such as cirrhosis of the liver (post-hepatitis, biliary atresia), extrahepatic portal vascular obstruction due to neonatal umbilical sepsis, Budd–Chiari malformation, hepatic vein webs. The usual mode of presentation is with a large haematemesis after the age of 2 years, although occasionally the initial clue is the incidental discovery of unexplained splenomegaly.

The diagnosis is made on endoscopy or barium study followed by a splenic portogram.

Treatment involves resuscitation with blood transfusion and occasionally IV pitressin. Gastro-oesophageal tamponade can be achieved with Sengstaken-type double lumen tube, inflated for 48 h. If bleeding recurs after deflation, the bag should be reinflated for a further 48 h. Surgical therapy must be selected from an array of palliative therapies which include sclerotherapy, shunting of portal blood, endoscopic or direct ligation of oesophageal varices.

# 12.9 Laboratory tests in gastroenterology

## STOOL

### *1 Inspection*

Consistency, odour, blood, mucus. Stools from patients with CHO malabsorption are frothy, liquid, acid and the perianal region is often excoriated. Fat malabsorption gives bulky pale offensive stools that are difficult to flush away. Blood and mucus are found in infectious colitis and inflammatory bowel disease.

### *2 Fatty acids and fat globules*

Place a match-head sized sample on three slides. The first may require an additional drop of water. Cover with coverslip and examine under 400 × magnification with narrow iris aperture. Fat globules are highly refractile. On the second slide, place 2 drops of 95% ethyl alcohol and 3 drops of Sudan Black III. Fat globules should stain easily. On the third slide, place several drops of Nile Blue Sulphate 0.1%. A pink colour indicates the presence of fatty acids. Fat globules are seen in steatorrhoeic faeces of children with pancreatic insufficiency (e.g. CF, Shwachman syndrome), whereas fatty acid in stools implies that fat malabsorption is occurring despite the presence of pancreatic lipase to hydrolyse the fat globules (e.g. coeliac disease).

### 3 Sugars

Clinitest: add 10 drops of water to 5 drops faecal fluid in a test tube or specimen bottle; add 1 Clinitest tablet. After 1 min, if the fluid is blue/green, <0.5% reducing sugars are present. Green/brown, yellow or orange indicate the presence of significant amounts (0.5% or more) reducing sugars. Sucrose is not a reducing sugar. It must first be hydrolysed by adding 2 parts water to 1 part stool and boiling for 30 s in 1 N HCl.

pH: Normal pH is 7–8. A pH <5.5 suggests the presence of organic acids (disaccharide intolerance). Stool pH >8 is seen in secretory diarrhoea. This is an unreliable test.

### 4 Blood

Haemoccult or guaiac test.

### 5 Leucocytes

Faecal leucocytes can be seen in a fresh smear, but are more readily identified after staining with Loeffler's methylene blue, or Wright's or Gram stains. Faecal leucocytosis is seen in *Campylobacter*, shigella, invasive *E. coli*, *Salmonella*, typhoid fever, *Clostridium difficile*, ulcerative colitis, and Crohn's disease.

### 6 Ova, cysts, parasites

Use saline and Lugol's iodine on a fresh specimen (see Section 12.15).

### 7 Stool culture

### 8 72-hour faecal fat collection

This is a cumbersome and frustrating test. A dietitian should arrange a measured fat intake. Infants should have 5 g/kg/day, young children 40–50 g/day and older children 70–80 g/day. In some centres, a red or blue carmine marker is given and collections begun with the appearance of the first coloured stool. The upper limit of normal for daily faecal fat excretion is 5 g. Faecal fat can also be expressed as a coefficient of absorption (CA):

$$\mathrm{CA} = \frac{(\text{Dietary fat} - \text{Faecal fat})}{\text{Dietary fat}} \times 100$$

| Normal CA: | | |
|---|---|---|
| | Term newborn | 80–85% |
| | <3 yr | 85–95% |
| | >3 yr | 95% |

### 9 Protein loss

Random sample for faecal alpha 1 antitrypsin. A high level suggests protein-losing enteropathy.

### *10 Electrolytes*

In congenital chloridorrhoea, the pathognomonic finding is a stool chloride concentration greater than the combined stool $Na^+$ and $K^+$ concentration.

## OTHER TESTS OF CHO MALABSORPTION

### *1 D-xylose test*

Fast overnight. Give 14.5 g/m$^2$ of oral xylose. Measure blood xylose at 1 h. A mucosal abnormality is suggested by a level of <1.6 mmol/litre (<25 mg/100 ml). This is an unreliable but nevertheless useful guide.

### *2 Breath hydrogen test*

For lactose and sucrose malabsorption. Undigested sugars are metabolized by colonic bacteria, releasing hydrogen which is absorbed and finally excreted in the breath. After an overnight fast, a loading dose of disaccharide is given. A nasal prong is inserted and 5 ml of exhaled air is collected at half-hourly intervals for 3 h. $H_2$ excretion of >20 p.p.m. above baseline suggests disaccharide malabsorption. No antibiotics should be given in the week preceding the test.

## OTHER TESTS OF FAT MALABSORPTION

### *Absorption of fat-soluble vitamins A, D, E, K*

Vitamin E level: 7.0–12.0 µmol/litre (0.3–0.5 mg/dl).
Vitamin A level: 0.7–2.1 µmol/litre (20–60 µg/dl).
Clotting profile: abnormal prothrombin time is a crude indicator of poor vitamin K status.
Vitamin D: serum Ca, $PO_4$, alkaline phosphatase, wrist x-ray, or vitamin D levels.

## HAEMATOLOGY

### *1 Full blood count and ESR*

Microcytic or macrocytic anaemias occur in haematinic deficiencies (iron and $B_{12}$/folate deficiencies, respectively).
Acanthocytosis is a feature of abetalipoproteinaemia.
Neutropenia is seen in Schwachman's syndrome. Lymphopenia occurs in intestinal lymphangiectasia.
A very high ESR or CRP is compatible with inflammatory bowel disease.

### *2 Serum and red cell folate*

Red cell folate is the better test. Serum folate may reflect recent dietary fluctuations. Low folate levels are seen with poor intake (goats' milk diet), or distal ileum disease.

### *3 Vitamin $B_{12}$ – Schilling test*

Two hour fast followed by 0.5 μCi of $^{57}Co$ $B_{12}$ oral. Two hours later, administer 1 mg non-radiolabelled $B_{12}$ IM to saturate body stores. Urine should be collected for 24 h before and after the test. $<12\%$ of $^{57}Co$ $B_{12}$ excreted in the urine indicates $B_{12}$ malabsorption. Repeat oral dose with intrinsic factor (IF) to differentiate ileal disease from IF deficiency.

## LIVER FUNCTION TESTS

Alkaline phosphatase, SGOT, bilirubin, albumin, total protein. Bilirubinuria and absent urinary urobilinogen in obstructive jaundice.

## SMALL BOWEL INVESTIGATIONS

### *1 Small bowel biopsy/Crosby capsule*

Check clotting profile. Fast the child 4 h prior to the procedure. One hour before the procedure administer oral chloral hydrate 50 mg/kg and insert an IV cannula. In the x-ray department one can administer 0.07–0.1 mg/kg midazolam IV (side effect: hypotension which responds to rapid infusion of normal saline). Ketamine 1 mg/kg IV is an acceptable alternative (see Section 4.4). With child lying on right side, pass a semi-rigid orogastric tube connected to a primed Crosby capsule. Under fluoroscopic control, ensure its passage into the small bowel. The biopsy provides useful information regarding coeliac disease, Whipple's disease, abetalipoproteinaemia, agammaglobulinaemia. A touch preparation (mucosal impression smear) should be inspected for *Giardia* trophozoites or cysts, as can the duodenal fluid. Brush border disaccharides can be quantified Initial investigation of possible giardiasis may be more easily done in the first instance by a String test (see Section 12.10 under 'Giardiasis').

### *2 GI endoscopy*

Increasingly used. Prepare the child as described for Crosby capsule. The main advantages over the Crosby capsule are that a biopsy is reliably obtained, the procedure is much faster and there is no radiation to patient or doctor.

### *3 Barium meal*

Useful for blind loop syndrome, Crohn's disease.

## PANCREATIC FUNCTION TESTS

### *1 Sweat test*

Obtain preferably >100 μl of sweat. Cystic fibrosis is diagnosed if sweat $Na^+$ >60 mmol/litre, $Cl^-$ >60 mmol/litre, osmolarity >200 mosm/litre.

### *2 Duodenal juice*

Collected by inserting a tube to the 4th part duodenum. A test meal or infusion of pancreozymin-secretin is given. Measure trypsin, lipase, esterase, amylase, pH, bile salt concentrations.

### *3 Others*

Bentioromide/PAS test of pancreatic function is not reliable in Schwachman's syndrome, but is easy and convenient (Puntis, J. W. L. *et al.* (1988) Simplified oral pancreatic function tests. *Arch. Dis. Child.,* **63**, 780–784). Faecal chymotrypsin assay is also a useful screening test (*Arch. Dis. Child.* (1988) **63**, 785–789). Stool trypsin activity is seldom performed because of its unreliability.

## LABORATORY TESTS OF NUTRITIONAL STATUS

The concentration of rapid turnover proteins such as transferrin, thyroxine-binding pre-albumin and retinol-binding protein are sensitive indicators of borderline protein intake (and the efficacy of TPN). The long half-life of albumin makes it a somewhat clumsy tool in assessing situations of rapid nutritional change (Burritt, M. F. and Anderson, C. F. (1984) Laboratory assessment of nutritional status. *Hum. Pathol.,* **15**, 130–133).

# 12.10 Chronic diarrhoea

Diarrhoea persisting for more than 2 weeks is considered to be chronic. There is no generally accepted clinical definition of diarrhoea other than the frequent passage of loose stools. It is a common complaint, especially in the toddler age group. In order to avoid over-investigation, it is important to distinguish between diarrhoea with failure to thrive, which suggests malabsorption or inflammatory bowel disease, from diarrhoea in a well, happy, thriving child.

## AETIOLOGY

1. Chronic non-specific (toddler's) diarrhoea.
2. Post-infective diarrhoea.
3. Milk allergy.
4. Chronic inflammatory bowel disease.
5. Malabsorption syndromes – coeliac disease, cystic fibrosis.
6. Chronic infective diarrhoea – e.g. *Giardia*.
7. Spurious diarrhoea – see Section 12.14.

## CLINICAL FEATURES

Document a thorough history, examination and current and previous growth centiles (see Sections 3.6 and 19.4).

## INVESTIGATION

This must be tailored to the individual situation (see Section 12.9).

## SOME SPECIFIC SYNDROMES

### *1 Chronic non-specific diarrhoea – toddler's diarrhoea*

This label is applied to the child usually between 12 months and 4 years of age, with loose stools especially by day, but in whom growth and general examination are normal. Stools are mucousy and contain undigested food. The mechanism is unknown, but it may represent immaturity of small bowel motility, food intolerance, excessive fluids, dietary fat restriction, or fruit juice carbohydrate malabsorption. Fruit juices are hyperosmolar, and in addition contain sorbitol (pear juice, 2%; apple juice, 0.5%), a non-absorbable sugar alcohol (Hyams, J. S. *et al.* (1988) *Pediatr.*, **82,** 64–68).

Management is largely confined to repeated reassurance, and avoidance of full-strength fruit juice. Elimination diets should be avoided. Drugs have no part to play. Investigations might include stool microscopy, culture, reducing and non-reducing sugars. The faeces will usually become firm by age 3 years or when the child is toilet trained.

### *2 Post-infective diarrhoea*

Most cases are due to lactose intolerance (uncommonly sucrose intolerance or cows' milk protein allergy). Intolerance to lactose is diagnosed with Clinitest tablets (see Sections 12.6 and 12.9). A trial of withdrawing the suspected offending substance may be required. A modified soya milk may be tried. Formula S has no disaccharides, whereas Wysoy contains sucrose. Pregestimil has no cow or soy milk protein, nor disaccharides, but it is unpalatable and expensive. Delact and Digestelac are humanified milks with added lactase. If antibiotics have been used, *Clostridium difficile* toxin may be causing prolonged diarrhoea. Diarrhoea usually resolves with cessation of the antibiotic. Full-strength fruit juice may cause an osmotic diarrhoea – see above.

### *3 Cows' milk allergy (CMA)*

This is a confused, controversial subject. According to Hill and co-workers (1986) there are several different groups.

Group 1: Predominantly urticarial and angio-oedematous eruptions within 45 min of ingesting cows' milk.

Group 2: Vomit, diarrhoea, abdominal pain, pallor, between 45 min and 20 h after milk ingestion. Some of these children will be relatively IgA deficient.

Group 3: Chronic eczematous eruptions, chronic diarrhoea, chronic bronchitis and wheezing, chronic ill health, failure to thrive.

In addition, there is cows' milk colitis.

**3.1 Investigations** These include radioallergosorbent testing (RAST), skin prick tests, and testing for eosinophilia and low IgA. Occult faecal blood and faecal leucocytosis suggest cows' milk colitis. Low total protein and serum albumin suggest protein-losing enteropathy. There is, however, no definitive test for CMA. Ultimately the diagnosis rests on clinical suspicion, response to withdrawal of milk and response to a milk challenge (this should not be attempted in those with angioneurotic oedema).

**3.2 Treatment** Once diagnosed, the child may be tried on a modified soya milk, but there is some cross-sensitivity in those with CMA. Exclusion of dairy products should be complete, although this can usually be substantially relaxed when the child approaches 3 years of age.

### *4 Sucrase isomaltase deficiency*

Although rare, this is an eminently treatable disorder. Children grow well, but suffer abdominal pain and profuse diarrhoea after a meal with high sucrose content (e.g. fruit juice). The diagnosis is made by testing faecal fluid with Clinitest (after prior hydrolysis with HCl), breath hydrogen testing, measurement of enzymes on biopsy and a sucrose exclusion diet. Treatment is lifelong. Inheritance is autosomal recessive.

### *5 Giardiasis*

This gut parasite is often asymptomatic; however, it can cause a wide range of symptoms including abdominal pain, chronic and recurrent diarrhoea and weight loss. Stools may be bulky and offensive. Steatorrhoea and malabsorption (including lactose) may occur.

**5.1 Diagnosis** Cysts may be seen in any stool, and motile trophozoites may be seen in fresh diarrhoeal stool or by direct examination of duodenal aspirate obtained by endoscopy or Crosby capsule. Alternatively, duodenal fluid may be obtained using the String test or 'Entero-test' (Hedeco, Palo Alto, California), in which a weighted gelatin capsule with an attached nylon string is swallowed and the string is taped to the face. Several hours later the string is withdrawn and the adsorbed duodenal contents are examined for trophozoites. Rapid antigen detection tests (ELISA and immunofluorescence) or CIE are available, with roughly 90% sensitivity and specificity.

**5.2 Treatment** Metronidazole 5 mg/kg/8 h (max. 750 mg/day) for 10 days, or 40 mg/kg once daily for 3 days (single dose tinidazole 50 mg/kg or quinacrine 2 mg/kg/8 h × 7 days are also effective).

### *6 Chronic inflammatory bowel disease* (see Section 12.11)

## Further reading

Hill, D. J., Firer, M. A., Shelton, M. J. *et al.* (1986) Manifestations of milk allergy in infancy: clinical and immunological findings. *J. Pediatr.*, **109**, 270–276

Pickering, L. K. and Engelkirk, P. G. (1988) *Giardia lamblia. Ped. Clin. N. Am.*, **35**, 565–577

# 12.11 Chronic inflammatory bowel disease (CIBD)

Ulcerative colitis (UC) and Crohn's disease (CD) are the two most notable forms of CIBD.

### DIFFERENTIAL DIAGNOSIS

All ages – infection: *Yersinia, Campylobacter, Shigella, Salmonella, Amoeba*, antibiotic-associated colitis (*Clostridium difficile* toxin).
Infants – Hirschsprung's disease, allergic colitis, intussusception.
Older children – Henoch–Schönlein purpura, haemolytic uraemic syndrome (HUS).

## 12.11.1 Ulcerative colitis

A chronic inflammatory disease of unknown aetiology. The pathology involves the colon, with continuous disease from the rectum, characterized by mucosal inflammation and crypt abscesses. Genetic, infectious, immunological and psychological factors have been implicated.

### *1 History*

Fifteen per cent of cases are aged <20 years. The disease is rare in early childhood. Presentation is with bloody diarrhoea, recurrent abdominal pain, tenesmus, failure to thrive. Systemic manifestations include arthritis, iritis, hepatitis, erythema nodosum and pyoderma gangrenosum.

### *2 Examination*

Growth failure, tender abdomen, examine for extracolonic manifestations.

### *3 Colonic complications*

Toxic megacolon, stenosis, perforation, internal fistulae.
Cancer – 3% in first decade, 20% per decade thereafter.

### 4 Investigations

**4.1 Stool culture and microscopy** For blood and faecal leucocytes, *Entamoeba histolytica*, and bacteria. Specifically request for *C. difficile* enterotoxin and, if HUS is a possibility, verocytotoxin-producing *E. coli*.

**4.2 Double contrast barium enema** May be normal early in the disease.

**4.3 Sigmoidoscopy and colonoscopy and biopsy** Colitis.

**4.4 FBC** Anaemia. Fragmented cells and high urea suggest HUS. ESR is often raised in UC.

### 5 Treatment

**5.1 Good nutrition** Vital. Low threshold for using TPN during an acute attack, or nocturnal NGT feeding, to boost caloric intake (Belli, D. C. *et al.* (1988) *Gastroenterology,* **94**, 603–610).

**5.2 Sulphasalazine (Salazopyrin)** Dose – acute attack 10–25 mg/kg/6 h; maintenance 10 mg/kg/6–8 h. Most useful in maintaining remission. Side effects: nausea, vomit, occasionally Heinz-body anaemia, reversible leucopenia, arthralgia, rash, Stevens–Johnson syndrome. For a mild attack, 5-aminosalicylic acid (5-ASA) enemas are an alternative. For more severe attacks, may need steroids.

**5.3 Steroids** For acute attack, methylprednisolone 0.5 mg/kg/6 h IV. For milder attack – prednisolone 1–2 mg/kg/day oral for inducing remission if sulphasalazine fails. If disease is limited, steroid enemas with or without 5-ASA enemas are preferred.

**5.4 Surgery** Total colectomy is used for intractable colonic manifestations, intractable FTT, unacceptable steroid side effects. Curative.

**5.5 Annual colonoscopy**

## 12.11.2 Crohn's disease (CD)

A segmental disease involving all bowel wall layers in a chronic inflammatory process with non-caseating granuloma. It usually involves distal ileum and colon, but may affect any part of the GIT from mouth to anus.

### 1 History

Thirty per cent of cases are <20 years of age. Presentation is extremely variable and includes abdominal pain with or without diarrhoea,

diarrhoea with or without blood/mucus, anorexia, weight loss, lethargy, pyrexia of unknown origin (PUO).
Systemic manifestations – similar to UC. PUO and clubbing are more common in CD.

### *2 Examination*

Growth failure, anaemia, clubbing (25%), delayed pubertal development, abdominal masses, perianal lesions.

### *3 Investigations*

Barium meal, follow through and enema.
Sigmoidoscopy and colonoscopy and biopsy.
FBC, ESR.
Albumin, folate, $B_{12}$, iron.

### *4 Colonic complications*

Bowel obstruction, fistulae, haemorrhage (uncommon).

### *5 Treatment*

**5.1 Good nutrition** Vital. TPN or elemental diet by nasogastric tube feeding should be considered.

**5.2 Site involved**

*Colon only involved* – sulphasalazine as per UC.
*Ileum only involved* – prednisolone 1 mg/kg/day (max. 40 mg/day) for 6 weeks, then taper. Azathiaprine and 6-mercaptopurine are second-line drugs.
*Colon and ileum* – try sulphasalazine first, and if it is unsuccessful try steroids or both.
*Perianal disease* – metronidazole.

**5.3 Surgery** Localized treatment of abscess, fistula or stricture. It may be of use in severe growth failure if there is localized disease in a prepubertal child. Surgery does not 'cure' Crohn's disease.

## 12.12 Malabsorption syndromes

The lumenal surface of the small bowel has villi and microvilli which give it a very large surface area through which absorption of food occurs. Crypt epithelial cells migrate up the villus and are eventually extruded into the gut lumen. Digestion is influenced by gastric, pancreatic, salivary and bile fluids and brush border enzymes. Absorption occurs through the epithelial cells and intercellular spaces to reach the lamina propria. Nutrients can then enter the circulation through the lymphatics or directly through the portal venous system. Malabsorption is best considered as defective absorption of fats, carbohydrates and protein.

For further explanation of the tests below, see Section 12.9.

## *Fat malabsorption (steatorrhoea)*

### *1 Physiology*

Triacyl glycerides (TAG) are broken down to free fatty acids (FFA) and 2-monoglycerides by pancreatic lipase. Cholesterol is hydrolysed by pancreatic esterase. These and other lipids (including fat-soluble vitamins) combine with lecithin and bile salts forming micelles which diffuse into enterocytes. The fats are then re-esterified, coated with lipoprotein phospholipid and cholesterol to form chylomicrons and enter the lymphatics heading for the thoracic duct. Some short- and medium-chain triglycerides (MCT) are absorbed directly into the portal venous system.

### *2 Causes of steatorrhoea*

Deficiency of:

| | |
|---|---|
| Lipase: | Cystic fibrosis – common.<br>Schwachman's syndrome – rare (FTT, bony dysostoses, neutropenia). |
| Bile salts: | Obstructive jaundice.<br>Ileal resection (diminished bile acid pool).<br>Blind loop, dysbiotic enteric flora (bile salt breakdown). |
| Enterocytes: | Coeliac disease – common.<br>Short gut, resection. |
| Chylomicrons: | Abetalipoproteinaemia (acanthocytosis, ataxia, neuropathy, retinopathy). |
| Lymphatics: | Whipple's, lymphangiectasia. |

### *3 Investigations*

**3.1 Confirmation of steatorrhoea** 3-day fat collection.

**3.2 Investigation of cause**

Sweat test.
Faecal fat globules, fatty acids.
FBC – acanthocytes, neutropenia.
Antigliadin antibodies.
Small bowel biopsy.

**3.3 Investigation of effects**
Vitamins E and A levels.
Prothrombin time (vitamin K).
Ca, P, alkaline phosphatase, wrist x-ray, or vitamin D levels.

## CARBOHYDRATE MALABSORPTION

### *1 Physiology*

Sucrose is broken down by sucrase in the brush border to fructose and glucose. Lactose is broken down by lactase to glucose and galactose. Starch, under the influence of amylase (saliva and pancreas), maltase and isomaltase (brush border), is broken down to glucose.

### *2 Causes of CHO malabsorption*

Deficiency of:

Lactase – secondary to mucosal damage (e.g. post-infective diarrhoea);
– physiological: seen in many non-Caucasians after 2–3 yr of age;
– congenital: very rare. Seen in Caucasians.

Sucrase isomaltase – see Section 12.10;
– secondary to mucosal damage;
– congenital.

Defective glucose/galactose transport – rare. Use fructose.

### *3 Investigation*

**3.1 Clinitest of faecal fluid** If sucrose is the main dietary sugar, then first hydrolyse faecal fluid by boiling in 1 N HCl for 30 s.

**3.2 Faecal pH** $<5.5$.

**3.3 D-xylose absorption.**

**3.4 Breath** $H_2$: >20 p.p.m.

## PROTEIN MALABSORPTION

### *1 Physiology*

Pepsinogen from gastric chief cells is the precursor of pepsin which initiates proteolysis. Trypsinogen, under the influence of brush border enterokinase, forms trypsin which in turn activates pancreatic zymogen so that peptides may be broken down. With the help of brush border peptidases and an active transport mechanism, amino acids can be absorbed into the portal circulation.

### *2 Causes of protein malabsorption*

N.B. Protein and fat malabsorption often go hand in hand.

**2.1 Mucosal damage** Decreased peptidases and enterokinase.

**2.2 Pancreatic insufficiency** Decreased proteases.

**2.3 Defect in amino acid transport** e.g. Hartnup disease with decreased tryptophan transport resulting in pellagrous rash, photosensitivity, ataxia, aminoaciduria. Treatment is with nicotinamide.

*3 Investigation*
Faecal nitrogen, radiolabelled albumin

### MISCELLANEOUS CAUSES OF MALABSORPTION

Blind loop syndrome.
Giardiasis.
Allergic enteropathy.
Immune deficiencies.
Abetalipoproteinaemia.
Histiocytosis X.
Acrodermatitis enteropathica.
Congenital chloridorrhoea.

## 12.13 Coeliac disease

A disease of permanent intolerance of gluten (wheat, barley, rye, ± oats). It classically presents at 9–18 months, with failure to thrive coinciding with the introduction of gluten-containing foods into the diet. Other problems are vomiting, diarrhoea (large, foul, pale stools), anorexia, irritability, lethargy. Examination typically reveals a miserable child with protuberant abdomen, wasted buttocks, pallor and, rarely, rickets. Occasionally an older child presents because of poor general health, short stature, pubertal delay or unexplained anaemia.

Continued ingestion of gluten in a gluten-sensitive person may lead to chronic malabsorption bone disease, infertility, intestinal lymphoma. The disease is associated with diabetes, atopy and IgA deficiency.

### INVESTIGATION (see Section 12.9 for details)

D-xylose absorption test (low blood levels).
3-day faecal fat balance.
Stool fat globules (usually absent), fatty acid (present).
Antigliadin antibodies.

In practice these are often bypassed in favour of intestinal biopsy.

## DIAGNOSIS AND MANAGEMENT

- *It is not possible to make a clinical diagnosis of coeliac disease – it must be proven histologically. Recommending an empirical trial of gluten-free diet is irresponsible.*

### *1 Small bowel biopsy*

Demonstrate villous atrophy, crypt hyperplasia and mononuclear infiltrate in lamina propria while on a gluten-containing diet.

### *2 Gluten-free diet*

For 2 years or until growth is completed, after which one should re-biopsy (some biopsy earlier), to document histological response.

### *3 Gluten challenge*

There is some question as to whether or not gluten challenge is justifiable (*J. Pediatr. Gastroent. Nutrit.* (1986) **5**, 565–569). If a challenge is considered worth while, then it is best done after 2 years or perhaps after growth is complete. Clinical evidence of relapse after gluten challenge should be confirmed with a further small intestinal biopsy. If, however, the child remains asymptomatic, then re-biopsy in any event 2 years after the challenge. A normal mucosa at this stage usually excludes the disease, although later relapses have been known.

### *4 Lifelong treatment*

A diagnosis of coeliac disease requires lifelong treatment, although some acquire the ability to withstand small challenges. There is an increased incidence of intestinal lymphoma and carcinoma in untreated and perhaps also in treated adults.

## Further reading

Ashkenazi, A. (1989) Living with celiac disease. *Child. Hosp. Quart.*, **1**, 265–270

Guandalini, S., Ventura, A., Ansaldi, N. *et al.* (1989) Diagnosis of coeliac disease: time for a change? *Arch. Dis. Child.*, **64**, 1320–1325

# 12.14 Constipation and encopresis

There is seldom a physical cause for constipation besides a painful anal fissure causing a reluctance to defaecate, resulting in faecal retention, hard stools, painful defaecation, and hence a vicious circle is set up. Hirschsprung's disease is unlikely if meconium was passed in the first 24 h of life. Children with neuromuscular handicap or hypothyroidism are predisposed to constipation.

Encopresis is the (usually involuntary) passage of stools into the underwear on a regular basis. Most encopretic children have chronic faecal retention as the underlying disorder, leading to chronic rectal dilatation and subsequent insensitivity to the normal urge to stool.

## CLINICAL FEATURES

There may be no apparent clinical features, or the child may have complaints of lacking in energy, poor appetite, abdominal pain, faecal soiling and spurious diarrhoea. Fresh blood in the stools suggests a fissure which might be seen on inspection of the anus. An impression of faecal loading of the colon can usually be obtained by abdominal examination, digital examination of the rectum (although constipation above the rectum may occur), or perhaps best of all, by plain abdominal x-ray (AXR). Urinary symptoms are common. Hirschsprung's disease classically gives an empty rectum, relatively tight anus. It need not be considered unless symptoms date back to early infancy.

## TREATMENT

Investigations are usually unnecessary apart from AXR. Explain to the child at an appropriate level that treatment aims to empower him to control his bowels and, in a sense, his own life. The child must regain confidence in his ability to pass a painless bowel motion.

### Aim

To empty the rectum and then keep it empty over many months.

Treatment should be aggressive and in chronic constipation or encopresis ideally should continue for at least 6 months to allow colonic calibre to return to normal and for the child to relearn the sensation of a full rectum. Regular follow-up is essential.

Treatment modalities include the following (N.B. Some drugs have more than one mode of action.)

#### *1 Dietary fibre*

Retains water and encourages bacterial growth, thus increasing faecal mass, gas and water and hence increasing peristalsis.

#### *2 Gut stimulants*

Senna is hydrolysed by colonic bacteria, and free anthracenes are absorbed and stimulate peristalsis. Onset of action is 8–12 h; hence it is given at bedtime. Bisacodyl (Dulcolax) is structurally related to the phenolphthaleins. Docusate sodium (Dioctyl) is only a weak gut stimulant with detergent-like actions. Danthron has been withdrawn because of possible carcinogenic potential.

### *3 Faecal softeners*

Many laxatives soften faeces. Liquid paraffin is useful in the short term, but may cause anal irritation and fat-soluble vitamin malabsorption in the long term.

### *4 Osmotic laxatives*

Lactulose exerts an osmotic effect and may encourage the proliferation of 'sachyrophilic' bacteria, thus increasing faecal mass. Magnesium hydroxide (with or without paraffin) or magnesium sulphate are traditionally prescribed for rapid bowel evacuation, not for treating constipation.

## SUGGESTED PROTOCOL

### *1 Therapeutic agents*

For mild–moderate constipation, use 1.1 and 1.2 ± 1.3, below. For more intractable problems also use 1.4 and 1.5.

**1.1 High-fibre diet education** Send to a dietitian if necessary. The whole family should change eating habits along with child.

**1.2 Bulk-forming agent** Fybogel, Normacol.

**1.3 Sennoside** 'Senekot' syr. 7.5 mg/5 ml. 1–6 yr, 1–5 ml nocte; 6 yr+, 5–10 ml nocte. This may temporarily worsen colicky abdominal pains.

**1.4 Lactulose** Initial dose: 1 yr, 3–5 ml; 1–5 yr, 5–10 ml; 6–12 yr, 15 ml, all given b.d. Doses may be doubled if ineffective.

**1.5 For severe constipation** or failure of simple medical treatment, use Microlette Microenema 5 ml daily or on alternate days over several days. Alternatively, admission to hospital and administration of 'phosphates' enemata may be required. Dose: 2–6 yr, 50 ml; 6 yr+, 128 ml. This can be repeated daily. After the initial catharsis, it is best to avoid rectal medications to minimize further anal fixation.

### *2 Encourage toileting*

This is done by the patient setting 10 min aside after breakfast daily to take advantage of gastrocolic reflex. Putting the feet up on a small foot stool will make defaecation easier.

### *3 Avoid punishment and emphasis on failure*

A relaxed attitude by the parents is needed. N.B. For chronic constipation, treatment should continue for many months.

### FAILED MEDICAL TREATMENT

1. Many behavioural problems and more complex psychopathologies are linked to constipation. Psychiatric expertise may be needed.
2. Short-segment Hirschsprung's disease may need to be excluded with rectal biopsy if symptoms date back from early infancy.

## Further reading

Anon. (1988) Laxatives: replacing danthron. *Drug Ther. Bull.*, **26**, 53–56

# 12.15 Parasitic infections

These include roundworms (nematodes), tapeworms (cestodes), flukes (trematodes) and protozoa.

Of the nematodes, threadworm (pinworm, *Enterobius vermicularis*) is the most common by far in the UK. Hookworm, *Ascaris*, whipworm and strongyloidiasis are rarely seen. Other parasitic worms (helminths) such as schistosomiasis, filariasis, trypanosomiasis and leishmaniasis are among the major world health problems but are not seen in the UK and will not be discussed.

Protozoal disease includes *Giardia, Amoeba, Toxoplasma*, Cryptosporidium, malaria, *Pneumocystis* and babesiosis, all of which are responsible for much morbidity or mortality in different parts of the world.

In this section we will discuss some nematode infestations.

The following tests may be useful in investigating suspected gut parasites.

### EOSINOPHILIA

Eosinophilia is a good clue to systemic invasion by intestinal helminths, whereas those remaining in the gut lumen evoke a mild response or none at all.

### STOOLS

Stools will often reveal helminth ova or protozoal cysts even in older specimens, but in order to identify living motile forms a 'hot specimen' is required.

#### *1 Stool microscopy*

It can be performed by placing a faecal sample the size of a small drop of water on each of 2 slides. Add 2 drops of saline to one and 2 drops of dilute iodine solution to the other, and cover with a coverslip. Examine under low power for helminth ova and high power/oil immersion for protozoal cysts. The unstained slide may reveal motile organisms (amoeba, trophozoites, larvae) under low or high power. Red cells are seen in the rare case of amoebic colitis. Leucocytes are best seen with Wright's or Gram stains, and suggest bacterial or inflammatory bowel disease.

### *2 'Sticky tape test'*

Lay a piece of clear adhesive tape, gummed side outwards, over a spatula and hold it in place with a rubber band around the spatula. Dab it on the perianal area first thing in the morning. Place the tape, sticky side down over a drop of toluene and examine under low power for threadworm (*E. vermicularis*) eggs.

## 12.16 Threadworms/pinworms (*Enterobius vermicularis*)

This is a relatively common gut parasitic infestation, affecting children more commonly than adults. It tends to occur in groups such as families living together. Humans are the only known hosts. The transmission is by ingestion of eggs from the hands or finger-nails of carriers.

### MORPHOLOGY

The male is 5 mm long and 0.1–0.2 mm in diameter. The female is 13 mm long, with a diameter of 0.3–0.5 mm. Eggs are 50–60 μm long and 20–30 μm in breadth.

### CLINICAL ASPECTS

Pruritus ani can be very troublesome and is often worse at night. Itching may lead to perianal inflammation and secondary bacterial infection. Rarely, the parasite lodges in the appendix causing appencititis. Insomnia, hyperactivity and nocturnal enuresis are not uncommon.

### DIAGNOSIS

See 'Sticky tape test' – Section 12.15.

Look for eggs around the anus with either a swab or adhesive tape. The eggs are not usually found in faeces. Intact worms may be passed on defaecation. Parents may see the worms if they inspect the perianal area while the child is asleep.

## TREATMENT

Treat all children in the household at the same time.

1. Pyrantel pamoate 10 mg/kg (max. 1 g) × 1. Repeat after 2 weeks.
   *Or*
2. Mebendazole 100 mg × 1. Repeat after 2 weeks. Not recommended under 2 years.
   *Or*
3. Pyrvinium pamoate 5 mg/kg (max. 350 mg). Repeat after 2 weeks.
   *Or*
4. Piperazine citrate 75 mg/kg/day for 2 days (max. 2.5 g/day) – seldom used.

## PREVENTION

Cutting finger-nails and hand-washing after defaecation may reduce transmission and self-reinfection.

# 12.17 *Ascaris lumbricoides*

This has a worldwide distribution, but is more frequent in moist warm climates (an unlikely contingency in the UK). Humans are the only susceptible hosts and are infected by faecal oral passage.

## MORPHOLOGY AND LIFE CYCLE

The round worm is easily recognizable to the naked eye and is 20–30 cm long. The female produces 200 000 ova per day which are passed in human faeces. The larva develops within an ovum in warm moist soil. Humans then ingest these 'live' ova which hatch in the jejunum, and the larvae penetrate the mucosa, after which they are carried by the blood to liver, heart and lungs. They escape into alveoli and are coughed up and swallowed again, finally reaching the intestine. This remarkable visceral round trip takes 2 weeks. Life span is 1–2 years.

## CLINICAL FEATURES

### *1 Pulmonary stage – within 2 weeks of ingestion*

Varying picture ranging from mild cough to severe pneumonia, with fever, haemoptysis and bronchospasm (Loeffler's syndrome).

*2 Intestinal stage – usually symptomless*
The wanderlust of the *Ascaris* can result in intestinal obstruction, appendicitis, regurgitation of worms, liver abscess.

## DIAGNOSIS

Ova in microscopic examination of faeces.
Worms seen in vomitus or stool.

## TREATMENT

*1 Pulmonary Ascaris – no treatment*
Dying larvae may make matters worse. Steroids may help.

*2 Intestinal Ascaris*
All cases should be treated because of the risk of complications.

**2.1 Mebendazole** 100 mg b.d. for 3 days if >2 yr. *Or*

**2.2 Pyrantel pamoate** 10 mg/kg × 1 (max. 1 g).

**2.3 Piperazine citrate** 75 mg/kg/day (max. 3.5 g) × 2 days is seldom used because of potential, neurotoxic and hepatotoxic side effects and hypersensitivity reaction.

## PREVENTION

Sanitary disposal of faeces.

# 12.18 Whipworm (*Trichuris trichiura*)

This too is seen commonly in the tropics. The human is the only natural reservoir and susceptible host. Transmission is by the faecal oral route.

## MORPHOLOGY AND LIFE CYCLE

The adult worm, 30–50 mm long, has a threadlike anterior portion and a broader posterior part. The females produce characteristic barrel-shaped eggs which are passed in the stool and then require 10 days to reach the infective stage. Ingested infective eggs attach in the duodenum and, when mature, migrate to caecum and colon.

### CLINICAL FEATURES

Light infections are asymptomatic. Heavier infections cause abdominal pain, tenesmus or bloody mucoid diarrhoea. Rare accompaniments include appendicitis, prolapsed rectum and malnutrition.

### TREATMENT

As per *Ascaris*.

## 12.19 Visceral larva migrans

This illness results from infection with tissue-dwelling nematodes, specifically the larvae of *Toxocara* spp. It usually occurs in children under 10 years, particularly those who have close contact with dogs and cats.

### LIFE CYCLE

*Toxocara canis* and *T. cati* are common parasites of dogs and cats. The adult worms lay large numbers of eggs in the intestines of these animals, which are then passed in the faeces. Ingestion of infective eggs by man is followed by larval penetration of the gut and migration to the liver, lungs and occasionally other sites. The larvae do not develop further in humans.

### CLINICAL MANIFESTATIONS

The typical history is one of fever, wheezing or seizures.
Examination may reveal hepatomegaly, wheezing, urticarial skin lesions and lymphadenopathy. Ocular toxocariasis is also reported.

### DIAGNOSIS

Eosinophilia (often up to 50 000/mm$^3$) – in all cases except ocular disease.
ELISA.

## TREATMENT

Usually none is needed as the disease is self-limiting over several weeks. Prednisolone 5 mg/kg/day may help severe respiratory symptoms. In severe cases, treatment is controversial. Some recommend none, others thiobendazole 25 mg/kg/12 h × 5 days (common side effect of nausea, vomit, dizziness).

# Further reading

Markell, E. K. (1985) Intestinal nematode infection. *Pediatr. Clin. N. Am.*, **32,** 971–986

Chapter 13

# Nephrology

## 13.1 Urinary tract infection (UTI)

The implication of diagnosing a UTI in a male or female child is that the urinary tract must be investigated; hence it is vital to prove rather than suspect a UTI, in order to avoid over- or under-investigation. Therefore, before commencing treatment ensure that an uncontaminated urine specimen has been taken. Accurate diagnosis and prompt treatment in children less than 5 years of age are important in order to minimize the chance of renal scarring.

Radiological abnormalities are found in approximately 50% of children with documented UTI of which about 75% are vesico-ureteric (VU) reflux. For significant VU reflux, low-dose chemoprophylaxis is increasingly being chosen over surgery.

### AETIOLOGY

*E. coli* – accounts for 80%
Others – *Proteus, Klebsiella, Pseudomonas, Streptococcus faecalis.*
Rarely – *Staphylococcus epidermidis, S. aureus.*

### PREDISPOSITIONS

Vesico-ureteric reflux.
Urethral valves.
Duplex system.
Ureterocele.
Pelvi-ureteric obstruction.
Uncircumcised infant (at least those <6 months).
Constipation.

### CLINICAL FEATURES

Symptoms and signs are usually non-specific, especially in a younger child. They include unexplained fever, vomiting, diarrhoea, abdominal pain, frequency, secondary enuresis. Most cases of dysuria or offensive urine are due to local vulvulitis or upper respiratory infection. Anxiety or tension may cause dysuria. Urge incontinence, especially when accompanied by abdominal pain, may be due to constipation, but constipation itself may predispose to UTI.

There is no simple technique that will reliably localize UTI in children, and clinical features can be misleading. Pyelonephritis is suggested by high fever (>39°C), toxic-looking child, loin pain and tenderness, and is commonly associated with VU reflux.

Examination should include measurement of BP, ballottement of the kidneys, palpation and percussion for a large bladder that suggests urethral valves, a careful inspection of genitalia and perineum, and attention to the degree of faecal loading of the colon which might suggest constipation.

## METHODS OF URINE COLLECTION

Always check for balanitis or vulvitis and interpret MSU or bag urine result with caution if present.

### *1 Mid-stream urine (MSU)*

It can usually be obtained in a child over 3 years of age.

### *2 Clean catch specimen*

May be obtained from children under 3 years, especially when undressing them prior to putting on a bag or performing a SPA.

### *3 Suprapubic aspiration (SPA)*

See Section 4.2. Always have a sterile container at the ready for a clean catch, in case the child voids spontaneously while being prepared for the SPA.

### *4 Bag specimen*

Useful in children under 3 years of age. The skin should be cleansed with sterile water, not antiseptic, and the urine bag removed as soon as possible after voiding. Colony counts of $< 10^4$ probably exclude infection, but higher counts may represent genuine UTI or merely bacterial contamination from skin or faeces, and therefore repeat collection with SPA or MSU is indicated. If the child is unwell, or if one wishes to commence antibiotic treatment, perform a SPA at the outset rather than first collecting a bag specimen and waiting 2 days for what is often an equivocal result.

### *5 Catheter specimen*

Performed on children with ileal conduit, i.e. a ‘conduit specimen’. Also after failed SPA when a specimen is urgently needed before starting treatment in a sick child.

**Axiom** Collecting bacteriologically uncontaminated urine is mandatory before commencing treatment for UTI.

## DIAGNOSIS

### *1 Cultures*

Urine and occasionally blood. Urine must be plated within 1 h of collection. If this is not possible, dipslides (Uricult) may be used.

**1.1 MSU or clean catch** A pure growth of $>10^5$ colony-forming units (CFU)/ml is significant; $10^4$–$10^5$ is equivocal, although probably insignificant if there is a mixed growth, but the test should be repeated. (N.B. Prior antibiotic treatment may give this result.)

**1.2 SPA** Any number of organisms is significant.

**1.3 Bag specimen** If specimen shows $< 10^4$ CFU/ml, then infection is probably excluded; $10^4$ CFU/ml or more indicates the need for repeat collection by MSU or SPA because of possible contamination from skin or faeces.

**1.4 Blood culture** Should be taken on all neonates (very high risk of septicaemia) and children with suspected pyelonephritis.

### *2 Microscopy*

Absence of pus cells does not rule out infection (Ginsberg and McCracken, 1982), although it makes it unlikely. Pyuria, although indicating possible infection, is not diagnostic. Sterile urine can give leucocyte counts of $>10/mm^3$, especially in vulvitis (*Lancet* (1975) **i,** 476–478). (N.B. Colony counts are in $cm^3$ and cell counts are in $mm^3$.)

Bacteriuria seen on stained uncentrifuged urine is a reliable indicator of infection (Ginsberg and McCracken, 1982). Granular casts suggest intrarenal disease.

### *3 Dipsticks*

The finding of urinary nitrites is very indicative of UTI, although there are many false negatives. The yield increases if the first morning voided specimen is used (*Arch. Dis. Child.* (1987) **62**, 138–140). Trace proteinuria as an isolated finding is meaningless.

## TREATMENT

### *1 Antibiotics*

N.B. *Has an adequate sample been taken for bacteriology*?

**1.1 Initial therapy for the severely ill child** Such a child may have accompanying septicaemia (especially neonates). Amoxycillin 25–40 mg/kg/8 h IV (or ampicillin 50 mg/kg/6 h), *plus*

Gentamicin 2–2.5 mg/kg/dose 8 hourly if renal function is normal.
*Measure drug levels.*
If renal function is abnormal adjust dosage interval:

$$\text{New interval} = \text{Standard interval (8 h)} \times \frac{\text{Patient's creatinine}}{\text{Normal creatinine}}$$

In the first 2 weeks of life give ampicillin /8 h and gentamicin /12 h with doses unchanged.

**1.2 Initial therapy for a relatively well child** Trimethoprim (TMP) 2.5–5 mg/kg/12 h for 5 days. Most urinary pathogens are resistant to sulphas. Cotrimoxazole has no advantage over monotherapy with TMP (White, 1987) and has more side effects. If used, the dose is nevertheless TMP 2.5–5 mg/kg/12 h in a 1:5 ratio with sulphamethoxazole.

**1.3 Duration of treatment** Treat according to sensitivities for 5–7 days in simple UTI, or for 10–14 days in suspected pyelonephritis.

**1.4 Alternative antibiotics include:**

*1.4.1 Amoxycillin* 10–15 mg/kg/8 h.

*1.4.2 Nitrofurantoin* Effective but causes nausea and vomiting, especially in young children who can only take the liquid preparation. Four doses (1--2 mg/kg/6 h) per day are recommended (two would probably suffice).

*1.4.3 Nalidixic acid* 10–15 mg/kg/6 h. Uncommonly causes severe headaches and vomiting due to a hypersensitivity reaction causing benign intracranial hypertension.

**1.5 Single dose therapy** There is evidence that one large dose works well in adults with cystitis in achieving bacteriological cure. In children, this is not as yet recommended because localizing the UTI is much more difficult, the dangers of renal scarring are much greater, and with single dose treatment higher recurrence rates have been noted (Madrigal, G., 1988, *Pediatr. Inf. Dis.*, **7**, 316–319).

## 2 Low-dose prophylaxis

**2.1 Indicated for:**

*2.1.1 Children under 5 years* who have a first UTI should have prophylaxis until radiological investigation is undertaken to exclude reflux.

*2.1.2 Significant reflux* of any grade that is managed non-operatively. Continue until reflux resolves, or age 7, or 2 years after last UTI.

*2.1.3 Obstructive uropathy* or neuropathic bladder with recurrent UTI.

*2.1.4 Prepubertal girls* with recurrent UTI despite normal urinary tract.

**2.2 Doses** Trimethoprim 2.5–5 mg/kg single daily dose (or cotrimoxazole at equivalent dose of TMP); nitrofurantoin 2 mg/kg single daily dose; nalidixic acid 20 mg/kg single daily dose.

**2.3 Breakthrough infections** These should be managed according to sensitivities. *Pseudomonas* infection can be managed with a single daily dose of IM aminoglycoside as an outpatient for 5 days. It gives very high urinary levels, and lasts $> 18$ h. The new fluoroquinolones probably should not be used in children because of adverse effects on growing cartilage in weight-bearing joints. *Candida* infection usually resolves with a brief interruption in antibiotic prophylaxis, although uncommonly oral ketoconazole or flucytosine may be needed.

### *3 General measures*

**3.1 Liberal fluid intake**

**3.2 Triple voiding** Especially for VU reflux. Effective but impractical.

**3.3 Perineal hygiene**

**3.4 Treat suspected constipation**

### *4 Circumcision*

There is evidence that uncircumcised boys are at far greater risk of UTI than their circumcised counterparts, at least in the first year of life (*Pediatr.* (1985) **75**, 901). Any boy with recurrent UTI should have circumcision considered whether the foreskin is tight or not (Winberg *et al.*, 1989).

## INVESTIGATIONS

All children with confirmed UTI need investigation, although there is controversy as to how this is best done. Below, a simple method is offered, although various grades of more elaborate investigation have their merits (Whitaker, R. H. and Sherwood, T. (1987) *Lancet,* **i,** 1266).

The micturating cystourethrogram (MCU) is the best way of diagnosing VU reflux. All agree that it should be done for children $< 1$ year old, and not done for those $> 8$ years. Some say that in the intervening years between 1 and 8, when chances of renal scarring are diminished, it is only needed if US or IVP are abnormal, or if infection recurs, whereas others hold that it should be done in any child until age 7 or 8, after the first UTI. It is an unpleasant experience for the child and involves gonadal irradiation.

### *1 Child <5 years*

Ultrasound and MCU and plain AXR. If any is abnormal or if US cannot be done, then perform an IVP. US should be carried out at the time of the infection, whereas MCU should be deferred for 4–6 weeks during which time the child should remain on antibiotic prophylaxis until reflux has been excluded.

### *2 Child >5 years*

US and AXR. An abnormal result or a second UTI indicates the need for IVP to obtain better definition of kidneys and ureters.

## CONTROVERSIES IN MANAGING VU REFLUX

Reflux nephropathy results from the reflux of infected urine into the renal parenchyma. Prevention of nephropathy must focus on preventing bacteria with antibiotic prophylaxis or surgical prevention of reflux by either reimplanting ureters or by endoscopic sub-ureteric injection of polytetrafluoroethylene. Of these, reimplantation of ureters is increasingly less favoured.

## Further reading


Alon, U., Berant, M. and Pery, M. (1989) Intravenous pyelography in children with urinary tract infection and vesicoureteric reflux. *Pediatr.,* **83,** 332–336

Alon, U., Pery, M., Davidai, G. and Berant, M. (1986) Ultrasonagraphy in the radiologic evaluation of children with urinary tract infection. *Pediatr.,* **78**, 58–64

Bailey, R. R. (1986) Single dose therapy of urinary tract infections. In *Recent Advances in Paediatrics* (ed. Meadow, R.), Churchill Livingstone, Edinburgh

Ginsberg, C. M. and McCracken, G. H. (1982) Urinary tract infections in young infants. *Pediatr.,* **69**, 409–412

Haycock, G. B. (1986) Investigation of urinary tract infection. *Arch. Dis. Child.,* **61**, 1155–1158

Herzog, L. W. (1989) Urinary tract infections and circumcision: a case-control study. *Am. J. Dis. Child.,* **143**, 348–350

McCracken, G. H. and Nelson, J. D. (eds) (1989) Symposium on genitourinary and gastrointestinal infections. *Pediatr. Infect. Dis. J.,* **8**, 547–563

O'Donnell, P. (1990) Management of urinary tract infection and vesicoureteric reflux in children. The case for surgery. *Br. Med. J.,* **300**, 1393–1394

Puri, P. (1990) Endoscopic correction of primary vesico-ureteric reflux by sub-ureteric injection of polytetrafluorethylene. *Lancet,* **335**, 1320–1322

White, R. H. R. (1987) Management of urinary tract infection. *Arch. Dis. Child.,* **62**, 421–427

White, R. H. R. (1990) Management of urinary tract infection and vesicoureteric reflux in children. Operative treatment has no advantage over medical management. *Br. Med. J.,* **300**, 1391–1392

Winberg, J., Bollgren, I., Gothefors, L. *et al.* (1989) The prepuce: a mistake of nature? *Lancet,* **i**, 598–599

Wiswell, T. E. *et al.* (1988) Effect of circumcision status on periurethral bacterial flora during the first year of life. *J. Pediatr.,* **113**, 442–446

# 13.2 Hypertension (HT)

Severe sustained HT in childhood carries a high risk of morbidity and mortality if untreated. In > 80% there is an underlying often remediable cause. The benefits of recognizing and treating mild–moderate HT are not so clear.

## MEASURING BLOOD PRESSURE (see Section 4.1)

## DEFINITION OF HYPERTENSION

See Figure 13.1 (more detailed charts can be found in the Report of the Second Task Force on Blood Pressure Control in Children (1987) *Pediatr.*, **79**, 5–6).

A BP above the 95th centile for age is by convention regarded as 'abnormal' (moderate–severe). Mild hypertension is defined as being between the 90th and 95th centile, although its significance is unknown. Fatter and taller children tend to have higher blood pressure than their peers; hence it would make more sense to define hypertension as being > 95th centile for height. To this end, tables of BP against height are

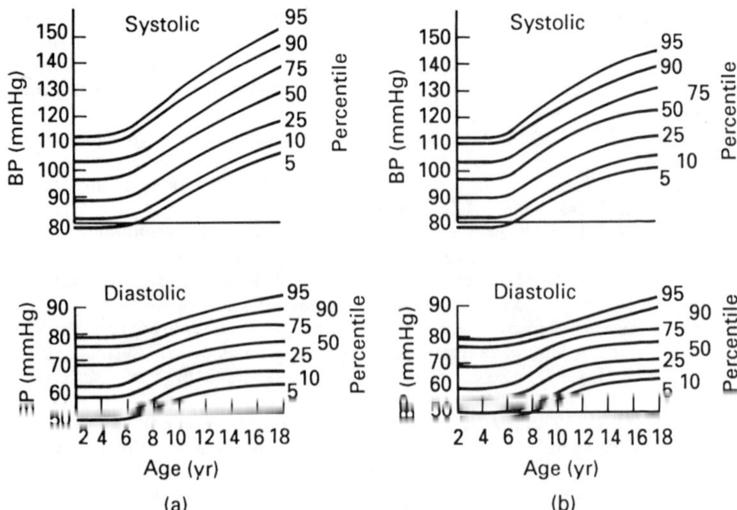


**Figure 13.1** Percentiles of blood pressure in children (right arm, seated): (a) males; (b) females) (From *Pediatrics* (1977) **59**, 803, with permission)

probably best of all in children between ages 2 and 14 years (de Swiet, M., Dillon, M. J., Littler, W. *et al.* (1989) Measurement of blood pressure in children. Recommendations of a working party of the British Hypertension Society. *Br. Med. J.*, **299**, 497). If the first recording is high, it should be remeasured on two or more occasions.

## AETIOLOGY

### *1 Primary or essential hypertension*

Mild hypertension (90–95th centile) is usually essential or primary in nature. Obese children feature prominently in this group (some of whom may have been misdiagnosed because of too small a cuff). More severe hypertension usually has a discernible cause.

### *2 Secondary hypertension*

Commonest causes are reflux nephropathy and chronic glomerulonephritis.

#### 2.1 Renal

*2.1.1 Renal parenchymal disease* Acute and chronic glomerulonephritis, reflux nephropathy, obstructive uropathy, congenital (polycystic, hydronephrosis), renal dysplasia.

*2.1.2 Renovascular disease* Renal vein thrombosis, renal artery stenosis including neurofibromatosis, renal artery aneurysm/thrombosis, arteritis.

*2.1.3 Renal tumours* Rarely cause HT – Wilms' tumour, sarcoma.

**2.2 Cardiovascular** Coarctation of the aorta.

#### 2.3 Endocrine

*2.3.1 Catecholamine excess* Pheochromocytoma, neuroblastoma.

*2.3.2 Excess corticosteroids* Cushing's syndrome, hyperaldosteronism, drugs (gluco- and mineralocorticoids, oral contraceptives), congenital adrenal hyperplasia with increased mineralocorticoid production (11β-OHase deficiency), adrenal carcinoma.

#### 2.4 Others

Autonomic neuropathy (Guillain-Barré, polio, dysautonomia).
Raised intracranial pressure.
Administration of excess blood, plasma, saline.
Burns.
Hypercalcaemia.

## CLINICAL PRESENTATION

### *1 History*

Mild–moderate HT usually does not cause symptoms, although it may occasionally cause lethargy, headache and vomiting. Severe HT may result in fits and neurological lesions.

Cardiovascular system (CVS) – breathlessness on exertion, cough.

Renal – nocturia, polyuria, oliguria or haematuria are due to renal involvement.

Episodes of pallor, sweating, tachycardia, flushing suggest pheochromocytoma.

### *2 Examination*

Measure BP in all four limbs – see Section 4.1. The cuff should be two-thirds the length of the upper arm and the bladder should completely encircle the arm.

Assess for possible fluid overload.

Weak femoral pulses or brachiofemoral delay suggest coarctation.

Fundi – narrowing and irregularity of arterioles followed later by haemorrhages, exudates and papilloedema.

Precordium – the left ventricle (LV) is usually enlarged. A third heart sound suggests left ventricular failure and a fourth heart sound left atrial hypertrophy. With worsening hypertension, normal splitting of S2 (i.e. P2 after A2 in inspiration) is lost and reverse splitting (i.e. A2 after P2 in expiration) may be heard, along with a loud aortic component of the S2.

Abdominal examination – palpate both kidneys and feel gently for suprarenal or other tumours and for an enlarged bladder. Pressure on a pheochromocytoma may precipitate a hypertensive episode. Auscultate over the kidneys, front and back, for the bruit of renal artery stenosis.

Inspect for – features of Cushing's syndrome and neurofibromatosis.

### *3 Acute (malignant) hypertensive crisis*

Presents with encephalopathy, seizures, headache, papilloedema, cardiac failure or a diastolic BP of >110 mmHg.

## POSSIBLE INITIAL INVESTIGATION

The sequence depends on clinical assessment. In acute hypertensive crisis, getting control of BP takes priority over investigating the cause.

### *1 Urine*

**1.1 Proteinuria and red cells** Suggest intrinsic renal disease or effects of hypertension. Heavy proteinuria and casts favour the former.

**1.2 Culture and sensitivity**

**1.3 24 h collection** For VMA and catecholamine estimation. Methyldopa interferes with this test. 24 h urinary free cortisol.

### *2 Blood*

**2.1 Urea and creatinine**

**2.2 $K^+$ and $Na^+$** Low $K^+$ and high $Na^+$ suggest hyperaldosteronism but may occur with renal disease. Low $Na^+$ and high $K^+$ suggest renal failure (or salt-losing congenital adrenal hyperplasia in which HT only occurs with overtreatment).

**2.3 High ASOT and low serum complement** Suggest post-streptococcal nephritis.

**2.4 FBC and haematocrit** May point to renal disease or fluid overload.

**2.5 Plasma renin activity**

**2.6 Endocrine** If there are features of Cushing's syndrome, then a.m. and p.m. cortisol levels will screen for Cushing's syndrome ± dexamethasone suppression test.

### *3 CXR*

Look for cardiomegaly, signs of coarctation.

### *4 ECG – LVH*

Increase in R-wave voltage in LV leads. With heart failure, ST depression and/or T inversion may occur.

### *5 US and DMSA scan*

If these are not available, an IVP is an acceptable but less sensitive alternative. US will detect abnormalities of renal structure (e.g. polycystic kidneys, hydronephrosis). DMSA scan is very sensitive in detecting regions of pyelonephritic scarring and localized ischaemic areas due to renovascular disease, and provides useful information concerning differential function.

### *6 Later investigations*

Should be carried out under the direction of a paediatric nephrologist.

## MANAGEMENT OF HT AND COMMENTS ON SOME HYPERTENSIVE DRUGS

### *1 Acute severe hypertension*

**1.1 Labetalol** Drug of choice: 1–3 mg/kg/h IV infusion. This is an alpha and beta adrenoreceptor blocker. Side effects include hypotension, heart failure, bronchospasm, GI upset, headache.

**1.2 Sodium nitroprusside** Drug of choice. Causes immediate vasodilatation. The effects disappear within 1 min of the drug being discontinued. Starting dose 0.5 μg/kg/min. Increase dose by increments of 0.5 μg/kg/min until desired effect is achieved. Should only be used if continuous BP monitoring is available, in an intensive care setting. Maximum dose 8 μg/kg/min. Put 3 mg/kg in 50 ml 5% dextrose: 1 ml/h = 1 μg/kg/min. Thiocyanate levels must be monitored if using >4 μg/kg/min. N.B. The prepared solution is inactivated by light; hence IV tubing should be covered in aluminium foil.

**1.3 Diazoxide** 2 mg/kg/dose IV stat (push dose over <10 s). Repeat every 15 min until BP is controlled, then 6 h p.r.n. This is a non-diuretic thiazide causing direct arteriolar dilatation. Side effects: profound hypotension, salt and water retention, hyperglycaemia. If more than 2 doses are given, use with frusemide to prevent salt and water accumulation.

**1.4 Phentolamine** An alpha blocker used primarily for managing pheochromocytoma.
Dose: 20–50 μg/kg/min infusion.

**1.5 Frusemide** Loop diuretic for use in salt and water overload, e.g. acute nephritis.

## *2 Moderate–severe hypertension*

**2.1 Hydralazine** Drug of choice. Dose: 0.2–0.4 mg/kg (max. 25 mg) slow IV or IM, then 0.1–0.2 mg/kg/4–6 h. Oral: 0.2 mg/kg/dose gradually increasing as necessary to max. of 2.0 mg/kg/12 h. It is a direct-acting arteriolar smooth muscle vasodilator. Side effects include tachycardia (may need prior beta-blockade with propranolol), nausea, vomit, headache and a rare dose-dependent lupus-like reaction.

**2.2 Propranolol** Drug of choice. Dose: 1–10 mg/kg/day orally in 2–4 divided doses, or 0.02–0.1 mg/kg/dose IV over 10 min, repeated as necessary, then 6 hourly. (N.B. Small IV dose.) This classical beta-blocker is a competitive antagonist of catecholamines on beta receptors in the heart, kidney, post-ganglionic nerve endings and in the CNS. Side effects include worsening heart failure, asthma or diabetes, some sodium and water retention, Raynaud's phenomenon, nightmares, lethargy.

**2.3 Atenolol** Dose 1–2 mg/kg/12–24 h oral. 0.05 mg/kg/dose IV every 5 min till response (max. 4 doses). It is a relatively cardioselective beta-blocker. Side effects as for propranolol.

**2.4 Angiotensin-converting enzyme inhibitors** Captopril – dose 0.25–1.0 mg/kg/8 h oral. Start with lower dose and gradually titrate increases in dose against response. It inhibits the enzymatic conversion of angiotensin I to highly vasoactive angiotensin II. Side effects include neutropenia, reversible renal failure in those with pre-existing renal disease, rashes, angio-oedema of face, taste disturbance and cough.

Enalapril – dose 0.2–1.0 mg/kg/day oral. Not yet widely used in children.

**2.5 Nifedipine** A calcium channel inhibitor. Dose 0.1–0.2 mg/kg/8 h orally (can be used sublingually). Dose may be increased to 0.3–0.5 mg/kg/8 h. Side effects include troublesome headaches and uncontrolled hypotension.

**2.6 Others** Diuretics should only be used for moderate HT associated with fluid overload as seen in acute nephritis/acute renal failure, otherwise the salt depletion may predispose to hyper-reninaemia.

### *3 Mild hypertension*

One needs to balance the risks of prolonged drug treatment against those of leaving mild HT untreated. Non-pharmacological therapy (diet, weight loss) should be tried initially, followed by a thiazide diuretic to which a diet rich in potassium or a potassium-sparing agent (e.g. spironolactone, amiloride) should be added. If unsuccessful, a beta-blocker or calcium channel inhibitor may be used.

**3.1 Conservative treatment** A low sodium diet coupled with weight loss is often helpful. Refer to a dietitian.

**3.2 Chlorothiazide** 10 mg/kg/12–24 h oral.

**3.3 Hydrochlorothiazide** 1 mg/kg/12–24 h oral.

Thiazides cause ECF volume depletion by inhibiting sodium transport in the distal tubule. There may also be other haemodynamic effects. The major side effect is hypokalaemia.

## Further reading

Dillon, M. J. (1984) Modern management of hypertension. In *Recent Advances in Paediatrics*, No. 7 (ed. Meadow, R.), Churchill Livingstone, London, pp. 35–55

Dillon, M. J. (1987) Investigation and management of hypertension in children. *Pediatr. Nephrol.*, **1**, 59–68

Dillon, M. J. (1988) Blood pressure. *Arch. Dis. Child.*, **63**, 347–349

Lauer, R. M., Burns, T. L. and Clarke, W. R. (1985) Assessing children's blood pressure – considerations of age and body size: the Muscatine study. *Pediatrics*, **75**, 1081–1090

# 13.3 Proteinuria and haematuria

## PROTEINURIA

### *1 'Normal' urine protein loss*

The normal concentration of protein in urine is <200 mg/litre, usually <50 mg/litre. Any child with >200 mg/litre should have an overnight and a 24 h collection for protein; <200 mg/day or <5 mg/m$^2$/h overnight or, in early infancy, <240 mg/m$^2$/day is normal. Trace proteinuria on routine commercial reagent strips is normal.

### *2 Mild–moderate proteinuria (200–500 mg/day)*

May occasionally be caused by fever, exercise, dehydration, heart failure, cystitis, orthostatic proteinuria. Some renal causes of mild proteinuria without haematuria include congenital renal anomalies, drug toxicity, and tubular or interstitial disease.

### *3 Mild proteinuria and haematuria*

Suggests focal nephritis (typically post-streptococcal, although Berger's disease can have mild–moderate proteinuria), vascular disease, renal tract infection.

### *4 Moderate – severe proteinuria (>1 g/day) with haematuria*

Renal vein thrombosis, significant GN, malignant hypertension.

### *5 Severe proteinuria (>2 g/day or >40 mg/m$^2$/h overnight) without haematuria*

Nephrotic syndrome (usually minimal change nephritis), membranous GN.

## MANAGEMENT

Trace proteinuria does not need investigation.

### *1 Clinical assessment*

Ask about a family history of renal disease and deafness (Alport's), and take a careful drug history. Measure BP, weight, height.

### *2 Urinalysis*

**2.1 Orthostatic proteinuria** Confirm the diagnosis by dipstick test of urine immediately upon waking, and again after walking or standing for >2 h. More formal testing can be done with a 12 h recumbent collection and a 12 h upright collection. Orthostatic proteinuria needs no further investigation.

**2.2 Microscopy of urinary sediment** White cells and bacteria suggest UTI, but white cells alone can indicate almost any genito-urinary inflammatory process. Haematuria – see above. The finding of casts strongly suggests a glomerular aetiology.

**2.3 Osmolarity and specific gravity (SG)** After 2 months of age, normal infants can concentrate urine to over 900 mosm/litre after overnight fast. Specific gravity usually parallels osmolarity, as they both mirror the body's need and ability to concentrate urine and conserve water. The presence of protein, glucose or urographic contrast in urine raises SG more than osmolarity, as these have relatively large molecular weight, but only contribute marginally to osmolarity. Under normal circumstances, SG >1.036–1.04 or <1.005 are considered abnormal.

### *3 Renal function*

**3.1 Blood urea, creatinine, electrolytes**

**3.2 Creatinine clearance ($C_{cr}$)** A good measure of GFR:

$$C_{cr} = \frac{U \times V}{P \times t} \times \frac{1.73}{SA}$$

where $U$ = urine creatinine (mg% or μmol/litre), $V$ = urine volume (ml) passed during a known period of time ($t$, usually expressed in minutes) which is usually 24 h (1440 min), $P$ = plasma creatinine, and SA = body surface area ($m^2$).

Age-related reference ranges in ml/min/1.73 $m^2$ corrected for body surface area are [mean (±2 SD)]:

| | |
|---|---|
| Newborn | 26 (±23) |
| 6–12 wk | 54 (±30) |
| 6–12 mo | 78 (±24) |
| 1–3 yr | 95 (±26) |
| > 3 yr | 117 (±24) |

A renal DTPA scan can very accurately determine GFR.

### *4 Further investigation*

The tests should be tailored to the child and the presentation. One should consider $C_3$, serum lipids, serum albumin, ASOT, and occasionally in the first instance a renal biopsy.

## ***Haematuria***

At least 5 red cells per high-powered field. The presence of casts in the urinary sediment indicates a renal cause.

### 1 Causes of haematuria

Glomerulonephritis: most commonly, acute post-streptococcal, HSP, Berger's/IgA disease, other GN (SLE, Goodpasture's syndrome, polyarteritis nodosa, Alport's syndrome).
Infection: pyelonephritis, endocarditis, acute haemorrhagic cystitis (adenovirus), TB.
Calculi.
Trauma.
Tumour: Wilms' tumour, bladder rhabdomyosarcoma.
Haematological: sickle cell anaemia, haemophilia (rare).
Drugs: cyclophosphamide, ifosfamide.

### 2 Other causes of red urine

**2.1 Neonates** Urates (in concentrated urine) – seen on nappy; *Serratia marcescens* (in nappy soiled for 24 h).

**2.2 All ages** Haemoglobinuria, myoglobinuria; dyes – phenolphthalein, senna, beeturia, food dyes; porphyria (congenital erythropoietic); drugs – rifampicin.

## 13.4 Glomerulonephritis (GN)

This is the result of immunological damage by:

(a) Antibodies to the glomerular basement membrane (BM) fixing to the BM.
(b) Deposition of circulating soluble antigen–antibody complexes on the BM (where the antigen is not glomerular).

The antigen–antibody interaction results in complement activation, liberation of chemotactic and vasoactive substances and the influx of polymorphs and macrophages. The result is a hypercellular glomerulus, with a leaky BM and decreased calibre of capillary lumens.

Glomerular nephritis is characterized by the nephritic syndrome (oliguria $<$350 ml/m$^2$/day, haematuria, oedema and hypertension), the nephrotic syndrome (see below), or a mixture of both.

The presence of proteinuria, haematuria and casts is very suggestive of GN. The diagnosis is made with renal biopsy; however, this is not considered necessary for *typical* cases of acute post-streptococcal nephritis, steroid-responsive nephrotic syndrome, Henoch–Schönlein nephritis, Berger's/IgA disease (moderate but otherwise asymptomatic haematuria).

## AETIOLOGY (see Table 13.1)

**Table 13.1 Causes of glumerulonephritis according to serum complement**

| *Normal $C_3$* | *Low $C_3$* |
|---|---|
| Berger's IgA nephropathy | Post-streptococcal (APSGN) |
| Henoch–Schönlein purpura | Membranoproliferative GN |
| Rapidly progressive GN | Bacterial endocarditis |
| Hereditary nephritis (Alport's) | Systemic lupus erythematosus |
| Goodpasture's syndrome | |
| Membranoproliferative GN | |

GN, glomerulonephritis; APSGN, acute post-streptococcal glomerulonephritis.

# 13.5 Nephrotic syndrome – most commonly minimal change nephritis (MCN)

## CLINICAL FEATURES

### *1 Proteinuria*

Selective, >1 g/day (often >3 g/day) *or* >40 mg/m$^2$/h.

### *2 Hypo-albuminaemia*

Also elevated $\alpha_2$ and $\beta$ globulin fractions. Clinical features consist of oedema, abdominal pain, vomiting, tachycardia, hypertension (rare in MCN).

### *3 Generalized oedema*

Due to hypo-albuminaemia with resulting interstitial fluid leak. Intravascular volume is *decreased*, giving increased renin–angiotensin and aldosterone, and eventual $Na^+$ retention and ADH secretion.

### *4 Hyperlipidaemia*

## AETIOLOGY

Usually (70%) MCN.
Others: Henoch–Schönlein, acute post-streptococcal GN, membranous, membranoproliferative, SLE, malaria, hepatitis B, renal vein thrombosis, drugs such as heavy metals and penicillamine, allergic reaction, lymphoproliferative disease, congenital.

## AGE

Seventy-five per cent are in children <5 years of age.

## INVESTIGATION

### *1 24 h collection for urinary protein*

If not possible, a timed overnight urine specimen will suffice. Children with nephrotic syndrome have >1 g/day (usually >3 g/day) or >40 $mg/m^2/h$ overnight.

### *2 Serum*

Urea, creatinine and electrolytes.
Albumin (decreased), lipids (increased), $C_3$ (normal).
Selective protein index (ratio of IgG:transferrin) is <0.2 in nephrotic syndrome, although it is not often used.

### *3 Renal biopsy*

It should not be performed unless MCN is unlikely. Some typical indications for biopsy are:

Moderate haematuria in addition to heavy proteinuria.
Failure to respond to corticosteroids.
Hypertension.
Age <1 year or >10 years.

## TREATMENT

### *1 Induce remission – prednisolone*

60 $mg/m^2/day$ in 2–3 divided doses – induces remission in 95% within 4 weeks. Continue until there is absent or trace proteinuria on first voided specimen for 3 consecutive days, then taper over 1 month by first going to alternate-day therapy, and then discontinue. If no remission within 1 month, biopsy is indicated. If the histology is that of MCN, continue steroids for another month.

### *2 Relapses*

Usually defined as at least ++proteinuria for 7 days.

**2.1 Steroids** Treat as above. If there have been more than 2 relapses within 6 months try alternate-day steroids at minimum dose required to maintain the remission. Avoid going above 1–2 mg/kg each alternate day.

**2.2 Cyclophosphamide** 3 mg/kg/day for 8 weeks. Used for steroid-dependent MCN with >3–4 relapses/yr. Risks: marrow suppression, sterility, late malignancy. Should only be used under supervision of nephrologist.

**2.3 Others** Chlorambucil. Cyclosporin has given encouraging results.

### *3 Ancillary treatment*

**3.1 Salt restriction** Used only in severe cases. Fluid restriction will be self-imposed if salt is restricted.

**3.2 Diuretics** Use with great caution because intravascular volume is already depleted and shock may be induced. Oral hydrochlorothiazide (1 mg/kg/12 h) can be tried in those with recurrent oedema, preferably with added spironolactone (1 mg/kg/day). Oral frusemide (1 mg/kg/12–24 h) may be added. IV frusemide may be given for severe ascites in the first few days of the illness while waiting for a response to steroids. If only minimal diuresis is observed, or tachycardia and hypotension develop, use albumin as well.

**3.3 Albumin** Used for hypovolaemia or severe oedema, both of which may lead to life-threatening venous and arterial thrombosis. Give 1 g/kg of 25% salt-poor albumin IV slowly over 3–4 h, every 12 h. Rapid administration can cause pulmonary oedema and CCF. Use in conjunction with 1 dose of frusemide 1 mg/kg IV.

**3.4 Antibiotics** Pneumococcal infection which may present as peritonitis may be life threatening. Some advocate prophylactic penicillin during the acute illness or alternatively vigorous early treatment of infection with IV penicillin.

**3.5 Home monitoring** Daily check of first voided urine specimen for protein.

## 13.6 Nephritic syndrome – commonly acute post-streptococcal glomerulonephritis (APSGN)

APSGN is the most common cause of the nephritic syndrome, usually occurring in children aged 4–11 years.

### CLASSICAL FEATURES

1. Haematuria – with mild proteinuria. Urine is often brown.
2. Hypertension.
3. Oliguria, renal failure.
4. Low serum complement ($C_3$).
5. Evidence of recent streptococcal infection: positive throat culture, high ASOT (in post-pharyngitis, not post-impetigo), antistreptococcal DNase B.

## AETIOLOGY

Group A beta haemolytic streptococcal infection.

## CLINICAL FEATURES

Variable.

### *1 Symptoms*

Haematuria – often macroscopic.
Malaise, anorexia, headache and loin pain.
Oliguria.

### *2 Signs*

BP – raised.
Oedema – mild, usually periorbital or pretibial.
Fever – occasionally.

## INVESTIGATIONS

$C_3$ – low.
Raised ASOT or antistreptococcal DNAase B.
Urea and electrolytes and creatinine – daily at least.
Accurate fluid balance, daily weight.

## NATURAL HISTORY

See Figure 13.2.

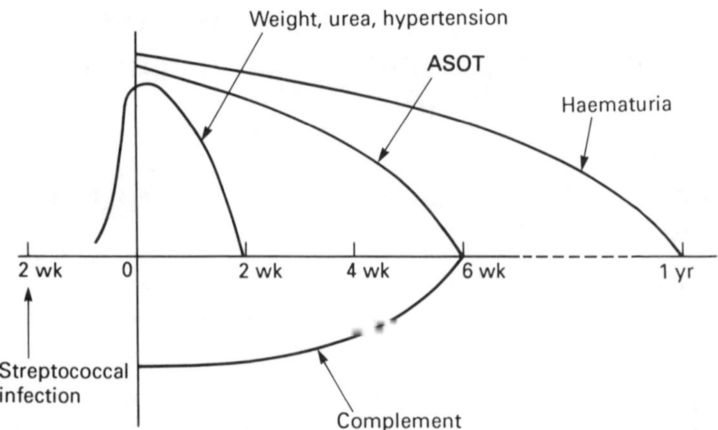


**Figure 13.2** Natural history of acute post-streptococcal glomerulonephritis (ASOT, antistreptolysin-O titre)

## COMPLICATIONS

1. Acute renal failure.
2. Hypertensive encephalopathy.
3. Heart failure – rare.

## MANAGEMENT

### *1 Frequent weight, BP, pulse, respiration*

### *2 Careful fluid management*

Great vigilance is required to recognize oliguria (warning bells should ring at <1 ml/kg/h) before it becomes anuria. Fluid restriction is imperative in the oliguric child. Give insensible losses (350 ml/m$^2$) plus urine output.

### *3 Salt restriction*

No longer considered to be a major part of the treatment.

### *4 Penicillin*

A 10-day course of penicillin V to eradicate streptococcal infection.

### *5 Acute renal failure* (see Section 13.7)

This involves careful management of fluids and electrolytes. The management of hyperkalaemia is discussed in Section 5.7. For early oliguria, one can give frusemide 1 mg/kg dose, and if there is no result give a single dose of 4–5 mg/kg. Dialyse for intractable oedema, hyperkalaemia, acidosis, hypertension.

### *6 Hypertension*

If salt and fluid restriction as well as frusemide have no effect, give hydralazine 0.2–0.4 mg/kg IV/IM. If hypertension is still difficult to control, try labetalol 1–3 mg/kg/h by infusion. See Section 13.2.

### *7 Cardiac failure*

If there is no response to the above diuretic and antihypertensive treatment, dialysis is indicated.

### *8 Renal biopsy*

Indicated for:

*Severe anuric renal failure* A nephritis requiring immunosuppression may be present.
*No evidence of recent streptococcal infection* (e.g. low ASOT).
*Failure of acute symptoms or renal function* To resolve by 4 weeks.
*Low $C_3$* Persisting longer than 2 months.
*Previous nephritis*
*Proteinuria, haematuria* Persisting beyond 1 year.

# 13.7 Acute renal failure (ARF)

## DEFINITION

### *1 Decreased glomerular filtration rate (GFR)*

Normal GFR is 80–150 ml/min/1.73 $m^2$ (see Section 13.3). Low GFR will usually cause oliguria, although non-oliguric ARF with low GFR is recognized.

### *2 Failure to clear renal solute load (RSL)*

Renal solute load comprises roughly 300 mosm/day of urea and electrolytes. If 1 litre of urine is passed per day it would therefore have an osmolality of 300 mosm/litre. If only 250 ml were passed, the urine would be at its maximum concentrating capacity of 1200 mosm/litre. If even less urine were passed, the RSL would not be fully excreted and would therefore accumulate. Oliguria causing retention of RSL occurs at approximately $<300$ ml/$m^2$/day.

## AETIOLOGY

### *1 Prerenal*

Water loss – e.g. diarrhoea, third space losses (ascites, peritonitis, leaky capillaries, peripheral vasodilatation of sepsis).
Plasma loss – e.g. burns.
Blood loss – trauma.
Poor cardiac output – myocardial insufficiency, hypotension/shock.

### *2 Intrinsic renal*

Glomerular – all glomerulonephritis, e.g. post-streptococcal, haemolytic uraemic syndrome (HUS), SLE, Henoch–Schönlein, rapidly progressive GN. Also DIC, septicaemia.
Tubular – acute tubular necrosis (ATN): any hypoxic ischaemic insult, progression of prerenal causes, drugs such as aminoglycosides, haemoglobinuria or myoglobinuria, DIC.
Vascular causes such as renal vein thrombosis and HUS.
Interstitial nephritis – allergic, post-infectious, pyelonephritis.

### *3 Post-renal*

Obstructive uropathy – if both kidneys are obstructed it implies a cause at or distal to the bladder, e.g. urethral valves, urethral stricture, phimosis, paraphimosis, bladder clots, tumour of bladder or kidneys.
Crystalluria ± stone formation – uric acid nephropathy (e.g. tumour lysis syndrome), high-dose methotrexate, Ca oxalate.

## CLINICAL FEATURES

### *1 Ask about:*

Haematuria, UTI, previous renal disease, diarrhoea with or without blood (HUS), features of dehydration or shock, nephrotoxic drugs.

Non-specific features of uraemia are nausea, anorexia, vomiting, drowsiness or convulsions.

### *2 Examine for causes*

Skin – petechial rash of HUS, Henoch–Schönlein purpura; SLE rash.
Large bladder – urethral valves.
Hydration status.
BP – ?hypotension.
Large kidneys – renal vein thrombosis, tumour, obstructive uropathy.

### *3 Examine for effects of ARF*

These are due to accumulation of:

| | |
|---|---|
| Water | – oedema; |
| $Na^+$ | – hypertension and expanded ECF volume; |
| $K^+$ | – arrhythmia, monitor with ECG; |
| Urea | – nausea, vomiting; |
| $H^+$ | – acidosis; |
| Phosphate | – hypocalcaemia, tetany. Acidosis will offset this by maintaining ionized calcium. |

## INVESTIGATIONS

### *1 Differentiate prerenal ARF from established ARF*

Prerenal ARF requires increased fluids and BP to better perfuse the kidneys. Established ARF is treated with severe fluid restriction. Differentiating between them is therefore important.

**1.1 Urinary sediment and ward test**

Distorted red cells or red cell casts – GN.
White cells – pyelonephritis.
Renal tubular cells, tubular cell casts – ATN.
Crystals – uric acid, calcium oxalate.
Normal microscopy – suggests a prerenal cause or post-renal cause other than stones.
Blood and protein – ATN, GN.

**1.2 Low CVP, hypotension** Suggests prerenal.

**1.3 Fluid and diuretic challenge** After correcting possible hypovolaemia with 15–20 ml/kg of colloid (see below), give frusemide 1 mg/kg which only works on a functioning tubule. If no effect, give another bolus of volume correction and give frusemide 4 mg/kg. If no result, assume established ARF and severely restrict fluids. N.B. It is important to obtain a sample of urine for urea, creatinine, and electrolytes and SG before giving frusemide.

**1.4 Tests of concentrating ability** In established tubular necrosis, the tubules cannot concentrate the filtrate, a feature which allows the tests in Table 13.2 to be used.

**Table 13.2 Tests to differentiate prerenal from established acute renal failure*†**

| | *Prerenal* | *Established ARF* |
|---|---|---|
| Urine $Na^+$ (mmol/litre) | <10 | >40 |
| Creatinine urine/plasma | >14 | <14 |
| Osmolality urine/plasma | >1.4 (>1.2) | <1.1 (<1.2) |
| Urea urine/plasma | >8 | <5 |
| Urine specific gravity | >1.015 | <1.015 |
| Urine osmolality (mosm/litre) | >500 (>400) | <350 (<400) |
| Fractional Na excretion | >1 (<2.5) | <1 (>2.5) |

* Results are meaningless if taken under the influence of frusemide.
† Figures in parentheses refer to neonates.

Fractional sodium excretion (FE Na):

$$\text{FE Na} = \frac{U\,\text{Na}}{P\,\text{Na}} \times \frac{P\,\text{Cr}}{U\,\text{Cr}}$$

where $U$ = urine, $P$ = plasma, Na = sodium concentration, and Cr = creatinine.

### *2 Blood chemistry*

Urea, creatinine, potassium, phosphate, magnesium – all increase.
$Na^+$, pH, $Ca^{2+}$ – all decrease.

### *3 Investigate the cause*

Assess renal perfusion – hydration, BP, CVP.
Blood film, clotting screen, fibrin degradation products – DIC, HUS.
ASOT – increase in post-streptococcal GN.
$C_3$ – decreased in post-streptococcal GN.
Abdominal ultrasound – the best way of excluding post-renal causes.
Pass urinary catheter to exclude urethral obstruction and to collect a sample for urinary electrolytes, urea, creatinine and SG.

## TREATMENT

### *1 Urinary catheter*

Important in monitoring urine output and excluding urethral obstruction.

### *2 Correct hypovolaemia, restore cardiac output*

Give plasma expanders if prerenal cause is suspected. Use normal saline, albumin or any colloid solution 15–20 ml/kg quickly and give frusemide

1 mg/kg fluid bolus (see above). If no response, consider repeat bolus and give frusemide 4 mg/kg. If oliguria persists, manage fluids as below and assume established ARF.

### *3 Fluid restriction*

Strict fluid balance. Restrict input to urine output plus insensible losses (350 ml/m$^2$/day). Use potassium-free solutions. Monitor body weight closely. When diuresis begins, the replacement solution should mirror the urine electrolytes, although potassium should initially be withheld.

### *4 Potassium*

Cease all $K^+$-containing fluids. Use ion exchange resins initially, but later give IV calcium gluconate, bicarbonate, glucose and insulin as necessary (see Section 5.7).

### *5 Diet*

High carbohydrate (CHO) to reduce catabolism. May give protein-free CHO additives to food. Caloreen powder (Roussel) contains 4 kcal/g, <0.02 mmol/g $Na^+$, and <0.003 mmol/g $K^+$. Other suitable alternatives include Polycal, Polycose, Hycal and others. Reduce protein to 1 g/kg/day but make it high quality. Refer to dietitian. May need parenteral nutrition.

### *6 Acidosis*

Prevent by providing adequate CHO for calories. The amount of $NaHCO_3$ needed for total correction of acidosis is:

$$HCO_3^- \text{ (mmol)} = 0.3 \times \text{Body weight (kg)} \times \text{Base deficit}$$

One normally gives only half-correction.
8.4% $NaHCO_3$ has 1 mEq/ml.
In severe acidosis, the sodium load of $NaHCO_3$ replacement may be excessive, in which case dialysis is indicated.

### *7 Dialysis*

Early dialysis before deterioration decreases mortality and may allow catabolic children to achieve adequate nutrition for healing. Only peritoneal dialysis (PD) will be described, although haemodialysis and continuous arteriovenous haemofiltration can also be used.

#### 7.1 Indications

Uncontrolled hyperkalaemia.
Severe uncontrolled metabolic acidosis.
CNS signs of uraemia.
Hyperammonaemia.

**7.2 Tests before insertion of PD** FBC, clotting profile, have cross-matched blood ready.

**7.3 Insertion of PD catheter** Disposable catheters are available, but if it is likely that PD will continue for >3–4 days, a Tenckhoff catheter should be inserted by a surgeon.

*7.3.1 Catheterize the bladder* to minimize risk of bladder perforation.

*7.3.2 Warm dialysate* to 37°C.

*7.3.3 Insert PD catheter* in midline, one-third the distance between umbilicus and pubic symphysis. Advance it to L or R iliac fossa.

**7.4 Dialysis fluids** Composition of dialysate is described in Table 13.3. Increasing degrees of hypertonicity will drag off correspondingly more body fluid. Add 0–3.5 mmol/litre potassium according to serum potassium. Add heparin 200 u/litre until peritoneal drainage is not blood stained. Some add antibiotics to the dialysate, e.g. cephazolin 250 mg/litre for the first 2 days.

**Table 13.3 Characteristics of dialysis fluids**

| *Glucose concentration (%)* | *Na* | *Ca* | *Mg* | *Cl* | *Lactate* | *mosm/litre* |
|---|---|---|---|---|---|---|
| | (mmol/litre) | | | | | |
| 1.5 | 140 | 1.8 | 0.75 | 100 | 45 | 360 |
| 2.5 | 132 | 1.8 | 0.50 | 96 | 40 | 398 |
| 4.25 | 132 | 1.8 | 0.50 | 96 | 40 | 485 |

**7.5 Cycles** Use aliquots of 40 ml/kg. In and dwell over 40 min. Drain fluid out over 20 min. In ventilated children, may need smaller volumes and shorter cycles.

**7.6 Monitor** Strict fluid balance, and at least once daily weight. Frequent check of electrolytes. If using 4.25% dextrose solution, check blood sugar frequently.

*8 Hypertension* (see Section 13.2)

*9 Convulsions*

Causes include hypertension, azotaemia, hypocalcaemia, hyponatraemia, hypomagnesaemia, dialysis disequilibrium syndrome.
Treat underlying cause. Anticonvulsants may be needed – see Section 8.3.

## Further reading

Gaudio, K. M. and Siegal, N. J. (1987) Pathogenesis and treatment of acute renal failure. *Pediatr. Clin. N. Am.*, **34**, 771

# 13.8 Haemolytic uraemic syndrome (HUS)

The HUS consists of a triad of acute nephropathy, thrombocytopenia and microangiopathic haemolysis, and is a major cause of renal failure in childhood. It must be suspected in all cases of acute renal failure (ARF), especially if preceded by gastroenteritis. It occurs in epidemic and sporadic forms.

## AETIOLOGY

The epidemic form has recently been linked to verocytotoxin-producing *E. coli* (VTEC), the most frequently reported serotype being 0157:H7. The toxin is sometimes produced by other organisms, e.g. *Shigella dysenteriae.*

## INCIDENCE

Reported at 0.3 per 100 000 children under 16 years of age per year, with a median age incidence of 2 yr 7 mo (*Br. Med. J.* (1986) **292,** 115–117).

## CLINICAL FEATURES

### *1 Prodrome*

Febrile illness with diarrhoea, usually bloody.

### *2 After several days*

Pallor, jaundice, bruises and petechiae, oliguria, brown or bloody urine. Oedema may be due to hypoalbuminaemia, salt or water retention due to poor GFR, or cardiac failure. Hypertension is recognized.

### *3 Atypical cases*

Mild or absent prodrome, and HUS presenting as severe ARF, hypertension and encephalopathy (altered conscious state, seizures).

## INVESTIGATIONS

FBC – fragmentation, thrombocytopenia, burr cells, helmet cells.
Other evidence of haemolysis – low haptoglobin, high indirect bilirubin, negative indirect Coombs' test.
Urea, creatinine – high.
Clotting profile – prolonged PT and PTT indicating DIC.
Urinalysis – haematuria, proteinuria, red cell and granular casts on microscopy.
Stool culture – culture for *E. coli, Shigella*, ask laboratory specifically for VTEC.

## TREATMENT

Manage as for acute renal failure. ?Role of plasmaphaeresis.
Early dialysis is important, as is regular blood transfusion.
Fluid overload leads to severe hypertension.
Manage consumption coagulopathy with 10 ml/kg boluses of fresh frozen plasma or cryoprecipitate 4 bags/$m^2$ for fibrinogen.
Anticoagulants, steroids, immunosuppressive drugs are of no use.
Unconvincing results have been obtained from intralipid, vitamin E, fibrinolytic agents, prostacyclin ($PGI_2$).

## PROGNOSIS

The sporadic cases with mild, non-diarrhoeal prodrome, and negative verotoxin, have a high mortality. Of those with 'classical' HUS, >90% will recover completely and the rest will have residual renal or rarely neurological impairment.

## COMMENT

It is likely that within the next few years much more will be known about HUS. The hope is that by understanding the pathogenesis of HUS and the mode of action of the verocytotoxin, more rational pharmacological approaches to the illness will be devised.

All cases in the UK should be notified to the Communicable Disease Surveillance Centre (tel. 081-200 6868), which will make arrangements for transport of stool specimens and the dispatch of a questionnaire.

## Further reading

Anon. (1986) British Paediatric Association – Communicable Disease Surveillance Centre: surveillance of haemolytic uraemic syndrome 1983–4. *Br. Med. J.*, **292**, 115–117

Anon. (1987) Unravelling HUS. *Lancet*, **ii**, 1437–1438

Cleary, T. G. (1988) Cytotoxin producing *E. coli* and the hemolytic uremic syndrome. *Pediatr. Clin. N. Am.*, **35**, 485–502

Kavi, J. and Wise, R. (1989) Causes of the haemolytic uraemic syndrome. *Br. Med. J.*, **298**, 65–66

# 13.9 Undescended testes (UDT)

Descent of the testes begins in the eighth *in utero* month under the influence of testosterone, and is usually complete by term. Only 0.8% of testes remain undescendced by 1 year of age. They must be differentiated from retractile testes. There is some evidence that cryptorchidism may be due to impaired gonadotrophin secretion. Cryptorchidism, especially when found with hypospadias, may be indicative of intersexuality, or of other major urogenital abnormalities.

## RETRACTILE TESTES

They can be coaxed to reach the bottom of the scrotum regardless of the position in which they are first located. Their ascent is due to the normal brisk cremasteric reflex of prepuberty.

## UNDESCENDED TESTES

Those which cannot be made to reach the bottom of the scrotum; 67% are ectopic and 33% are arrested in the normal line of descent.

### *1 Ectopic testes*

Most are locked in the superficial inguinal pouch and can be felt by gently stroking along the course of the inguinal ligament. They are usually of normal size, with good length of spermatic cord. Others include inguinoperineal and perineal.

### *2 Arrest in normal line of descent*

Most are near the pubic tubercle, in the inguinal canal, or intra-abdominal. They tend to be small and ill-formed.

## COMPLICATIONS

### *1 Decreased spermatogenesis*

UDT for >2 years results in decreased germ cell numbers, although some UDT are dysgenetic anyway. Bilateral UDT is more strongly associated with azoospermia and infertility.

### *2 Tumours*

UDT for >6 years has an increased risk (30 × normal) of testicular cancer. Operative descent may not eliminate this possibility but will facilitate its detection.

### *3 Increased incidence of torsion and trauma*

## TREATMENT

### *1 Surgery*

Treatment of choice. Advised at age 2–3 years.

### *2 Hormonal therapy – LHRH or HCG*

Not widely recommended in the UK. Claims for its efficacy vary widely. It will not work in ectopic testes.

## Further reading

Anon. (1986) The undescended testis: is there a role for LHRH? *Lancet*, **i**, 1133–1134

Colodny, A. H. (1986) Undescended testes – is surgery really necessary; *New Engl. J. Med.*, **314**, 510–511

---

# 13.10 Wetting

---

Wetting may occur only at night, by day, or both. Nocturnal wetting seldom has an organic cause. Daytime wetting is more likely to have an organic cause.

## AETIOLOGY

Nocturnal enuresis – functional developmental delay.
Neurogenic bladder – overt: meningomyelocele; hidden: spina bifida occulta, spinal dysraphism, cord tumour.
Urinary tract infection.
Structural urinary tract abnormalities – ectopia vesicae, ectopic ureter, epispadias, urethral valves.
Functional.
Polyuria – includes diabetes mellitus and insipidus, chronic renal failure.

## CLINICAL FEATURES

### *1 History*

Establish the following features:

Pattern of wetting – dribbles all of the time? Some of the time? Relationship to exercise or giggling? Has the child always wet himself or is it only recent? Number of days or nights per week?
Dysuria, polyuria, polydypsia.
Family history of wetting.
Recent family or personal stresses.
Sleep abnormalities.
Associated constipation.
How does the wetting affect the child, especially in relation to peers?

### *2 Examination*

Blood pressure.
Observe the child voiding if history suggests abnormal stream.
Locate urethral meatus – ? epispadias.
Palpate and percuss for enlarged or expressible bladder – suggests obstructed or neurogenic bladder.

Neurological examination – leg reflexes, patulous anus, perineal sensation, peripheral sensation, foot drop.
Inspect lower back – sacral dimpling, patch of hair or pigmentation, or other cutaneous abnormality suggesting spinal abnormality.
Assess psychosocial status and look for evidence of physical or sexual abuse.

## INVESTIGATION

All children who wet must have a MSU taken for microscopy and culture. Other investigations to consider include:

Urea, creatinine.
Urine specific gravity.
Abdominal ultrasound.
Radiology – micturating cystourethrogram, IVP, vertebral x-ray.

## SOME SPECIFIC CONDITIONS

### *1 Neurogenic bladder*

Usually associated with flaccid paralysis of bladder, resulting in uncontrolled day and night dribbling. Examination may reveal an expressible distended bladder, patulous anus, perineal anaesthesia.

### *2 Urinary tract infection*

Causes increased sensory stimulation of the bladder mucosa, and is accompanied by frequency and urgency. Wetting disappears rapidly with treatment.

### *3 Structural abnormalities*

Incontinence in epispadias is due to the dorsal urethral defect extending into the sphincter. Ectopic ureters cause incontinence only when they open distal to the internal urethral sphincter into the urethra vestibule or vagina. The wetting occurs every few minutes, but normal micturition also occurs independently. It is almost always associated with duplex ureters in girls. A simple test is to insert indigo carmine dye into the bladder through a catheter and ask the child to refrain from voiding for 2 h. During this time, wetting with dye-free urine suggests an ectopic ureter.

### *4 Functional wetting*

No organic abnormality can be demonstrated. Wetting may be associated with giggling or occasionally the 'sham' syndrome in which the child has urgency and occasionally dysuria, with no abnormality. Oxybutynin (anticholinergic, antispasmodic) 10 mg nocte is being used with success.

### *5 Others*

Sexual abuse may present with wetting, as may sleep and seizure disorders. There are numerous causes of polyuria which may present as wetting, notably diabetes mellitus and insipidus, chronic renal failure.

# 13.11 Nocturnal enuresis

Thirty per cent of 4 year olds and 7% of 7-year-old children still wet the bed at night. It is therefore sensible to wait until after the 2nd year of schooling before considering treatment. Prior to that, most parents wish for reassurance about the absence of organic pathology, rather than aggressive attempts at preventing wetting. Boys are affected more often than girls, in a ratio of 1.5–2:1. Enuresis is more common in those of lower birth weight, shorter stature, delayed bone age, or with delayed sexual maturation. It is more common in those with psychiatric disturbance, although most children with enuresis do not have psychiatric disease.

## AETIOLOGY

### *1 Primary enuresis*

Defined as never having had a prolonged period of night dryness, although in practice parents often describe short periods of dryness. It is assumed to be a genetically determined predisposition to a maturational delay in bladder control. There is usually no obvious cause. Often either or both parents will have been enuretic in childhood.

### *2 Secondary enuresis*

Such children have previously achieved a period of nocturnal continence. A sudden recurrence of enuresis may be due to organic causes (see Section 13.10), or a response to a recent psychological stress (birth of sibling, divorce, new school).

## CLINICAL FEATURES (see Section 13.10)

A history regarding the type of enuresis, any daytime voiding problems, previous UTI, and any psychosocial or family problems should be elicited. Examination should include a complete neurological examination, especially the low back, perineal and leg sensation and reflexes. The bladder and kidney should be palpated, and the urethra inspected closely.

## INVESTIGATIONS

Urinalysis.
Mid-stream urine – microscopy and culture.

If physical examination and these urine tests are normal, then organic pathology is very unlikely and no further evaluation is indicated.

## TREATMENT

None is needed until at least age 6–8 years. Explain that many other children (and perhaps the child's own parents) have or had this problem.

### *1 Tricyclic antidepressants*

Imipramine: 25 mg 1–2 h before bed. Can be increased to 50–75 mg in older children or adolescents. Cease after 1 month if ineffective. Continue for 4 months if effective, then gradually wean by decreasing dose and frequency (i.e. every other night) over 1 month. Relapse rate is high. Long-term cure rates are approximately 25%.

### *2 Conditioning alarm*

This has the highest reported cure rates and lowest relapse rates. Various machines are available which have in common the triggering of an alarm and a light when urine makes contact with a sensor. The time-honoured system is a pad (on which the child lies) and buzzer system. Recent transistorized modifications of the system use a smaller sensor attached to the child's underwear, whereas the alarm may be attached to the child's wrist or pyjama collar. 70–90% respond, although 20–30% relapse but will often respond well to retreatment. Average duration of treatment is 6 weeks, or 1 month after response.

### *3 Desmopressin*

It achieves cure in 12–40% of reported cases, although up to 80% derive some benefit. Long-term treatment may be needed. There are virtually no side effects. The dose is 10–40 μg given intranasally. A week's treatment with imipramine costs in the vicinity of 10p, whereas desmopressin may cost up to £10. It may well have a use for 'one off' special occasions (staying over at a friend's house) or short-term use.

### *4 Other treatments*

**4.1 Bladder training** Involves conscious attempts at bladder 'stretching', by voluntarily prolonging the intervals between voidings.

**4.2 Motivational therapy** An approach heavily dependent on counselling. The child is encouraged to assume responsibility for learning control of bladder function. The child keeps progress record (gold star on a chart). A positive relationship is promoted between child and parents, and the removal of blame and guilt is addressed. The success rate is small, however; many of the principles should be applied to pharmacological or conditioning therapies.

**4.3 Miscellaneous treatments** Psychotherapy, hypnotherapy, diet therapy. These do not play a major role.

### *5 Ineffective or harmful treatments*

Fluid restriction in the evenings, or random wakening of the child to void are ineffective, Oxybutynin (an anticholinergic) is probably of no use (*Pediatrics* (1988) **81**, 104–106). Shame, blame or punishment are at best ineffective, and should be avoided.

## Further reading

Crawford, J. D. (1988) Treatment of nocturnal enuresis: proceedings of a symposium held 6 August 1988. *J. Pediatr.*, **114**, 687–726

Forsythe, W. I. and Butler, R. J. (1989) Fifty years of enuretic alarms. *Arch. Dis. Child.*, **64**, 879–885

Gil Rushton, H. (1989) Nocturnal enuresis: epidemiology, evaluation, and currently available treatment options. *J. Pediatr.*, **114**, 691–696

Meadow, S. R. and Evans, J. H. C. (1989) Desmopressin for enuresis. *Br. Med. J.*, **298**, 1596

Chapter 14

# Endocrine

## 14.1 Normal pubertal development

| *Stage* | *Male genitalia* | *Mean age at onset* (± SD) |
|---|---|---|
| 1 | Pre-adolescent | |
| 2 | Slight enlargement and reddening of scrotum and testes | 11.4 ± 1.1 yr |
| 3 | Penis lengthens | 12.9 ± 1.0 yr |
| 4 | Broader penis with development of glans; testes larger; scrotum darker | 13.8 ± 1.0 yr |
| 5 | Adult | 14.9 ± 1.1 yr |

Peak male height velocity: 14.1 yr ± 0.9 yr.
Testicular volume >4 ml = puberty is initiated. Best assessed with standard volumes of the Prader orchidometer.

| *Stage* | *Female breast* | *Mean age at onset* (± SD) |
|---|---|---|
| 1 | Pre-adolescent | |
| 2 | Breast bud; elevation of breast and papilla as a small mound | 11.2 ± 1.1 yr |
| 3 | Breast and areola enlarge further as a single contour | 12.2 ± 1.1 yr |
| 4 | Areola and papilla project to form a secondary mound | 13.1 ± 1.2 yr |
| 5 | Adult | 15.3 ± 1.7 yr |

Menarche: 13.5 yr ± 1.0 yr.
Peak female height velocity: 12.1 yr ± 0.9 yr.
By bone age 15 yr <1% of growth remains – this is useful in reassuring tall adolescent girls.

| *Stage* | *Pubic hair – male and female* | *Mean age at onset* (± SD) | |
|---|---|---|---|
| | | Male | Female |
| 1 | Pre-adolescent | | |
| 2 | Fine downy hair | 12.0 ± 1.0 yr | 11.7 ± 1.2 yr |
| 3 | Darker coarser hair | 13.9 ± 1.0 yr | 12.4 ± 1.1 yr |
| 4 | Adult quality | 14.4 ± 1.1 yr | 13.0 ± 1.1 yr |
| 5 | Adult distribution including medial thighs | 15.2 ± 1.1 yr | 14.4 ± 1.1 yr |

# 14.2 Precocious puberty

## DEFINITION

Isosexual precocity refers to the early onset of sexual characteristics appropriate to the child's sex. True precocious puberty is associated with an elevation of gonadotrophins, whereas pseudoprecocious puberty is due to sex hormone secretion independent of pituitary gonadotrophins.

Puberty is thought to be precocious if sexual development is >2 SD advanced for age, i.e. <8 yr in girls, <9.5 yr in boys.

## AETIOLOGY

### *1 Central causes*

**1.1 Idiopathic (constitutional)** Can be sporadic or familial. More common in girls than in boys (testes are always enlarged). Presumably the normal hypothalamic mechanism that initiates puberty is precociously activated.

**1.2 Pathological** CNS tumours and trauma, hydrocephalus, post-encephalitis, neurofibromatosis, tuberous sclerosis, other CNS abnormalities, chronic severe hypothyroidism.

### *2 Non-central causes*

Increased adrenal sex hormones – congenital adrenal hyperplasia, adrenal adenoma or carcinoma, ovarian or testicular tumours, non-pituitary gonadotrophin (beta-HCG from tumours), exogenous sex steroids, syndromes such as McCune–Albright, Russell–Silver.

## INVESTIGATIONS

Oestradiol (girls), testosterone (boys).
24 h urinary FSH and LH.
Thyroid function test ± LHRH stimulation.
Bone age.
Skull x-ray or brain CT scan.

## MANAGEMENT

Refer to a paediatric endocrinologist.

## CONDITIONS RESEMBLING PRECOCIOUS PUBERTY

### *1 Premature thelarche (early breast development)*

Thirteen per cent of girls under 2.5 years have palpable breast tissue >1 cm diameter. It is most commonly seen in the neonatal period, and may persist or regress and reappear. It is also common around 18 months to 2 years. It can be unilateral, and it is almost invariably benign. Plasma gonadotrophins and prolactin are normal. The fear is that it may be the first sign of pseudoprecocious or true precocious puberty. Observation and reassurance are all that is needed provided that:

1. Growth is normal (i.e. not accelerating).
2. No other secondary sex characteristics are noted.
3. Vagina is not oestrogenized.

If one is concerned, it is reasonable to perform bone age assessment (normal or only slightly advanced in premature thelarche) and serum oestradiol.

### *2 Premature pubarche or adrenarche (early development of pubic hair)*

Females much more commonly affected than males. It is usually due to harmless premature activity of the adrenal cortex. Affected children are usually tall and some may be cerebrally damaged.

**2.1 Differential diagnosis** True precocious puberty, adrenal hyperplasia, adrenal tumours.

**2.2 Investigations** 17-Hydroxyprogesterone, testosterone, androstendione, dihydroepiandrosterone, 24 h urinary 17-ketosteroids, to exclude adrenal hyperplasia or tumour. Bone age may be slightly advanced; however, if markedly so, true precocious puberty is more likely.

## Further reading

Pescovitz, O. H. (1990) Precocious puberty. *Pediatr. in Rev.*, **11**, 232–237

Van Winter, J. T., Noller, K. L., Zimmerman, D. and Melton, L. J. (1990) Natural history of premature thelarche in Olmsted County, Minnesota, 1940 to 1984. *J. Pediatr.*, **116**, 278–280

# 14.3 Short stature

Growth is a complicated process influenced by genetic, hormonal, nutritional and environmental factors. Endocrine causes of short stature are rare, but are important by virtue of the fact that they are eminently treatable. Normal variants are common.

## AETIOLOGY

### *1 Normal variants*

**1.1 Familial** Remain small.

**1.2 Maturational delay (often familial)** Will get there eventually. Usually have delayed puberty as well.

### *2 Organic causes*

**2.1 Intra-uterine growth retardation (IUGR)** For example, placental insufficiency, intra-uterine infection, alcohol consumption, poor maternal nutrition, chromosomal abnormality, Russell–Silver syndromes.

**2.2 Skeletal dysplasias** For example, achondroplasia.

**2.3 Systemic disease** For example, chronic renal disease, inflammatory bowel disease.

**2.4 Nutritional** For example, malabsorption syndromes, coeliac disease, anorexia nervosa.

**2.5 Psychosocial deprivation**

**2.6 Iatrogenic** Steroids, irradiation.

**2.7 Chromosomal** For example, Turner's (XO) syndrome, Down's syndrome.

**2.8 Endocrine** For example, growth hormone and thyroid hormone deficiency, excess corticosteroids.

## CLINICAL FEATURES

### *1 History*

Features of IUGR – low birth weight for gestational age, maternal smoking and alcohol intake, TORCH infections.

Family history – parental height, age at onset of puberty and growth spurt in parents.
Systematic questioning – chronic illnesses; CNS disease – headache, visual disturbance; diarrhoea; thyroid disease – constipation, poor appetite, lethargy; medications.
How does this affect the child? – Is the child teased at school, is it the parents' problem?

### *2 Examination*

#### 2.1 Plot the following:

Weight.
Height – use stadiometer or other similar device. Apply gentle upward pressure on the mastoids; heels should remain touching the floor. Height age is the age for which the child's current height is considered to be the 50th centile.
Child's previous heights and centiles (less than 5 cm growth per annum in a prepubertal child >7 yr is <25%ile).
Mid-parental centile = (Father's centile + Mother's centile)/2. Plot this centile on child's chart to estimate expected adult height. Mid-parental centile ±8.5 cm indicates expected mean ± 2 SD for adult height of the children of this couple.

#### 2.2 Body proportions

Arm span:height ratio – <0.9 suggests skeletal dysplasia. Span should roughly equal height at all ages.
Inspect for unusual proportions.
Measure upper segment/lower segment ratio. Lower segment is the distance from pubic symphysis to floor via medial maleolus.
Alternatively, measure sitting height to lower segment ratio. Normal values are 1.7 at birth, 1.4 at 6 yr, 1.2 at 8 yr, 1.0 at 11 yr. The ratio remains high in hypothyroidism.

**2.3 Appearance** Cushingoid, myxoedema, Turner phenotype, i.e. square build, webbed neck, cubitus valgus, dysplastic nails, trident posterior hairline, 'shield' chest.

Assessment of pubertal stage (see Section 14.1).

**2.4 Cardiovascular** BP is high in chronic renal disease and Cushing's syndrome. Brachiofemoral delay (coarctation in Turner's).

**2.5 CNS** Fields and fundi (pituitary tumour).

**2.6 Dentition** ? Delay (see Section 3.3).

## INVESTIGATIONS TO CONSIDER

### *1 Bone age*

Indicates skeletal maturity. Estimated from x-ray of left wrist and hand as compared to a series of standards in the Greulich and Pyle atlas. If it is less than chronological age, then it suggests degree of future growth potential. If it is also less than height age, hypothyroidism or other pathology must be considered.

**1.1 Estimated mature height (EMH)** Radiologists will give this, if they know the child's height:

$$\text{EMH} = \frac{\text{Ht} \times 100}{\%\ \text{Skeletal maturation}}$$

### *2 Biochemistry*

Thyroid function.
Urine pH and blood acid-base status – renal tubular acidosis.
Serum urea, creatinine and electrolytes.

### *4 Karyotype*

Must be done in short females. Turner's syndrome is often difficult to diagnose clinically.

### *5 Others*

MSU.
FBC.
Skull x-ray – pituitary fossa size.
Growth hormone stress tests – clonidine stimulation, exercise, insulin/arginine infusion.

## MANAGEMENT

### *1 First clinic visit*

Generally, if one does not find an obvious organic cause it is reasonable to do few or no investigations. A bone age is often reassuring in that, if it is delayed, it will indicate future growth potential. Observation is all that is required unless the height velocity proves inadequate. A healthy short child with height within the parental target area, normal height velocity and bone age equal to chronological age has familial short stature.

### *2 Second visit – usually 6 months later*

If growing at rate >5 cm/yr (>25th centile of growth velocity in a prepubertal child), do nothing and remeasure in 6 months. If <5 cm per year, embark on the above investigations with the possible exception of growth hormone tests. If still concerned after a further 6 months, perform a dynamic test of growth hormone secretion.

### *3 Endocrinopathies*

These are an uncommon cause of short stature. Suspect them if the child was of normal size at birth and later began to deviate from expected growth line, bone age less than height age, delayed dentition, previous cranial irradiation or pituitary surgery, prolonged neonatal jaundice, micropenis and cryptorchidism. Such children need endocrinological evaluation.

## Further reading

Lippe, B. and Frasier, S. D. (1989) How should we test for growth hormone deficiency and whom should we treat? *J. Pediatr.*, **115**, 585–586

# 14.4 The child on steroids

The three major problems encountered in children on long-term steroids are retardation of linear growth, accelerated weight gain, and an inability of the pituitary-adrenal axis to respond adequately to stresses such as infection and operations. Other problems include cosmetic effects, hyperglycaemia, immunosuppression, peptic ulcer, behaviour disturbance, cataracts. Myopathy and osteoporosis are uncommon.

## ASSESSMENT AT EACH ADMISSION/CLINIC VISIT

### *1 BP*

### *2 Height and weight*

Plot centiles.

### *3 Urine*

Glycosuria.

### *4 Ask about:*

**4.1 Diet** All children on steroids should have a low-calorie, high-satiety diet involving low-calorie sweeteners, high-bulk/unprocessed foods.

**4.2 Exercise** Reasonable exercise appropriate to the child's age is to be encouraged.

**4.3 Any infections**

**4.4 Cosmetic difficulties** Cushingoid appearance may increase peer ridicule.

### *5 Examination*

Note any Cushingoid features – 'lemon on a stick' appearance, moon face with red cheeks, buffalo hump, thin skin, striae, truncal obesity, poor muscle bulk, easy bruisability, poor wound healing, hirsuitism.

## Acute adrenal stresses

The child on steroids who is subjected to stresses such as an operation or infection may be unable to respond normally. Without additional steroids there is a risk of an acute life-threatening adrenal crisis. The pituitary-adrenal axis may remain suppressed for up to 6 months after discontinuing high-dose steroid therapy, during which time steroid cover for such stresses should be given. The cortisol secretory rate of the normal adrenal gland is 12.5 ± 2.5 (SEM) mg/m$^2$/day. A simple febrile illness increases the secretion 2–3-fold. Severe infections or operations increase it 4–6-fold. Increases in steroid doses to cope with stress should be infrequent and done with good cause in the case of intercurrent illness because growth retardation may occur.

### *1 Steroid cover for operations*

Hydrocortisone 50–100 mg/m$^2$ with premedication. Repeat intraoperatively if the procedure lasts >4 h. Gradually wean back onto maintenance steroids over 3 days.

### *2 Steroid cover for infections*

For a simple febrile illness (e.g. URTI), increase normal steroid dose by a factor of 2–3 during the period of stress. More significant illnesses (e.g. meningitis, pneumonia) require a 4–5-fold increase. The height of the fever has no bearing on the normal cortisol response to illness.

## Acute adrenal crisis

### *1 Clinical features*

Sudden onset of cold, clammy, ashen grey skin, rapid weak pulse, hypotension, rapid laboured respiration. A clinical clue may be the presence of Cushingoid features, or perhaps a talisman around the neck or wrist. Hypoglycaemia and hyponatraemia may occur.

### *2 Treatment*

**2.1 Insert IV**

**2.2 Take blood** for glucose and give IV bolus (0.5 g/kg or 1 ml/kg of 50% dextrose) stat, without waiting for result.

**2.3 Give normal saline** 10–20 ml/kg IV stat to expand circulating blood volume.

**2.4 Hydrocortisone** 100 mg/m$^2$ (about 3 mg/kg) IV stat. Give the same dose up to 4 hourly over the next 24 h according to the clinical progress.

**2.5 Check electrolytes and glucose** Calcium may be needed to counteract hyperkalaemia.

**2.6 Further correction of hypoglycaemia** After initial volume expansion, change to 5–10% dextrose + 10 ml of 30% NaCl/litre.

**2.7 Treat any underlying infection**

### *Vaccinating the child on steroids*

1. A child on alternate-day steroids or <2 mg/kg/day of prednisolone should have unrestricted immunization.
2. A child on 2 mg/kg/day of prednisolone should not receive live virus vaccines (MMR, live polio). Inactivated polio vaccine is preferred. All other vaccines can be given without restriction. Once steroids have been discontinued for >3 months, then the child is regarded as a normal vaccination candidate.
3. Contact with infectious disease – see Chapter 6.

## Further reading

Hughes, I. A. (1987) Steroids and growth. *Br. Med. J.*, **295**, 683–684

Joint Committee on Vaccination and Immunisation (1988) *Immunisation Against Infectious Disease*, HMSO, London

Nickels, D. A. and Moore, D. C. (1989) Serum cortisol responses in febrile children. *Pediatr. Inf. Dis. J.*, **8**, 16–19

# 14.5 Obesity

Since obesity is usually associated with moderately advanced skeletal maturation, a fat child who is small for his age should be suspected of having a pathological cause of obesity. Most obesity, however, is 'simple' obesity which is due to an imbalance between energy intake and expenditure, although there is no overwhelming evidence that the obese eat more than their peers. Genetic and emotional factors play a significant part. Many fat children become fat adults which often has unfortunate medical and social consequences. There are no obvious preventative or novel treatment options in obesity, except diet and exercise. Success is limited.

## PATHOLOGICAL CAUSES OF OBESITY

### *1 Endocrine*

Cushing's syndrome.
Growth hormone deficiency.
Craniopharyngioma.

Hypothyroid (muscular appearance is more common).
Hyperinsulinaemia – nesidioblastosis, Beckwith syndrome, insulinoma (may be normal height or tall).

### *2 Hypothalamic*

Prader–Willi syndrome (PW).
Laurence–Moon–Biedl syndrome (LMB).
Others – Carpenter's and Alstrom's syndromes, pseudohypoparathyroidism.
Acquired – TB, sarcoid, neoplasia, trauma.

### *3 Chromosomal*

Down's syndrome.

### *4 Drugs*

Steroids.
Valproate/clonazepam.
Pizotifen.

### *5 Reduced activity*

Spina bifida.
Duchenne muscular dystrophy.

## HISTORY

Birth weight.
Family history of obesity.
Age at onset of obesity.
Social assessment – school and family stresses.
Detailed dietary history.
Sleepy, constipated, mental decline – hypothyroid.
Tetany – pseudohypoparathyroidism.
Drugs.

## PHYSICAL EXAMINATION

In most cases there are no specific physical features.
Plot height and weight centiles.
Urinalysis for glycosuria.
Inspect for – Cushingoid features (striae commonly seen in simple obesity), dysmorphic features (Down's).
BP (? cuff too small) – raised simple obesity and Cushing's syndrome.
Visual fields, fundi (pituitary tumour, retinitis pigmentosa of LMB).
Mental assessment – retardation seen in PW, LMB.
Hypotonia – PW, Down's.
Hyporeflexia – hypothyroid.
Hands and feet – small in PW, polydactyly in LMB.

| | |
|---|---|
| Skin | – dry, cool in hypothyroid. |
| Genitalia | – cryptorchidism and small penis in PW. The external urethra may appear small in simple obesity, but the subcutaneous track will be normal. |
| CVS | – loud P2, R ventricular hypertrophy (Pickwickian pulmonary hypertension). |

Pubertal assessment.

## INVESTIGATIONS

- *An obese child with normal intellect who is tall or of normal height, usually does not need further investigation.*

Karyotype.
Urinalysis – glycosuria.
Thyroid function tests.
Cushing's assessment – very rarely needed in this context:
- plasma cortisol a.m. and p.m.;
- 24h urinary free cortisol.

Lateral skull x-ray.
Bone age.
Serum lipids if has vascular disease.

## COMPLICATIONS OF EXTREME OBESITY

Hypertension.
Cholelithiasis.
Psychosocial problems.
Heart disease.
Diabetes.
Pickwickian syndrome.
Increased postoperative morbidity.
Arthritis.

## MANAGEMENT

Do not force (usually unsuccessful) measures on a reluctant child. Self-help groups (e.g. Weight Watchers) are more successful than hospital clinics.

### *1 Motivation*

Explain that obese people eat more than they need, although not necessarily more than that eaten by their slimmer peers.

### *2 Reduce energy intake*

Refer to a dietitian. Slimming can only be achieved by reducing energy intake. Dietary advice should be aimed at the whole family; parental participation is a useful therapeutic tool. Eliminate snack foods which are high in energy and low in satiety.

Confine eating to meal times.

Avoid fried or fatty foods – grill, roast, steam or boil instead.

No added sugar to cereals, drinks, or cooking.
Low-calorie fruit squash and carbonated drinks.
Consume high-fibre foods.

The consequences of even moderate caloric restriction may include an impairment of structural or brain growth. Therefore, diet should be directed against slowing the rate of fat accretion until body composition is normalized, rather than restricting energy to the point of weight loss.

### *3 Increase energy output*

Increased exercise is important.

### *4 Follow-up*

Frequent encouragement; be positive. If linear growth outstrips weight gain this is relatively speaking 'weight loss' – explain this to parents and child. Avoid despair and a sense of failure.

## Further reading

Epstein, L. H., Wing, R. R. and Valoski, A. (1985) Childhood obesity. *Pediatr. Clin. N. Am.*, **32**, 363–379

Poskitt, E. M. E. (1987) Management of obesity. *Arch. Dis. Child.*, **62**, 305–310

Rosenbaum, M. and Leibel, R. L. (1989) Obesity in childhood. *Pediatr. in Rev.*, **11**, 43–55

Van Itallie, T. B. (1986) Bad news and good news about obesity. *New Engl. J. Med.*, **314**, 239–240

# 14.6 Diabetes

## 14.6.1 Ketoacidosis

A minority of diabetics now present with severe ketoacidosis which retains a significant morbidity. Known diabetics may become ketoacidotic with infection, other stresses, steroids, poor compliance or increased endogenous requirements for insulin. The primary disturbance is an inability to utilize glucose due to insulin deficiency. Hyperglycaemia develops, and fat is used for energy with resulting ketoacidosis. The overwhelming majority of children have type I diabetes which is insulin dependent. HLA DR3 and/or DR4 haplotypes are present in about 90%.

### CLINICAL FEATURES

#### *1 Symptoms*

Polydypsia, polyuria, weight loss, enuresis, vomiting.

### *2 Signs*
Deep sighing (acidotic) breathing. Ketotic (fruity) breath.
Decreased conscious state.
Evident dehydration and shock occur relatively late.

## INVESTIGATIONS – URGENT

Blood glucose.
Urine ketones.
Acid-base status.
Electrolytes.
MSU – consider any other possible infections.

## INITIAL MANAGEMENT

To be commenced without waiting for results.

### Principles
Rehydrate – gradually rather than suddenly.
Correct hyperglycaemia – gradually, using insulin.
Correct potassium loss (even though may not be hypokalaemic).

### *1 On admission*
Weigh the child; unless the child is fully conscious, insert a NGT to empty the stomach, insert 1 or 2 intravenous lines.

### *2 Fluids*
If patient is shocked give 20 ml/kg of plasma, Hemaccel or normal saline over the first half-hour. Reassess and repeat if necessary. Assume 12% dehydration if unwell (i.e. 120 ml/kg). Rehydrate using normal saline initially (+ 25 mmol KCl/500 ml once urine flow is established).

For example, a 20 kg child, 12% dehydrated:

Deficit = 2400 ml – to be corrected over 48 h, i.e. 1200 ml 1st day
Maintenance = 100 ml/kg/day for first 10 kg;
50 ml/kg/day for 2nd 10 kg;
25 ml/kg/day thereafter.
Therefore maintenance = 1000 + 500
= 1500 ml 1st day

*Total daily fluids* 1200 ml + 1500 ml = 2700 ml on each of days 1 and 2.

However, if the child is polyuric, additional fluids should be given because of excessive ongoing losses.

### *3 Regular (fast-acting) insulin* (see Table 14.1)
N.B. Potassium must be added to the IV fluids before commencing insulin.

**Table 14.1 Insulin preparations**

| *Insulin** | *Compatible when mixed with* |
|---|---|
| *Fast-acting* | |
| Actrapid MC (P) | Protaphane MC |
| Actrapid HM (H) | Protaphane HM |
| Velosulin (P) | Insulatard |
| Velosulin Human (H) | Insulatard Human |
| Humulin R (H) | Humulin NPH |
| *Intermediate-acting* | |
| Protaphane MC (P) | Actrapid MC |
| Protaphane HM (H) | Actrapid HM |
| Insulatard (P) | Velosulin |
| Insulatard Human (H) | Velosulin Human |
| Humulin NPH (H) | Humulin R |
| Monotard MC (P) | Actrapid MC |
| Monotard HM (H) | Actrapid HM |

* All fast-acting insulins start to have an effect within half an hour, have peak effect at about 4 h, and cease to have an effect at about 6–8 h. For intermediate insulins, the figures are 2–4 h, 4–20 h and 16–24 h, respectively. P, porcine; H, human.

Administer insulin through a 'Y' connector or through a different IV line, at 0.1 u/kg/h initially. This can be made up by adding 50 u regular insulin to 500 ml 0.9% saline (0.1 u/ml) and running it at 1 ml/kg/h. Titrate rate against hourly blood sugar. A gradual reduction in blood sugar is preferable to a sudden lurch. Avoid reducing blood glucose to <12 mmol/litre in the first 24 h.

### *4 KCl*

Add 20–25 mmol/500 ml of IV fluid. Aim for 6–8 mmol/kg/day (occasionally need more). Monitor plasma $K^+$ frequently as it may fall quickly. An ECG monitor of T-waves in lead II (or V2) is helpful.

### *5 Bicarbonate*

Avoid using it unless patient is dangerously acidotic (pH <7.00). Acidosis self-corrects with normoglycaemia and rehydration.

### *6 Exclude/treat any infection*

## SUBSEQUENT MANAGEMENT

Hourly blood glucose.
4-hourly electrolytes and acid-base – continue until conscious and oral fluids are tolerated.

Careful, frequent observation of clinical condition and fluid balance.
Calculate serum osmolarity: 2 ($Na^+$ + $K^+$) + Glucose + Urea.
As blood glucose descends to <12 mmol/litre, change to 4% dextrose/0.18% saline + 20–25 mmol KCl/500 ml. If serum osmolarity is >340 mosm/litre, use 0.45% saline with added glucose. If blood glucose is <6 mmol/litre, halve the insulin infusion rate. Commence oral fluids as early as possible, then manage as below.

## 14.6.2 Diabetes without severe acidosis or dehydration – including the newly diagnosed diabetic

*1 Admit*

An IV line is not necessary.

*2 Regular (fast-acting) insulin* (see Table 14.1)

The initial predicted dose is 0.25 u/kg SC 6–8 hourly. Aim to keep blood sugar between 5 and 10 mmol/litre. Response to this initial dose of insulin is in fact unpredictable, hence a 6-hourly 'sliding scale' of insulin against blood glucose may be of use:

<4.9 mmol/litre: administer predicted dose minus 1 or 2 u;
5.0–9.9 mmol/litre: administer predicted dose (0.25 u/kg);
10.0–14.9 mmol/litre: administer predicted dose plus 1 or 2 u;
15.0–19.9 mmol/litre: administer predicted dose plus 2 or 3 u;
>20 mmol/litre: administer predicted dose plus 4 or 5 u.

*3 Planning a maintenance dose*

Add up previous day's total insulin. Give two-thirds of that total in the morning and one-third in the evening. Each dose should in turn consist of two-thirds intermediate-acting and one-third fast acting (see Table 14.1). Final insulin stabilization is only possible at home. There may be a 'honeymoon' period in new diabetics in which insulin requirement may temporarily fall, sometimes even to zero. Once daily intermediate-acting insulin may be adequate in this period.

*4 Diet*

A dietitian should be involved from the outset. 10 g carbohydrate = 40 kcal = 1 portion. Daily caloric requirement is very roughly 1000 kcal + 100 kcal extra for each year of life until puberty. More specifically, one could offer 65 kcal/kg ideal body weight until after the pubertal growth spurt and 35 kcal/kg thereafter; 45–50% of the calories should be carbohydrate (primarily complex), 20% protein and 30% fat (primarily unsaturated). Approximately 30% of the daily allowance should be consumed at each major meal, with the remainder for snacks. Increasingly, active well children are being offered an unrestricted diet that consists largely of unprocessed carbohydrates.

### 5 Education/involving other members of the team

Patient and parental education is the foundation of successful diabetic care. Initial explanation and education should be slow, in small 'portions', and should be couched in optimistic language as the family must contend with the normal grief reaction. Diabetic sister, dietition and social worker should form part of the management team. Time spent at this stage educating child and parents may well prevent a host of management problems in the future. While in the ward, the child and parents will learn much about self-administering insulin, diet, monitoring blood glucose, the recognition and management of hyper- and hypoglycaemia, insulin requirement during illness, and who to contact if there are problems.

## ELECTIVE AND MINOR SURGERY

If possible, it should be performed in the morning.
Withhold breakfast.
Insert IV line and run 5% dextrose and electrolytes at maintenance rates.
Give one-half the normal morning intermediate-acting insulin SC.
Aim to keep blood glucose between 5 and 12 mmol/litre.
Check blood glucose before leaving the ward, immediately postoperatively, and 1–2 hourly thereafter, until child resumes eating and drinking (usually later that afternoon).
That evening, return to normal diet and normal insulin regimen.

## EMERGENCY AND MAJOR SURGERY (lasting >1 h)

For elective procedures, admit the previous day and assess diabetic control. For emergency procedures, assess clinically and biochemically for ketoacidosis or dehydration (blood glucose, acid-base, electrolytes, urinary ketones, urine output, blood pressure). Insert IV line and infuse 5% dextrose/0.18% saline, and omit normal subcutaneous insulin dose.

Commence infusion of fast-acting insulin at 0.05 u/kg/h through a 'Y' connector or different IV line.

Adjust rate of insulin infusion to maintain blood glucose between 5 and 15 mmol/litre. Continue infusion until oral feeding is resumed.

### Intercurrent illness

#### 1 Vomiting

Check blood glucose, urine ketones, and assess hydration.

**1.1 Normal blood glucose without urinary ketones** Continue normal insulin regimen. One can substitute easily tolerated, sugar-containing fluids such as soft drinks or fruit juice for usual meals. Mild hyperglycaemia can be managed with small increases in fast-acting insulin.

**1.2 Low blood glucose** Halve normal insulin dose. Oral fluids as above. Monitor blood glucose 2–4 hourly and as blood glucose rises give increased amounts of fast-acting insulin.

**1.3 High blood glucose** If there is no ketonuria, increase normal daily fast and intermediate-acting insulin dose by 10%. If ketonuria is present, or if hyperglycaemia persists, give additional supplments of fast-acting insulin (10% of total daily insulin dose) 4 hourly according to blood sugar. As soon as there is an improvement in the illness, insulin dose must be rapidly cut back to normal to prevent hypoglycaemia.

Monitor urinary ketones and blood sugar 4 hourly.

Oral fluids should be continued as above.

There should be a low threshold for admission if there is any doubt about the child's clinical condition, or about the parents' ability to cope, especially if vomiting appears to be continuing into the night.

### *2 Other intercurrent illness*

Any illness poses the threat of hypoglycaemia (decreased intake), or hyperglycaemia ± ketosis (insulin resistance).

**2.1 Frequent monitoring of blood glucose and urinary ketones** These will determine subsequent management.

**2.2 Treat any infection**

**2.3 Maintain carbohydrate intake** Simple carbohydrate-containing foods, or sugar-containing fluids as above.

**2.4 Insulin** If hyperglycaemia develops, increase fast- and intermediate-acting insulin dose by 10%. If hyperglycaemia persists or ketonuria develops, give additional supplements of fast-acting insulin (10% of total daily insulin dose) 4 hourly according to blood sugar.

As soon as there is an improvement in the illness, insulin dose must be rapidly cut back to normal to prevent hypoglycaemia.

## HYPOGLYCAEMIA

### *1 Mild hypoglycaemia*

Many diabetic children will have symptoms of mild hypoglycaemia with strenuous activity or prolonged periods without food, although they should not occur with normal day-to-day activities. Most children and their parents can recognize these symptoms early and self-administer food or drink with easily absorbed sugars, e.g. fruit juice, soft drinks, sweets, honey, milk. Frequent episodes suggest that an adjustment in diet and/or insulin is needed.

### 2 Severe hypoglycaemia

Hypoglycaemia associated with altered consciousness such that another person must render the child assistance is classified as severe. Parents should have available glucagon 1 mg which should be given SC. If the child presents to hospital with convulsions or loss of consciousness, take a blood sugar and give 0.5 g/kg of 50% dextrose IV (1 ml/kg) without waiting for the result. Repeat × 1 if necessary. Continue an IV infusion of 5% dextrose for several hours.

The reason for the attack should be explored. If none can be found, a change in insulin or diet may be required.

## OUTPATIENT EVALUATION (some suggestions)

Inspect records of home insulin requirements and blood sugar control.
Height, weight, growth centiles, sexual maturation.
Blood pressure, peripheral pulses.
Neurological examination – deep tendon reflexes, sensory nerves, touch and position sense.
Ophthalmological assessment – every other year in prepubertal and yearly thereafter.
Laboratory tests to consider: urine culture (especially in girls), blood urea, creatinine, creatinine clearance, $HbA_1C$, cholesterol and triglyceride levels and lipoprotein fractions.

## Further reading


Baum, J. D. and Kinmouth, A. (1985) *Care of the Child with Diabetes*, Churchill Livingstone, Edinburgh

Ginsberg-Fellner, F. (1990) Insulin-dependent diabetes mellitus. *Pediatr. in Rev.*, **11**, 239–247

Harris, G. D., Fiordalisi, I. and Finberg, L. (1988) Safe management of diabetic ketoacidemia. *J. Pediatr.*, **113**, 65–67

Chapter 15

# Cardiology

## 15.1 ECG interpretation

Normal ECGs may change radically from the neonatal period, through infancy, childhood, adolescence and finally adulthood. This is not a comprehensive discussion on ECGs, but several useful points will be stressed to facilitate ECG interpretation.

### *Things to know before interpreting an ECG*

1. Age (in days) – waves in the R precordial leads change from positive to negative within the first 5 days.
2. Medications – especially digoxin.
3. BP.
4. Reason for doing the ECG.
5. Any electrolyte disorder.

### *Systematic approach to the interpretation of ECGs*

1. Rate.
2. Rhythm.
3. Axis.
4. P-wave morphology.
5. PR interval, QRS duration, QT interval.
6. ST or T-wave abnormalities.

### *Rate*

5 large squares (25 mm) = 1 s.
1 beat per 5 squares = 60/min
1 beat per 4 squares = 75/min
1 beat per 3 squares = 100/min
1 beat per 2 squares = 150/min
1 beat per 1 square = 300/min

For normal rate according to age, see Table 15.1.

**Table 15.1 Normal heart rate according to age**

| | *Awake* | *Asleep* | *Fever/agitation* |
|---|---|---|---|
| Newborn | 100–180 | 80–160 | < 220 |
| 1 wk–3 mo | 100–220 | 80–200 | < 220 |
| 3 mo–2 yr | 80–150 | 70–120 | < 200 |
| 2–10 yr | 70–110 | 60–90 | < 200 |
| > 10 yr | 55–90 | 50–90 | < 200 |

## *Rhythm*

Sinus arrhythmia is the commonest 'rhythm disturbance' of childhood.

## *Axis*

Finding the QRS axis is the pivotal point of paediatric ECG interpretation:

1. Normal cardiac axis – changes with age (Figure 15.1).
2. Abnormal cardiac axis.

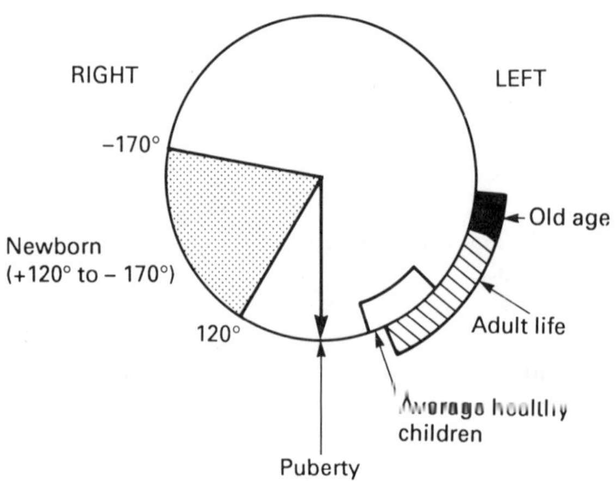


**Figure 15.1** Normal trends of QRS axis from birth to old age (From Harris, L. C. and Feinstein, E. (1979) *Understanding ECGs in Infants and Children*, Little, Brown and Co., Boston, with permission)

R axis deviation (RAD) suggests R ventricular hypertrophy (RVH).
L axis deviation suggests LVH (but not as strongly as RAD and RVH).
Typical axes of some congenital anomalies – see Figure 15.2.

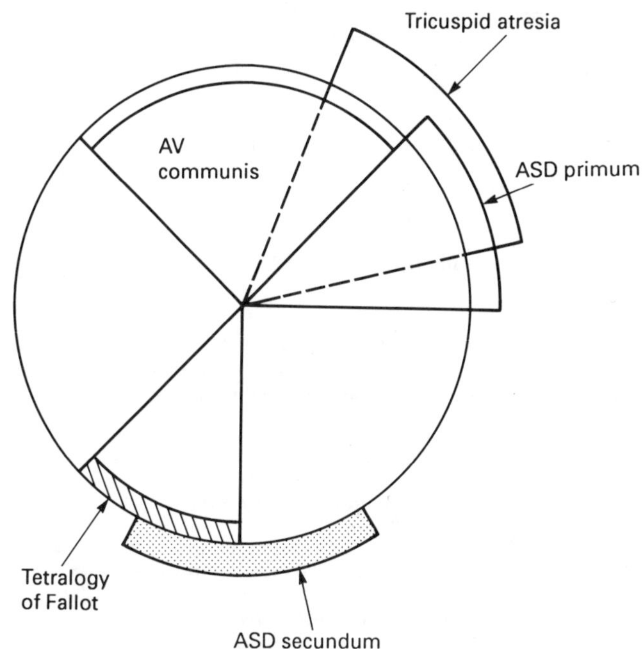


**Figure 15.2** Typical cardiac axis of some congenital anomalies (From Harris, L. C. and Feinstein, E. (1979) *Understanding ECGs in Infants and Children*, Little, Brown and Co., Boston, with permission)

## *P-wave morphology*

Normal height: <2.5 mm (<3 mm in neonates).
P-waves in any lead that are above these voltages indicate R atrial enlargement (P pulmonale). In rheumatic carditis, broadening of the P-wave suggests L atrial enlargement (P mitrale). Maximum normal P-wave breadth is 0.08 s (2 small squares). Best seen in lead I or II.

## *PR interval*

Usually best assessed in lead II.
Normal PR interval – see Table 15.2.

**Table 15.2 Normal PR interval according to age***

| | *PR interval in children* (s) | | |
|---|---|---|---|
| | Min. | Max. | Mean |
| Infants (6–12 mo) | 0.07 | 0.15 | 0.10 |
| Child (4–8 yr) | 0.09 | 0.19 | 0.13 |
| Child (8–13 yr) | 0.09 | 0.20 | 0.14 |

* Prolongation of the PR interval indicates a first-degree heart block (? digoxin, ? rheumatic carditis).

## *The QRS complex*

Anterior chest/precordial leads (i.e. $V_{1-6}$ and $V_4R$ or $V_3R$).

### *1 Normal complex*

In the newborn there is right ventricular dominance which is reflected in large R-waves in $V_4R$ and large S-waves in $V_6$. As the child progresses through infancy and childhood, the converse occurs (Figure 15.3).

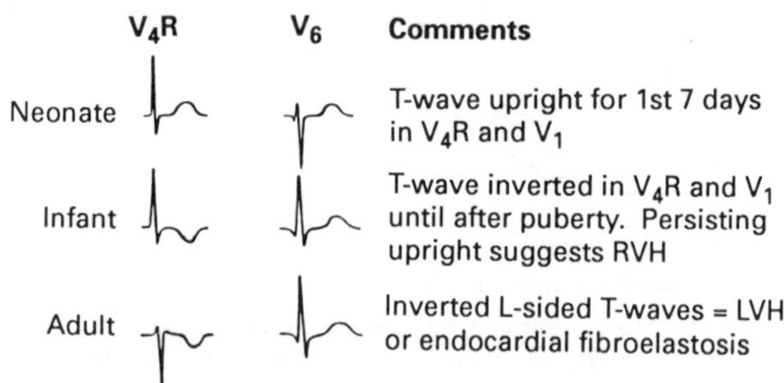


**Figure 15.3** The changing QRST complex in infancy

### *2 Broad QRS*

Bundle branch block can be considered to be present at any age when the QRS complex is >0.10 s (2.5 small squares); however, one should consider it in an infant with QRS duration >0.07 s or in a child with >0.08 s.

### *3 rsR′ pattern*

R′ indicates the taller of the two waves designated r and R′. The rsR′ pattern may be seen in normal infants in the right chest leads or may signify an atrial septal defect (ASD), in which case the R′ will have a much greater amplitude than r. If the QRS interval is within normal limits, bundle branch block is excluded.

## QT interval

The normal QT interval is influenced by heart rate, hence a QT index or corrected QT interval (i.e. QTc) needs to be calculated as follows:

$$QTc = \frac{\text{QT interval (s)}}{\sqrt{\text{R–R interval (s)}}} \quad \text{Normal value is} <0.425\,\text{s}$$

Prolonged QT interval has been linked to syncope and sudden death.

### *1 Causes of prolonged QTc*

Myocardial disease especially myocarditis.
Electrolyte disturbance:
Low $K^+$ (also see U-waves after the T), $Mg^{2+}$, $Ca^{2+}$ (also gives a flat ST segment).
Drugs – phenytoin, quinidine.
CNS damage.
Syndromes:
Jervell–Lange–Neilsen syndrome of long QT plus congenital deafness.
Romano–Ward syndrome is characterized by a dominantly inherited prolonged QT without deafness.

### *2 Short QT*

Hypercalcaemia.

## Left ventricular hypertrophy (LVH)

### *1 ECG criteria*

R in $V_5/V_6$ >20 mm in a child <3 months;>25 mm in a child >3 months.
S in $V_1$ of >25 mm.
$S_{V1} + R_{V5-6}$ >50 mm (suggestive).
Inverted T in $V_6$ (suggestive).
Q >4 mm in $V_{5-6}$ (suggestive).

### *2 Causes*

VSD, PDA, aortic stenosis and incompetence, coarctation of the aorta, mitral incompetence, cardiomyopathy, endocardial fibroelastosis.

## Right ventricular hypertrophy (RVH)

### *1 ECG criteria*

R in $V_4R$ >15 mm in a child <3 months; >10 mm in a child >3 months.
S in $V_6$: 0–7 days >14 mm; 8–30 days >10 mm; 1–3 months >7 mm; 3 months–11 yr >5 mm.
R in $V_2$ >30 mm (suggestive).
rsR′ in $V_4R$ and V1 (suggestive).
Upright T-wave in $V_4R$ and $V_1$ after the first week of life until 12 yr old.
R-axis deviation (suggestive).

*2 Causes*

Pulmonary stenosis, Fallot's tetralogy, pulmonary hypertension, transposition of great arteries.

### ***Biventricular hypertrophy***

*1 ECG criteria*

Independent criteria for LVH and RVH.
R + S in $V_3$ or $V_4$ >50 mm (infants); >60 mm (children).
Criteria for LVH present and either $R_{V1}$ >10 mm or $S_{V6}$ >$R_{V6}$.
Criteria for RVH present and either Q of 3 mm or more in $V_{5-6}$, or inverted T in $V_{5-6}$.

*2 Causes*

Large VSD.

### ***Effects of electrolyte disturbance on the ECG***

Hypokalaemia – prolonged QT, ST depression, flat T-waves, prominent U-waves*, arrhythmias.
Hyperkalaemia – broad P-waves, broad QRST, peaked tall T-waves, arrhythmia.
Hypocalcaemia – prolonged QT.
Hypercalcaemia – shortens QT.

*Abnormal U-waves have an amplitude of at least 1 mm and are best seen in the middle chest leads in the same direction as T-waves.

## Further reading

Feinstein, E. and Harris, L. C. (1979) *Understanding ECGs in Infants and Children*, Little, Brown and Co., Boston

# 15.2 Prophylaxis against infective endocarditis

## COMMON PREDISPOSITIONS TO ENDOCARDITIS

Congenital heart disease.
Prosthetic cardiac valves, patch repairs, Gor-Tex shunts.
Rheumatic/acquired valve disease.
Idiopathic hypertrophic subaortic stenosis.
Past history of bacterial endocarditis.
Surgically constructed systemic–pulmonary shunts.
Mitral valve prolapse if associated with murmur.

## PROPHYLAXIS IS NOT NECESSARY FOR:

Isolated secundum ASD.
Secundum ASD repaired without a patch more than 6 months ago.
Ligated PDA.

## PREDISPOSING PROCEDURES

### *1 Standard risk*

**1.1 Dental procedures likely to cause gingival bleeding** Extractions, scaling or gum treatment.

**1.2 Trauma to respiratory mucosa** Tonsillectomy, adenoidectomy, bronchoscopy.

### *2 High risk*

**2.1 Colorectal and urinary tract surgery**

**2.2 Urethral catheter if urine infected**

**2.3 Cystoscopy, colonoscopy**

### *3 Negligible risk*

Tooth filling, liver biopsy, in/out urinary catheter (if urine is sterile), upper GI endoscopy.

## ANTIBIOTIC PROPHYLAXIS (see Table 15.3)

**Table 15.3 Antibiotic prophylaxis against infective endocarditis**

| *Category* | *Antibiotic* | *Regimen* |
|---|---|---|
| STANDARD RISK | Penicillin V (oral) | 50 mg/kg 1 h before and 25 mg/kg 6 h after procedure |
| | *or* | |
| | Amoxycillin | 40 mg/kg 1 h before procedure |
| Penicillin-allergic patients or patients already on penicillin | Erythromycin | 20 mg/kg (max. 1.0 g) 1 h before and 10 mg/kg (max. 500 mg) 6 h after procedure |
| | *or* | |
| | Clindamycin | 6 mg/kg 1 h before procedure |
| HIGH RISK | Ampicillin IV | 50 mg/kg |
| | + | |
| | Gentamicin IV | 2.5 mg/kg 30 min before procedure; repeat after 8 h |
| Penicillin allergic | Vancomycin IV | 20 mg/kg up to 1.0 g given over 30 min |
| | + | |
| | Gentamicin IV | 2.5 mg/kg 60 min before procedure; repeat after 8 h |

## Further reading

Dajani, A. S. (1985) Prevention of bacterial endocarditis. *Pediatr. Inf. Dis.*, **4**, 349–352

Working Party of British Society for Antimicrobial Chemotherapy (1990) *Lancet*, **335**, 88–89

# 15.3 Tetralogy of Fallot spells

Infundibular shutdown or increased pulmonary resistance gives a sudden increase in R to L shunting. These spells can resolve within minutes to hours or result in worsening hypoxia, acidosis and occasionally death.

## CLINICAL FEATURES

Agitated, blue child, progressing to limpness, loss of consciousness, and in severe cases convulsions, cerebrovascular accidents, and death. There may be no lung findings, but may be tachypnoeic with increased depth of breathing.
Normal volume pulse.
Murmurs of VSD or pulmonary stenosis – ejection murmur may be quieter or shorter than usual.

## INVESTIGATIONS

None is usually needed to make the diagnosis.
Arterial gases – hypoxaemia, acidosis.
ECG – increased P-wave voltage.
Chest x-ray (rarely done during the episode) – pulmonary oligaemia.

## MANAGEMENT

### *1 Posture*
Children with Fallot's will classically squat during these turns. Holding the child in the knee–chest position will mimic this posture and hopefully increase L to R shunting by increasing systemic vascular resistance.

### *2 Oxygen*
Hood or mask at 6–8 litres/min.

### *3 Morphine*
0.1 mg/kg IV.

*4 Propranolol*
0.03 mg/kg IV over 5 min. Repeat up to × 5, at 5-min intervals.

*5 Correct metabolic acidosis*
Bicarbonate deficit (mEq) = Base excess × Weight (kg) × 0.3.
Give half this amount initially and then review.
Do not give bicarbonate if there is also respiratory acidosis, i.e. if $P\text{CO}_2$ is high.

*6 Metaraminol*
0.01 mg/kg stat, repeat p.r.n., then 0.1–1.0 μg/kg/min infusion and titrate against BP. Rarely used.

*7 Blood transfusion*
Give 5 ml/kg if Hb <15 g%.

*8 After the child recovers*

**8.1 Propranolol** 0.5–1.0 mg/kg/8 h oral.

**8.2 Consider** Corrective or palliative surgery.

PREVENTION

*1 Treat hypovolaemia*
Generous rehydration in diarrhoeal or febrile illnesses.

*2 Propranolol*
0.5 mg/kg/8 h oral long term.

## 15.4 Paediatric cardiac surgical procedures

| *Operation* | *Description* |
|---|---|
| *1 To increase pulmonary blood flow (TOF, PS, tricuspid atresia, transposition of great vessels)* | |
| Blalock–Taussig | Subclavian artery–pulmonary artery anastomosis |
| Potts | Descending aorta–pulmonary artery anastomosis |
| Waterston | Ascending aorta–pulmonary artery anastomosis |

| | |
|---|---|
| Central | Aorta–pulmonary artery anastomosis (with graft) |
| Glenn | SVC–pulmonary artery anastomosis |
| Brock | Pulmonary valvotomy and infundibulectomy (closed) |
| Outflow patch | Right ventricle–pulmonary artery outflow tract patch |
| Rastelli | Right ventricle–pulmonary artery anastomosis (valved conduit) |

*2 To decrease pulmonary blood flow (AV canal, truncus arteriosus, tricuspid atresia, large VSD, complex congenital cardiac defects)*

| | |
|---|---|
| Pulmonary artery banding | Constrictive band around pulmonary artery |

*3 To increase pulmonary–systemic mixing (transposition of great vessels)*

| | |
|---|---|
| Rashkind (balloon septostomy) | Rupture of membrane of fossa ovale |
| Park | Atrial septostomy using catheter blade |
| Blalock–Hanlon | Atrial septectomy (closed) |
| Mustard or Senning (palliative) | Intra-atrial venous transposition without closure of septal defect |

*4 Corrective operations*

| | |
|---|---|
| Jatene (TGV) | Arterial switch |
| Fontan (tricuspid atresia) | Right atrium–right pulmonary artery (aortic valve homograft) |

## 15.5 The blue child

Peripheral cyanosis is not uncommon in neonates and infants. It may merely signify that the child is cold, or it may be a sign of sepsis, polycythaemia or acrocyanosis (autonomic).

Central cyanosis is always a serious sign. It is due to the presence of more than 5 g of reduced haemoglobin per 100 ml of blood. Anaemia can make cyanosis difficult to detect. Apart from the rare situation of methaemoglobinaemia (familial or due to alanine dyes), the sign implies reduced arterial oxygen saturation. Clinical suspicion should be confirmed with a pulse oximeter (using different absorption of 2 wavelengths of red light, it calculates the ratio of oxygenated to deoxygenated haemoglobin) and an arterial blood gas estimation. The cause is usually either pulmonary or cardiac. The hyperoxic test will differentiate the two. Cardiac causes of central cyanosis involve conditions with a R to L shunt and reduced pulmonary flow, transposition of the great arteries, or common mixing situations. Echocardiography has contributed greatly to pre-catheter diagnosis, although much can be learned from clinical examination, chest x-ray and ECG (see Figure 15.2 for clues from cardiac axis).

### *The hyperoxic test*

This test helps to differentiate cyanotic (R to L shunt) congenital heart disease from lung disease, and other causes of hypoxaemia (CNS depression, etc.).

An arterial blood gas analysis is taken from the R arm if possible (preductal circulation), and then repeated after administration of 100% $O_2$ for 10 min. Oxygen is best delivered via an enclosed head box, an anaesthetic bag and mask T-piece circuit with high flow of $O_2$, or an endotracheal tube.

## AETIOLOGY OF CYANOSIS

First perform the hyperoxic test.

### *1 $Pa_{O_2}$ is $<100$ mmHg*

The cause is a right to left cardiac shunt. A rise to 75–100 mmHg may be seen in transposition of the great vessels with VSD, or total anomalous pulmonary venous return.

### *2 $Pa_{O_2}$ is $>100$ mmHg*

Possible causes are:

**2.1 Primary lung disease** (Hyaline membrane disease of the newborn, pneumonia, aspiration, many others).

**2.2 Others** Sepsis, non-cyanotic heart disease with heart failure, CNS lesion, polycythaemia.

## INVESTIGATIONS

Acid-base, arterial blood gases.
Hyperoxia test.
Haemoglobin.
Chest x-ray.
ECG.

Once cyanotic heart disease is confirmed with the hyperoxic test, the probable cardiac cause of the cyanosis can be decided according to the chest x-ray, ECG and clinical examination.

### *1 Decreased pulmonary blood flow*

**1.1 Right ventricular hypertrophy (RVH)**
Tetralogy of Fallot – boot-shaped heart, pulmonary murmur with single $S_2$.
Pure pulmonary stenosis – late pulmonary murmur, widely split $S_2$, faint $P_2$.
Eisenmenger syndrome – features of pulmonary hypertension.
Ebstein's anomaly – severe cardiomegaly, occasionally split $S_1$, murmur of tricuspid insufficiency.

**1.2 Left ventricular hypertrophy (LVH)** Tricuspid atresia or pulmonary atresia – single $S_2$.

**1.3 Combined ventricular hypertrophy (CVH)** Transposition of the great vessels (arteries) (TGV) with pulmonary stenosis ± ventricular septal defect (VSD). Stenotic ± pansystolic murmur. Truncus arteriosis and hypoplastic pulmonary arteries.

### *2 Increased pulmonary blood flow*

**2.1 LVH or CVH**
Truncus arteriosis – mixing occurs at arterial level. Often systolic ejection click, single $S_2$, systolic murmur.
Single ventricle.
TGV with VSD – the VSD allows the child to be only partly desaturated, resulting in later presentation in the first weeks of life with heart failure, and a pansystolic murmur.

**2.2 RVH**
TGV with intact septum – usually presents on the first day of life with marked cyanosis. There is no murmur.
Total anomalous pulmonary venous drainage (TAPVD) – mixing occurs at atrial level. Occasionally widely split $S_2$.
Occasional 'snowman' appearance on chest x-ray.
Hypoplastic L heart – marked cardiac enlargement, congestive heart failure, diminished peripheral pulses, within the first few days of life.

### Eisenmenger syndrome

This occurs when a L to R shunt reverses, and blood flows from R to L, because pulmonary pressure exceeds systemic arterial pressure. Any child with a L to R shunt (e.g. VSD, ASD, PDA) has increased pulmonary blood flow and may eventually run the risk of developing irreversible pulmonary hypertension and R to L shunting with cyanosis. It should be suspected when a previously pink child with a cardiac murmur becomes cyanosed. The early warning signs are a cardiac murmur of diminishing intensity with persistence of a loud pulmonary second sound and a RV heave. Once the Eisenmenger syndrome is established, operative repair is no longer possible.

### Secondary pulmonary hypertension

Children with Down's syndrome have a predisposition to developing pulmonary hypertension and R to L shunting, as do those who suffer from extreme obesity (Pickwickian), obstructive sleep apnoea, kyphoscoliosis and other restrictive lung diseases. All heart diseases with high flows from L to R may develop pulmonary hypertension. Surgery may be life saving if it is performed before the Eisenmenger syndrome develops.

Chapter 16

# Dermatology

## 16.1 Bacterial skin conditions

### *Impetigo – school sores*

This is a contagious skin infection caused by *Staphylococcus aureus*, *Streptococcus pyogenes* or both. In infants, bullous lesions may erupt. Usually, lesions are bright and yellow with crusting and occasional ooze. It may be a primary infection or else conditions such as scabies or eczema may become 'impetiginized', i.e. secondarily infected. Glomerulonephritis may result from streptococci M-type 49 or 50. Rheumatic fever is not a sequela of cutaneous infection.

#### *1 Clinical features*

Multiple lesions, often on face or extremities, with characteristic yellow crusts. Regional lymphadenopathy is common.

#### *2 Treatment*

**2.1 Topical** Crusts can be bathed off with simple soap and water or hexachlorophane 3 times daily. A topical antiseptic may be used. Topical antibiotics are no better than simple bathing.

**2.2 Systemic antibiotics** Most cases respond rapidly to antibiotics. Penicillin V or erythromycin are the drugs of choice. Oral first-generation cephalosporins (cephalexin) are a sensible alternative.

#### *3 Patient education*

Good handwashing techniques should be emphasized because of the contagious nature of the illness. Prevent scratching by cutting finger-nails.

### *Erysipelas*

A rapidly spreading superficial cellulitis with distinct borders, accompanied by prominent systemic signs and symptoms (although bacteraemia is rare). The skin is shiny, warm and indurated. Most commonly affected site is the face. Infection penetrates the skin through minor skin abrasions. It is caused by group A streptococci. Rarely, other beta haemolytic streptococci or *Staphylococcus aureus* produce a similar picture.

### 1 Treatment

IV benzyl penicillin 60 mg (100 000 u)/kg/6 h.
Erythromycin for penicillin-hypersensitive patients.

## Cellulitis

Cellulitis is a more deep-seated infection, largely caused by *S. aureus* or *Streptococcus pyogenes*. It lacks distinct elevated borders (cf. erysipelas). Lymphangitis and enlarged regional nodes are common. Facial and orbital cellulitis may be caused by *Haemophilus influenzae* and are considered in Section 10.9.

### Treatment

Penicillin as for erysipelas. Consider adding flucloxacillin.
Alternatively, one can use a first-generation cephalosporin (cefazolin 10–35 mg/kg/8 h IV, or cephalexin 10–15 mg/kg/6 h oral). In those with hypersensitivity to penicillin, use erythromycin.

## Staphylococcal scalded skin syndrome (Ritter's disease)

This serious disease is a result of exotoxin production from certain staphylococcal phage types (group II, type 55 or 71), causing widespread intra-epithelial splitting of the stratum granulosum. It occurs in children <8 yr of age.

### 1 Clinical features

Sudden onset fever, irritability and generalized erythema developing over 2–3 days. Soon bullae and a positive Nikolsky sign (separation of a layer of skin with a minor degree of friction) develop, followed by spontaneous sheet-like separation of the skin leaving a moist denuded area. Often the child is surprisingly well or has only a minor primary staphylococcal infection, which is not surprising given that it is the toxin rather than the infection itself which causes the clinical picture.

### 2 Differential diagnosis

Scarlet fever, toxic shock syndrome, Kawasaki syndrome, erythema multiforme/Stevens–Johnson syndrome, toxic epidermal necrolysis (usually drug induced – sulphonamides and barbiturates), sunburn. The dramatic rapid superficial peeling, coupled with sparing of the mucous membranes and the absence of recent drug ingestion, usually establish the diagnosis.

*3 Complications*
Profound protein loss.
Hypovolaemia.
Secondary infection (uncommon).

*4 Treatment*

**4.1 IV/oral flucloxacillin** For 10 days to eliminate primary focus.

**4.2 Careful attention** To fluids and electrolytes. Fluid loss may require management similar to that of severe burns.

# 16.2 Viral skin infections

## *Herpes simplex*

Major morbidity occurs with gingivostomatitis (see Section 18.2).

## *Warts*

Caused by human papilloma viruses.
They give rise to:
 common warts – commonly on fingers;
 plantar warts;
 genital warts (condylomata acuminata);
 plane warts;
 filiform warts.

Genital warts are transmitted by sexual contact and tend to be of types 6–11, 16 and 18.

Warts on hands and feet tend to be types 1 and 2 (Priestly, B. (1988) Child Abuse Forum, BPA annual meeting, York).

Warts are usually benign, resolving spontaneously over years.

Plantar warts are often troublesome and may need help from a dermatologist.

*1 Possible treatments*
Recurrence rates for all treatments are high. The natural history of warts is variable, but most spontaneously resolve in 12–24 months. These points should be considered before embarking on any treatment.

**1.1 Wart paints** For example, 16.7% salicylic acid with 16.7% lactic acid in flexible collodion (salactol paint). The wart must be pared or filed off each day before each application.

**1.2 Cryotherapy** A cryosurgery probe or copper bar cooled in liquid nitrogen may be used. Most commonly, a cotton swab with a loose, pointed tip is dipped in a Thermos flask containing liquid nitrogen (−195°C) and the saturated swab is applied to the centre of the wart until a white 'ice ball' extending 1–3 mm beyond the margin of the wart is formed. The freeze is maintained for 20–30 s. After 1 week it may be necessary to de-roof the blister and re-freeze.

**1.3 Other treatments** Excision, retinoic acid 1% cream. Podophyllum should not be applied to extensive areas of mucosa. X-ray and electrocautery should not be used in children because of high recurrence rate and high incidence of side effects.

**1.4 Some unconventional treatments**

1. Hypnosis.
2. Rubbing with potato peel prior to throwing the peel over one's shoulder and burying it where it lands (Tunnessen, W. W. (1983) *Pediatr. Clin. N. Am.*, **30**, 515–532).
3. Enshroud finger in adhesive tape, wrapped first longitudinally then circumferentially. Remove tape once a week for 12 h, then reapply. Works within 4 weeks (Litt, J. Z. (1978). Don't exercise, exorcise. *Cutis,* **22**, 673).
4. The sap of the radium weed (*Euphorbia peplus*, petty spurge). Scrub the wart with soap and water and dry it. Apply a bead of sap daily (Grounds, M. (1980) Radium weed. *Family Med. Progr. Newsl.*, Victorian Post Graduate Medical Foundation, March; 18–19).

There are many other unconventional treatments.

## *Molluscum contagiosum*

These are highly contagious smooth asymptomatic papules 1–3 mm in diameter, many having a characteristic central punctum. They occur in crops and are caused by poxvirus. Usually no treatment is required, as they resolve spontaneously over several years. If parents or child are unwilling to wait for spontaneous resolution, a drop of cantharidin (0.7%) or trichloroacetic acid 25% can be applied to the central umbilication with a wooden toothpick. Liquid nitrogen or curettage can also be used. Repeated treatment every 2–3 weeks is often necessary as new crops arise.

# 16.3 Fungal infections

## DIAGNOSTIC METHODS

### *1 Skin scrapings – microscopy and culture*

Scrape the scaly border of a skin lesion with a scalpel blade to collect fine scales, or collect hair stubs and place on some black paper. Transfer some of the material onto a glass slide. Put 1 drop of 10–20% KOH (for keratolysis) on the slide and cover with coverslip. Warm over a light bulb for 5 min and wait a further 5 min. Examine for fragments of mycelia. Send the black paper to the microbiology laboratory for culture of fungi, which may take up to 6 weeks.

### *2 Wood's light (long-wave ultraviolet light)*

In a darkened room, involved hairs of scalp show brilliant green fluorescence at their bases if *Microsporum* is the responsible agent; however, many cases of tinea capitis are caused by *Trichophyton* and will not fluoresce.

## ***Tinea capitus***

An infection of scalp and hair with any of the dermatophytes.

### *1 Diagnosis*

KOH examination under light microscopy, or culture of affected hairs. Wood's lamp – most species (especially *Microsporum*) fluoresce.

### *2 Treatment*

Topical antifungals usually will not work.
Griseofulvin (micronized form) 10–15 mg/day (in 1–2 divided doses) orally with milk or a meal for 6–12 weeks plus shampoo with selenium sulphide suspension (Selsun).

## ***Tinea corporis (ringworm)***

Caused by several species of dermatophyte, most commonly *Microsporum canis* or *Trichophyton rubrum*. It usually appears as a complete or partial annular or ring-like configuration of red papular scaly border with a clear centre.

### *1 Diagnosis*

KOH preparation of scrapings from the border of the lesion.

### *2 Treatment*

Topical antifungals – clotrimazole 1%, miconazole, haloprogin and tolnaftate are all efficacious against about 90% of dermatophyte species. Apply twice daily, as a cream or solution, to the whole affected area until the lesions have cleared.

If *Microsporum canis* is the pathogen, the household pet may need treatment by a veterinarian.

## 16.4 Scabies

*Sarcoptes scabei* completes its life cycle in humans. Fertilized mites burrow into the skin, laying several eggs per day during their 1–2-month lives. The eggs take up to 2 weeks to reach adulthood. Spread is by direct skin contact, commonly within families or between children (also between sexual contacts).

### CLINICAL FEATURES

The typical skin lesions are not unique to scabies and include papules, pustules and vesicles distributed over hands, feet, skin folds, finger-nails and genitalia. Head and neck may be affected in infants. Babies can occasionally have very bullous eruptions. Pruritus (especially at night) is very common. Pathognomonic linear or S-shaped burrows less than 1 cm long are found in less than 10% of scabetic children. They are most commonly seen on wrist, palm, interdigital webs or genitalia. Examining other family members may be illuminating.

### DIAGNOSIS

Skin scrapings of an unscratched papule should be taken from interdigital webs, linear lesions or intensely pruritic areas. Put a drop of immersion oil on a slide, add skin scraping, and place a coverslip over the oil. Mites, ova or faecal concretions are best seen with × 10 magnification. If a burrow is seen, gently put a needle into it; the mite often grips onto it and can then be put on a slide.

### TREATMENT

Treat all skin from neck down including genitalia, palms and soles.
Treat face as well in infants.
Conventional wisdom is that clothing and bedding are sources of reinfestation and therefore must be aired, changed or washed. Some claim

that this is not so and that reinfestation from these sources is not a risk (*Drugs Ther. Bull.* (1988) **26,** 19–20).
Treat all close contacts.
Itching may persist for 4–8 weeks after successful treatment. Patients should be forewarned of this so that expectations are lowered and despair avoided.
Repeat treatment before then, only if burrows reappear or if the mite or her products are seen on repeat scrapings.
Transmission of mites ceases within 24 h of effective treatment.

*1 Gamma benzene hexachloride 1% lotion (Lindane)*
Apply on dry skin for only 6 h, then wash off. It has a pleasant odour and is non-irritant. Do not use in children less than 3 yr of age because of the risk of neurotoxicity when applied to large areas of skin.

*2 Malathion*
0.5% lotion – used for children <3 yr. Apply once and wash off after 24 h.

*3 Benzyl benzoate 25%*
Dilute 1:1 with water. Apply once for 24 h and then again 2 days later. It is a skin irritant, has an unpleasant odour and cures only two-thirds of cases (*Br. Med. J.* (1986) **292**, 1172). Despite widespread use it is not the best drug.

*4 Others*
10% crotamiton (Eurax) has antipruritic properties but is less effective than Lindane. Sulphur formulations (e.g. 6–10% sulphur in petrolatum) are malodorous and stain clothing.

## 16.5 Head lice (pediculosis)

### DIAGNOSIS

The major symptom is pruritus. Adult lice may be seen on the scalp. Nits (ova) will be cemented to the hairs. They fluoresce a pearly colour under Wood's light (may be difficult to interpret). If in doubt, place a plucked hair with attached nit on a glass slide with a drop of oil, and examine under a microscope.

### TREATMENT

*1 Gamma benzene hexachloride 1% shampoo (Lindane)*
It should be rubbed in and left *in situ* for 5 min before rinsing and drying. Leaving it for 10 min may be more effective (*Pediatr. Dermatol.* (1984) **2**, 74–79). Repeat treatment after 1 week.

Following the shampoo, gelatinous nits will remain, hence leave scalp wrapped in a warm damp towel for 30 min, and mechanically remove nits with a fine-toothed comb. Alternatively, remaining nits can be removed with vinegar (acetic acid 5%) followed by combing.

Treat all household members.

Soak combs and brushes in Lindane shampoo for 10 min.

Parents should notify the school which in turn should notify all parents of potentially involved children. The community stigma associated with having head lice is totally unjustified. It crosses all class and socioeconomic boundaries. Children can return to school the morning after the first treatment.

**1.1 Complications** Neurotoxicity has been reported when the whole body of a scabetic infant was covered with Lindane. For the local treatment of pediculosis, it is safe.

It may sting the eyes and cause mild skin irritation.

**1.2 Resistance in the UK** Reported in the 1970s. It may have been due to non-compliance, reinfection or use of the 0.2% lotion.

### *2 Others*

Malathion 0.5% lotion (*Br. Med. J.* (1980) **280**, 546), or pyrethrins (e.g. A-200 Pyrinate) can be used as above instead of Lindane.

## 16.6 Napkin dermatitis

A very common problem of early infancy.

### MAIN CAUSES

Contact dermatitis.
Candidiasis.
Seborrhoeic dermatitis.

### *Contact dermatitis*

This is due to prolonged skin contact with urine and faeces. It is an erythematous and occasionally ulcerating rash that spares the flexures. Bacteria convert urea to ammonia which is an alkaline irritant. Plastic or rubber nappy covers lead to increased penetration of these irritants. The rash may be complicated by *Candida* or seborrhoeic dermatitis.

### *Treatment*

1. Ideally one would keep the nappies off for as long as possible during the day to avoid the contact irritant, although this is not a practical proposition for incontinent infants in the cool UK climate.
2. Frequent nappy changes – by day and night.
3. Careful washing with warm water at each nappy change. Putting the child's bottom in warm running tap water ensures the removal of chemical irritants of urine and faeces from the skin.
4. Thick frequent application of protective (barrier) cream, e.g. Metanium cream, or zinc oxide creams or ointments. In addition, 0.5–1% hydrocortisone is often used with good results, especially if eczema, seborrhoeic dermatitis or psoriasis are present. Nystatin is often recommended because of the frequent association with *Candida.*
5. Boil nappies when washing them and rinse thoroughly.
6. Use disposable nappy liners.
7. Avoid plastic or rubber pants.

### *Candidiasis (thrush)*

Often superimposed on napkin dermatitis. It causes a bright red rash involving the flexures, and has 'satellite' patches. Often associated with oral thrush.

### *Treatment*

1. Nystatin cream 100 000 u/g or one of the imidazole creams (Canesten, Daktarin). Apply with each nappy change.
2. Also manage as for ammoniacal dermatitis.
3. If oral thrush is present, treat it to prevent reinfection from the gastrointestinal tract.

### *Seborrhoeic dermatitis*

See Infantile seborrhoeic dermatitis ('cradle cap') – Section 16.7.

## 16.7 Some neonatal rashes

### *Strawberry naevus (capillary haemangioma)*

Single or multiple vascular lesions, often on the face, becoming conspicuous in the first month of life. Involution occurs spontaneously by age 6 or 7 yr, with the first signs often appearing by age 1. Strenuously avoid surgical intervention.

### *Milia*

Seen in the newborn. They are small sebaceous cysts giving pearly yellow-white specks on the nose and face. Disappear spontaneously over 4–6 weeks.

### *Milaria*

Very common. Crops of papules or papulovesicles over face, trunk and napkin area.
Possibly due to overheating.
Rarely becomes secondarily infected.
Resolves with more appropriate clothing and time.

### *Infantile seborrhoeic dermatitis ('cradle cap')*

It is an erythematous scaling of scalp ('cradle cap'), nappy area, forehead, eyelids, retro-auricular region, neck, axillae. The onset is usually in the first week or two of life. Unlike infantile eczema, itching is absent or very mild and the child presents as happy and untroubled. The rash clears spontaneously over 2–3 months.

#### *Treatment*

1. None – if mild.
2. For more severe forms use hydrocortisone 0.5–1.0% applied sparingly 1–2 times daily.
3. The thick scaling of 'cradle cap' may be removed with arachis oil, baby oil or olive oil massaged into scalp prior to the use of a mild shampoo.

### *Erythema toxicum*

Blotchy erythematous macules 2–3 cm in diameter, with a tiny central vesicle or pustule (filled with eosinophils). They develop in up to 50% of term infants, usually within the first 1–4 days of life, and fade by about 7 days of age. Lesions are seen on chest, back, face and extremities. A smear of the central vesicle contents will reveal numerous eosinophils on Wright-stained preparations.

No treatment is needed.

## 16.8 Atopic eczema (AE) – or atopic dermatitis

About 3% of children between 2 and 18 months of age suffer from this condition which is associated with atopy in the child and family. Its cause is unknown. The face is often affected in infants, with flexures becoming more involved with advancing age. Spontaneous improvement is common after 2–3 years of age. Of all infants with AE, one-third will still have it in mid-childhood, and one-third of those will still have it in adolescence. Significant complications include impetigo, and primary herpes infection precipitating Kaposi's varicelliform eruption (eczema herpeticum).

## CLINICAL FEATURES

### *1 Distribution*

**1.1 Infancy** Face, trunk and extensor surfaces of arms and legs.

**1.2 Older children** Flexor surfaces of limbs.

**1.3 Eyelids** The presence of Dennie–Morgan folds (an extra crease of the lower lid) may help make the diagnosis.

### *2 Rash*

Erythema, scaling with or without crusting, dry skin, with pathognomonic lichenification. Itching is both common and irritating.

### *3 Aggravating factors*

Abnormal sweating, contact sensitivity (commonly to wool), occlusive clothing, stress and anxiety, secondary bacterial infection.

## TREATMENT

### *1 General measures*

Wear long-sleeved and trousered nightwear. Hands may have to be bandaged, gloved or splinted during acute episodes. Keep nails short. Wear loose, cool, cotton clothing. Avoid wool. Avoid frequent soaping of skin.

### *2 Baths and bland emollients (moisturizers)*

Baths should be short and only lukewarm. They provide a good opportunity to cleanse the skin of debris and crusts. Dispersible bath oil should be added to bath water, e.g. 'Alpha Keri', 'Oilatum', 'Balneum', 'Hamiltons' or baby oil. The use of soap is contraindicated; use a dispersible emollient as a soap substitute and bath additive, e.g. Emulsifying Ointment BP, Aqueous Cream BP or Unguentum Merck. These are applied to the wettened skin, massaged in and rinsed off.

Emollients can also be applied frequently at other times, especially last thing at night. An ideal preparation for such a purpose is equal parts of White Soft Paraffin BP and Liquid Paraffin BP. This is cheap and non-irritant. Among other good emollients are Locobase ointment, Unguentum Merck, Ultrabase, Nutraplus, Aquatain, Aquadrate and E45 cream.

### 3 Topical steroids

Use minimum possible potency (i.e. 0.5–1% hydrocortisone) and avoid fluorinated steroids. Ointments are preferable to creams. It is usually adequate to apply it once or twice a day, ideally immediately after a bath. For acute exacerbations, increase the frequency or use stronger (fluorinated) steroids (not on the face).

### 4 Antibiotics

For 'impetiginized' eczema use penicillin V or erythromycin after taking a swab for culture and sensitivity. Cloxacillin or first-generation cephalosporins are reasonable alternatives.

Topical antibiotics may be irritant and encourage the emergence of resistant strains, and therefore should not be used.

### 5 Antihistamines

Useful only as a sedative at night.

### 6 Diet

Breast feeding does not confer major protection, but a small beneficial effect cannot be excluded. All studies addressing this issue have their flaws (Kramer, 1988).

Elimination diets must be considered only as second-line treatment. A 4–6-week trial avoidance of cows' milk and eggs may be justified, although it should be abandoned if it has not worked by then. More stringent measures are difficult to implement and are unlikely to help many more children. Advise parents that any particular dietary avoidance is likely to be temporary.

### 7 Coal tar

For severe cases. It can be applied in the form of paste bandages (Ichthopaste and Icthaband bandages). Suitable for use on limbs overnight or for a 24-hour period. They are wound around the affected limb and secured with a stretch bandage (e.g. Coban 3M).

## Further reading

David, T. J. (1989) Dietary treatment of atopic eczema. *Arch. Dis. Child.*, **64**, 1506–1509

Kramer, S. (1988) Does breast feeding help protect against atopic disease? Biology, methodology, and a golden jubilee of controversy. *J. Pediatr.*, **112**, 181–190

# 16.9 Psoriasis

It is thought to be an hereditary disorder that requires an interplay of genetic and environmental factors for full clinical expression. It tends to occur in children older than 4 years who have a positive family history for psoriasis.

## CLINICAL FEATURES

The eruption consists of erythematous macular or papular lesions that develop a thick, silvery scale. Sites of predilection include scalp, ears, eyebrows, elbows, knees, gluteal crease, genitalia and nails.

Guttate (discrete scaly papules) psoriasis is an eruption of widespread small scaling lesions, often commencing after a streptococcal sore throat. Scalp involvement with psoriasis results in accumulation of thick scales throughout the scalp, with thickened scales along the frontal hairline and behind the ears. Hair loss does not occur. Genital involvement (perineum, penis, inguinal folds, labia) is common. Nail signs include pitting, onycholysis (separation of nail from nail bed), thickening of the distal nail, and crumbling of the entire nail. The Koebner phenomenon, whereby psoriasis develops in areas of skin trauma, is well recognized.

Itching is infrequent. Arthritis is seldom seen in childhood.

## TREATMENT

### *1 Initial treatment*

Keep treatment to a minimum initially. Two per cent sulphur and salicylic acid ointment or coal tar and salicylic acid ointment are good initial therapy. Therapy may be enhanced by ultraviolet light such as sunbathing or artificial sources.

### *2 Topical steroids*

Should be regarded as second-line drugs if above measures fail. Most benefit is obtained from fluorinated steroids. Systemic steroids are contraindicated.

### *3 Penicillin V*

? Helpful for confirmed streptococcal infection.

### *4 Dithranol*

Treatment of choice for difficult psoriasis. Lassar's paste 0.1% (= salicylic acid, zinc oxide and dithranol 0.1%) is an appropriate preparation initially, but 0.25%, 0.5% or 1% dithranol may later be needed. Apply accurately to affected areas.

Antimetabolites and other therapies should only be used under the guidance of a dermatologist.

## Further reading

Anon. (1988) Treating scabies. *Drugs Ther. Bull.*, **26**, 19–20
Finch, R. (1988) Skin and soft tissue infections. *Lancet,* **i**, 164–167
Gurevitch, A. W. (1985) Scabies and lice. *Pediatr. Clin. N. Am.*, **32**, 987–1018
Harper, J. I. (1988) In (eds Clayden, G. S. and Hawkins, R. L.) *Paediatrics: Treatment and Prognosis,* Heinemann, London, pp. 250–261
Honig, P. J. (1983) Bites and parasites. *Paediatr. Clin. N. Am.*, **30**, 563–571
Milner, A. D. and Hull, D. (1984) *Hospital Paediatrics*, Churchill Livingstone, London
Rook, A. *et al.* (1986) *Textbook of Dermatology*, Blackwell, Oxford
Stein, D. H. (1983) Fungal infection. *Pediatr. Clin. N. Am.*, **30**, 545–562
Tunnessen, W. W. (1983) Cutaneous infections. *Pediatr. Clin. N. Am.*, **30**, 515–532
Weston, W. L. (1985) *Practical Pediatric Dermatology*, Little, Brown and Co, Boston

Chapter 17

# Neonates and infants

## 17.1 Infant feeding

### *Breast milk*

Human placental lactogen secreted in pregnancy prepares the maternal breast such that lactation can be stimulated by prolactin from the anterior pituitary. Sucking triggers the expulsion of milk under the influence of oxytocin from the posterior pituitary. It is no surprise, given the delicate neurohormonal control of breast milk supply, that having to breast feed furtively or cope with anxiety, stress, illness or regimented feeding schedules will suppress lactation.

#### ADVANTAGES OF BREAST FEEDING

It is warm, cheap, requires no preparation, and provides comfort and security to mother and child. It has numerous anti-infective properties such as secretory IgA, lysozymes, macrophages and lactoferrin. There are no foreign proteins, the bioavailability of the iron is relatively high and the fact that the composition of the milk varies both during a feed and from one feed to the next, may be of importance to the infant. Fats, proteins, calcium, phosphorus and solute load are present in optimum quantities and form. Boiling, pasteurizing, freezing and thawing eliminate some of the advantages of human milk. Preterm babies benefit from special formulae which may be supplemented by expressed breast milk.

#### THE BREAST-FED INFANT

Ideally a child is solely breast fed for at least [illegible] months, after which 'solids' should progressively be introduced in addition to ongoing breast feeding. Such solids include cereal, broth, puréed fruit and vegetables, rusks, meat, egg (some advise not before 7 months). Salt and sugar should be used sparingly if at all. Vitamin C-containing juice can be introduced at 3 months. Heating inactivates vitamin C. By 6 months nearly all normal children can make chewing movements and accommodate lumpy solids.

Foods should be introduced one at a time to enable identification of intolerance.

At 8 months, a regular eating pattern often emerges, coarser foods can be introduced and training to cup feed should commence. Night-time breast feeds can be discontinued. By 12 months a smooth transition to eating the family's diet has usually been effected.

## Artificially-fed infants

Aproximately two-thirds of UK babies are breast fed at birth and about one-seventh are still breast fed at 4 months of age. For the overwhelming majority of artificially-fed term infants there are cheap, safe milks available that allow optimum growth and development. Many mothers feel a sense of failure if they are unable to breast feed – they should be reassured.

### 1 Volume

Day 1: 60 ml/kg/day. Increase by 30 ml/kg/day until 150 ml/kg/day and continue at that rate.

### 2 Preparation of formula

In developing countries, the unsanitary use of bottles, teats and formula contribute greatly to the ubiquity of diarrhoea. In developed countries, the issue is not as clear. The American Academy of Pediatrics advocates aseptic technique (sterilization of water, containers and utensils by boiling for 5 min) or terminal sterilization (with formula already in the bottle). Formula should be used within 4 h of preparation. Manufacturers recommend aseptic technique and refrigeration and use within 24 h of preparation.

In societies with 'safe' water supplies, refrigeration and high general hygiene, aseptic technique for the first month of life is perhaps prudent, but thereafter the use of tap water and cleaning of equipment with detergent seems to be adequate (Little, G. A. (1988). Preparation of infant formula. *Pediatr. Inf. Dis.*, **7**, 529–530).

Formula and other foods may be served at room temperature. The hole in the teat should be of a size that allows that infant to feed in under 15 min. Microwave heating of infant formula may be a risky practice because the bottle may feel warm, while the liquid is hot and may result in palatal burns (*Pediatr. Alert* (1988) **13**, 78–79).

### 3 Artificial milks

**3.1 Cows' milk** Compared with human milk (HM), cows' milk (CM) contains more protein which is less digestible, more saturated fat, more Ca and P and a lower Ca:P ratio which may predispose to hypocalcaemia in the neonatal period. The iron has a lower bioavailability and the renal solute load is higher. The use of unmodified CM in early infancy may be

**Table 17.1 Composition of various infant feeds per 100 ml**

| Product (company) | % Soln | Protein Tot. (g) | Protein L (%) | Protein C (%) | Carbohydrate Tot. (g) | Carbohydrate Type | Fat Tot. (g) | Fat Sat. | Fat Unsat. |
|---|---|---|---|---|---|---|---|---|---|
| Human milk (mature) | Liquid | 1.3 | 60 | 40 | 7.2 | Lactose | 4.1 | 50 | 47 |
| Human milk (transitional) | Liquid | 2.0 | 60 | 40 | 6.9 | Lactose | 3.7 | 50 | 47 |
| Cows' milk | Liquid | 3.3 | 18 | 82 | 4.7 | Lactose | 3.8 | 61 | 35 |
| Goats' milk | Liquid | 3.3 | – | – | 4.6 | Lactose | 4.5 | – | – |
| WHEY-BASED MODIFIED MILKS (powder or ready to feed) | | | | | | | | | |
| Gold Cap SMA (S26) (Wyeth) | 13 | 1.5 | 60 | 40 | 7.2 | Lactose | 3.6 soyalecithin veg. and beef fat | 47 | 53 |
| Premium (Cow and Gate) | 12.5 | 1.5 | 60 | 40 | 7.3 | Lactose | 3.6 veg. and butter fat | 41 | 56 |
| MODIFIED SOYA MILKS | | | | | | | | | |
| Formula S (Cow and Gate) | 12.7 | 1.8 | Soy isolate and L-methionine | | 6.7 | Glucose syrup | 3.6 veg. oils | | |
| Wy soy (Wyeth) | 13.5 | 2.1 | Soy isolate and L-methionine | | 6.9 | Sucrose corn syrup | 3.6 oleic beef corn and coconut | | |
| HYDROLYSED PROTEIN FORMULAE | | | | | | | | | |
| Pregestimil (Mead Johnson) | 15.0 | 1.9 | Hydrolysed casein and cystine, tyrosine, tryptophan | | 9.1 | Corn syrup Tapioca starch | 2.7 corn MCT and soyalecithin | | |
| Nutramigen (Mead Johnson) | 15.0 | 2.3 | Hydrolysed casein | | 8.9 | Sucrose Tapioca starch | 2.7 corn oil | | |

L, lactalbumin and whey as percentage of total protein; C, casein as percentage of total protein; MCT, medium-chain triglycerides.

complicated by hyperosmolar dehydration, hypocalcaemic fits, casein curd bowel obstruction, vitamin deficiency (D and C), iron deficiency, GI blood loss. Goats' milk is deficient in folic acid. Unmodified cows' and goats' milk should not be used in infants under 6 months of age.

**3.2 Proprietary milks** (see Table 17.1) Numerous milk formulae are available that mimic the composition of human milk, including Gold Cap, Premium, Nan and Osterfeed. They are virtually identical to one another in their composition. There are no indications for changing from one to the other in an attempt to find one that 'best suits the child'. Modified soya milks can be used in the uncommon cases of cows' milk protein allergy or lactose intolerance. Formulae made with hydrolysed proteins are expensive (Table 17.2). They are of use in infants with fat malabsorption, cows' milk and soy protein allergy.

| *Energy* (kJ/kcal) | *Osmolality* (mmol/kg) | *Renal solute* (mmol/100 ml) | *Minerals* (mmol) | | | | | | | | |
|---|---|---|---|---|---|---|---|---|---|---|---|
| | | | Na | K | Ca | P | Mg | Fe | Cu | Zn | Cl |
| 289/69 | 264 | 8.4 | 0.6 | 1.5 | 0.9 | 0.5 | 0.1 | 1.3 | 0.6 | 4.3 | 1.2 |
| 281/67 | – | 14.2 | 2.1 | 1.7 | 0.6 | 0.5 | 0.1 | 1.3 | 0.6 | – | 2.4 |
| 272/65 | – | 22 | 2.2 | 3.9 | 3.0 | 3.1 | 0.5 | 0.9 | 0.3 | 5.4 | 2.7 |
| 296/71 | – | 23 | 1.7 | 4.6 | 3.3 | 3.5 | 0.8 | 0.7 | 0.8 | 4.6 | 3.7 |
| 274/65 | 300 | 9.1 | 0.7 | 1.4 | 1.1 | 1.1 | 0.2 | 12.0 | 0.8 | 7.6 | 1.2 |
| 275/66 | 290 | 9.6 | 0.8 | 1.7 | 1.4 | 0.9 | 0.2 | 8.9 | 0.6 | 6.1 | 1.3 |
| 280/67 | 165 | 10.8 | 0.8 | 1.7 | 1.4 | 0.9 | 0.2 | 8.9 | 0.6 | 6.2 | 1.1 |
| 280/67 | 242 | 12.2 | 0.9 | 1.9 | 1.6 | 1.4 | 0.3 | 12.1 | 0.8 | 5.7 | 1.0 |
| 287/68 | 338 | 12.5 | 1.4 | 1.9 | 1.6 | 1.4 | 0.3 | 23.0 | 0.9 | 6.0 | 1.6 |
| 290/69 | 443 | 13.8 | 1.4 | 1.8 | 1.6 | 1.6 | 0.3 | 23.0 | 1.0 | 6.6 | 1.4 |

**Table 17.2 Cost of artificial milks***

| *Milk* | *Unit* (= tin powder) | *Cost* |
|---|---|---|
| SMA Gold Cap | 450 g | £1.43 |
| Premium | 450 g | £1.43 |
| Formula S | 450 g | £2.38 |
| Wysoy | 430 g | £2.42 |
| Nutramigen | 450 g | £7.00 |
| Pregestimil | 450 g | £8.01 |

* August 1988 prices.

All the formulae (except Nutramigen) are suitable for infants less than 3 months of age. All contain sufficient amounts of iron, fat-soluble vitamins, vitamins C, B group and folic acid, for the term infant not to require supplements (assuming that solids are commenced by about 6 months). The addition of some vitamin C (fruit juice) into the diet will increase the absorption of iron.

## *Introduction of solids and unmodified cows' milk*

By 4–6 months of age the infant will tolerate purèed or lumpy food. CM can be substituted for formula or HM after 6 months of age. By 12 months, milk is usually no longer the mainstay of the child's nutrition; however, it should nevertheless be a staple in the child's diet. Semi-skimmed milk may be used after 2 years if the overall diet is adequate.

## *Breast feeding and prevention of atopic disease*

This is a controversial question to which there are no clear answers. All studies examining the issue have serious methodological problems. It seems likely that if HM confers some protection, it is only small (Kramer, 1988). It is worth reiterating that mothers who abandon breast feeding should not be made to feel guilty, because in developed countries the objective benefits of HM are slender.

## *Maternal aspects of breast feeding*

Feed scheduling is a recent Western notion with no scientific basis and has the potential to disturb the normal physiology of lactogenesis. Demand feeding has anthropologically demonstrated its soundness. It is important that a mother be allowed time and tranquillity to learn how best to feed her child. Addresses of some helpful organizations:

### *1 United Kingdom*

The National Childbirth Trust, 9 Queensborough Terrace, Bayswater, London W2 3TB (tel. 071-221-3833).

La Leche Great Britain, Box 3424, London WC1 6XX.

### *2 Australia*

Nursing Mothers' Association of Australia, National Headquarters, 99 Burwood Road, Hawthorn, Victoria (tel. 03-8188031)

Childbirth Education Association of Australia (NSW), Box N206, Grosvenor St., Sydney NSW 2000.

### *3 New Zealand*

The Federation of New Zealand Parents' Centres Inc., Box 11310, Wellington (tel. 766-950).

## Breast-feeding problems

### 1 Prevention

Babies will normally 'fix on' or take the areola and nipple into their mouths, and the lower jaw is used to express milk from the lactiferous ducts behind the nipple. Proper education and help by experienced attendants is most useful in preventing mechanical difficulties. Retracted nipples should be prepared during pregnancy, but occasionally nipple shields may be needed during feeding.

### 2 Sore/cracked/bleeding nipple

Often the result of inadequate 'fixing' or not getting enough of the nipple and areola into the baby's mouth, with the result that the baby drags on the nipple stem. An experienced attendant may be of help to the mother in getting the child to adequately fix on the areola, i.e. really breast feeding rather than nipple sucking. Nipple soreness is at its most severe before the let-down reflex has occurred, after which it tends to disappear quickly. Feeding should continue until and beyond the occurrence of the reflex. If one finds that the let-down reflex is delayed (? anxiety, ? pain), stimulation of the breast prior to a feed may be a good idea. Sore nipples may also benefit from local heat (hot water bottle or hot bath), avoiding synthetic bras and plastic-lined nipple pads, going topless about the house, thus allowing nipples to dry in air, and nipple shields while feeding. A novel idea (Kitzinger, 1987) is to insert small plastic tea-strainers with the handles cut off under the bra, thus allowing air to circulate over the nipples while dressed. A wide range of creams are in common use, although there is little to suggest that they do anything to prevent or treat sore nipples.

If the nipple is very cracked or bleeding, cease feeding for 24–36 h, but express milk either by hand or with a pump. Continue to demand feed on other side. Expressed milk may be given by teaspoon.

### 3 Breast engorgement

Many need an experienced assistant in helping baby fix onto the breast. Hot flannels, or expressing a small amount of milk before the feed, may soften the areola and allow the child to fix.

### 4 Mastitis and breast abscess

Mastitis should be treated with regular frequent feeding to keep the milk flowing, hot nappies applied over the sore area, and antibiotics (flucloxacillin). Established abscesses require incision and drainage. Usual advice is for the child to not receive milk from that breast temporarily, although pumping milk from the breast may be helpful.

## Breast feeding and AIDS

The risk of HIV transmissions via breast milk is unknown, but is probably extremely low compared with antenatal and intrapartum vertical transmission.

### *1 HIV-positive mother*

Most clinics in developed (not in developing) countries agree that the mother should be discouraged from breast feeding.

### *2 High-risk mothers who are HIV negative or not tested*

These mothers could be HIV negative, HIV positive, or in the process of seroconverting. The issue is complex, however. If a mother in this category is keen to breast feed, on balance it seems that she should not be dissuaded. There is, however, a school of thought that advocates pasteurizing her milk before giving it to the baby (this diminishes but does not eliminate risk) and repeating HIV serology after 3 months. If it is negative, then normal breast feeding can be resumed.

## Further reading

Acheson, D. and Poole, A. A. B. (1989) HIV infection, breastfeeding and human milk banking in the United Kingdom. DoH Communication PL/CMO(89)4. Department of Health, London

Anon. (1987) Advice about milk for infants and young children. *Lancet,* **i**, 843–844

Anon. (1988) HIV infection, breastfeeding and human milk banking. PL/CMO(88)13, PL/CMO(88)7. DHSS, London

Francis, D. (1986) *Nutrition for Children*, Blackwell, London

Kitzinger, S. (1987) *The Experience of Breastfeeding*, Penguin, Harmondsworth

Kramer, M. S. (1988) Does breast feeding help protect against atopic disease? Biology, methodology and a golden jubilee of controversy. *J. Pediatr.*, **112**, 181–190

Lawrence, R. A. (1989) Breast-feeding. *Pediatr. in Rev.*, **11**, 163–171

Lissauer, T. (1989) Impact of AIDS on neonatal care. *Arch. Dis. Child.*, **64**, 4–7

Oxtoby, M. J. (1988) HIV and other viruses in human milk: placing the issues in broader perspective. *Pediatr. Inf. Dis. J.*, **7**, 825–835

Pencharz, P. B. (1985) *Pediatr. Clin. N. Am.*, **32**, 335–362

# 17.2 Ophthalmia neonatorum/neonatal conjunctivitis

## AETIOLOGY

*Staphylococcus aureus*.
*Chlamydia trachomatis*.
*Neisseria gonorrhoeae*.
Others – *Haemophilus influenzae, Streptococcus pneumoniae*, beta-haemolytic streptococci, *Streptococcus viridans*, coliforms (in other countries – chemical conjunctivitis due to silver nitrate prophylaxis).

## CLINICAL FEATURES

The clinical characteristics are not distinct enough to enable one to make an aetiological diagnosis. The time of onset of the conjunctivitis may be of some help. Chemical conjunctivitis starts on the first day of life, *Neisseria* on days 2–5, *Chlamydia* between days 5 and 26 and it may be associated with pneumonia. Other bacteria may start from the first week to the first month.

## COMPLICATIONS

Usually none. The infection may spread to the cornea (especially with gonococci, thus causing blindness), lachrymal apparatus, orbit, cavernous sinus.

## PREVENTION

In some countries (not the UK), 1% silver nitrate drops are applied at birth. This not effective against *Chlamydia trachomatis* and may cause chemical conjunctivitis. 0.5% erythromycin (combats *Chlamydia*) or 1% tetracycline have been used.

## INVESTIGATION

### *1 Gram stain*

Sterile cotton-tipped swabs or sterile loop:

(a) Polymorphs and Gram-positive intracellular diplococci = *N. gonorrhoeae*.
(b) Polymorphs with no bacteria = *C. trachomatis* or partially treated infection.
(c) Polymorphs and bacteria = neither of the above, i.e. other infection.
(d) No polymorphs or bacteria = ?partially treated infection.

### *2 Eye swab*

Take to laboratory immediately for bacterial culture. Specifically request culture for gonococcus.

### *3 Giemsa stain of conjunctival scrapings*

Detects intracytoplasmic inclusions of chlamydial infection. Nowadays one can also use fluorescein conjugated monoclonal antichlamydial antibodies.

## TREATMENT

Mild conjunctivitis may respond to regular eye toilet with cotton wool and boiled water 4–6 hourly for several days. Removal of pus must precede the instilling of antibiotic drops or ointment. Neomycin is the initial treatment of choice (some use chloramphenicol or gentamicin). Ointment is used 8 hourly and is more practical than drops which should be applied 1–2 hourly.

Gonococcal ophthalmitis – procaine penicillin 50 000 u/kg/day IM for 7 days (*J. Pediatr.* (1987) **317**, 18–22) or IV crystalline penicillin 30 mg (50 000 u)/kg/6 h. Penicillinase-producing *N. gonorrhoeae* requires parenteral cefotaxime. Endocervical swab of mother with contact tracing should be carried out in a clinic for sexually transmitted diseases.

Chlamydia – 1% chlortetracycline drops 6 hourly or erythromycin ointment, or 10% sulphacetamide for 2 weeks, plus oral erythromycin 10 mg/kg/dose q.i.d. for 14 days.

## Further reading

Friendly, D. S. (1983) Ophthalmia neonatorum. *Pediatr. Clin. N. Am.*, **30**, 1033–1042

Winceslaus, J., Goh, B. T., Dunlop, E. M. *et al.* (1987) Diagnosis of ophthalmia neonatorum. *Br. Med. J.*, **295**, 1377–1379

# 17.3 Umbilical sepsis

## INTRODUCTION

Systemic infection may result from umbilical infection (notably *Staphylococcus aureus*) spreading up the falciform ligament to cause a portal pyaemia and septicaemia. Other problems are necrotizing fasciitis, acidosis, shock, coagulopathy, secondary haemorrhage and, in the long term, portal hypertension.

## CLINICAL

### *1 Localized infection*

Minor purulent umbilical stump discharge or peri-umbilical redness.

### *2 Systemic infection*

Peri-umbilical redness or induration radiating in streaks towards the liver, or systemic illness.

## INVESTIGATION

Umbilical stump culture.
Blood culture.
FBC.

### TREATMENT

#### *1 Local infection*

Frequent cleaning with 70% isopropyl alcohol ('Sterets'). Alternatively, painting with Gentian Violet or application of topical antibiotic powder have been advocated.

#### *2 Systemic infection*

If suspected, one must administer IV cloxacillin 25–50 mg/kg/8 h (1–4 weeks of age), or /6 h (over 4 weeks of age) and gentamicin 2.5 mg/kg/12 h (<2 weeks of age) or /8 h (>2 weeks).

### Further reading

Mason, W. H., Andrews, R., Ross, L. A. and Wright, H. T. (1989) Omphalitis in the newborn infant. *Pediatr. Inf. Dis. J.*, **8**, 521–525

## 17.4 Umbilical granuloma

This usually is a result of chronic low-grade infection at the site of cord separation. Cautery with silver nitrate sticks, carefully applied, will usually resolve the problem.

## 17.5 Congenital dislocation of the hips (CDH)

CDH can be found in approximately 1.3 per 1000 live births with 70% occurring in girls and 20% in infants born in breech position. Early recognition and treatment of this problem has met with spectacular success. The longer CDH remains unrecognized and untreated, the worse the eventual outlook for normal acetabular and femoral head development. Routine screening for CDH with Ortolani and Barlow tests should be an integral part of the examination of all infants before discharge from hospital, and those seen in the first 3 months of life.

## DIAGNOSIS

### The Ortolani test

With hips and knees in 90° of flexion, grasp the thigh with middle finger over the greater trochanter and the thumb over the distal femur. Examine one hip at a time. The manoeuvre involves simultaneous gentle traction on the thigh, with abduction of the hip, in an attempt to reduce the femoral head back into the acetabulum from its (presumed) posterior dislocated position. A positive test is a distinct 'clunk', not merely a noise such as when cracking one's knuckles. Outside of the neonatal period, the Ortolani test may be unreliable, as the femur remains trapped outside the acetabulum.

### The Barlow test

This is Ortolani in reverse. The femoral head is assumed to be reduced and this manoeuvre detects if the hip is able to be dislocated. With the hip and knee flexed, the same grip as above is adopted and the femur is adducted while the thumb attempts to push the femur posteriorly out of the acetabulum. This test, if performed repeatedly, may actually predispose the hip to dislocation, and therefore clinicians increasingly consider the test to be ill-advised.

## INVESTIGATIONS

### *1 X-ray*

Not reliable in first 2–3 months of life.

### *2 Ultrasound of hips*

Very good in experienced hands, even in the neonatal period. Some advocate routine screening of the newborn.

## MANAGEMENT

### *1 Referral*

All suspected CDH at any stage should be seen by a paediatrician and referred to an orthopaedic surgeon with experience in managing this condition.

### *2 Double nappies*

While waiting for an orthopaedic consultation, the use of double cloth nappies will (unreliably) keep the hips flexed and abducted. Triple nappies are probably better.

### *3 Pavlik harness*

A device which keeps the hips flexed and abducted. Other devices are the Aberdeen and Von Rosen splints and Frejka pillow.

### *4 Duration of treatment*

The earlier the dislocation is discovered, the shorter the period required to achieve clinical stability. CDH detected in the neonatal period is usually treated for 6–12 weeks and then reviewed.

### *5 Surgery*

If CDH is detected in the neonatal period, surgery (adductor tenotomy) is rarely required.

## Further reading

Berman, L. and Klenerman, L. (1986) Ultrasound screening for hip abnormalities: preliminary findings in 1001 neonates. *Br. Med. J.*, **293,** 719–722

Dunn, P. M., Evans, R. E., Thearle, M. J., Griffiths, H. E. D. and Witherow, P. J. (1985) Congenital dislocation of the hip: early and late diagnosis and management compared. *Arch. Dis. Child.*, **60**, 407–414

MacEwen, G. D. and Millet, C. (1990) Congenital dislocation of the hip. *Pediatr. Rev.*, **11**, 249–252

# 17.6 Neonatal jaundice in the term infant

Jaundice is more frequent in the neonatal period than at any other time during life. Although generally a trivial problem, it poses two main clinical problems. First, unconjugated bilirubin may cause irreversible brain damage; secondly, jaundice may be a sign of underlying disease. Jaundice may become clinically apparent when the serum bilirubin exceeds 85 μmol/litre; about 50% of normal term infants achieve such a level.

**Axioms** (a) Jaundice appearing in the first 24 h of life is pathological; (b) jaundice which persists for longer than 10 days in a term baby should be investigated; (c) jaundice which reaches a level at which treatment is considered in a term baby should be investigated (bilirubin level 300–340 μmol/litre after 48 h of age).

### *Physiological jaundice*

Jaundice is common in newborn babies, beginning on the 2nd day, reaching a peak on the 3rd day and fading by 10 days. It occurs because of:

1. The haemoglobin load from the placenta.
2. Immaturity of glucuronyl transferase and relative absence of ligandin (Y protein) in the liver.
3. Failure of the GI tract to clear the meconium load.

Such jaundice is *unconjugated* and harmless, i.e. it does not reach a degree at which there is a risk of bilirubin crossing the blood brain barrier and causing kernicterus. The tendency to treat such jaundice with phototherapy should be discouraged: in a well, term baby there seems little risk of kernicterus at levels below 350 µmol/litre of unconjugated bilirubin, and therefore phototherapy is not usually used until the level reaches at least 300 µmol/litre.

## 17.6.1 Other causes of unconjugated hyperbilirubinaemia

### *1 Haemolytic*

*Bruising, cephalhaematoma, exaggerated physiological jaundice.*
*Polycythaemia* Small for gestational age, late clamping of cord, cord stripping, maternal–fetal transfusion.
*Isoimmune haemolysis* Rh, ABO, minor blood group incompatibility.
*RBC metabolic disorders* G-6-PD deficiency, pyruvate kinase deficiency.
*RBC morphology disorders* Hereditary spherocytosis.

### *2 Infections*

Bacterial sepsis – always consider meningitis, septicaemia, UTI, omphalitis.
TORCH (intra-uterine) infections.

### *3 Metabolic disorders*

Galactosaemia, Crigler–Najjar disease, breast milk jaundice, familial neonatal jaundice (Lucey–Driscoll syndrome), infant of diabetic mother, hypothyroidism.

### *4 Others*

Toxins (too much vitamin K), high GIT obstruction.

## *Evaluation of the jaundiced infant*

### *1 History*

Birth weight, gestation, complications of pregnancy, delivery or immediate postnatal period.
Parents' assessment of baby's well-being (feeding well, vomiting, etc.).
Breast or bottle fed?
Family history of neonatal jaundice – haemolytic disease, breast milk jaundice, Lucey–Driscoll syndrome.
Onset of jaundice <36 h of age – suggests a pathological cause.

### *2 Examination*

Assess general well-being and alertness.
Bruising, cephalhaematoma, petechiae.
Degree of prematurity.

Poor feeding.
Obesity (infant of diabetic mother).
Microcephaly – associated with intrauterine infection.
Hepatosplenomegaly – haemolytic anaemia, congenital infection, liver disease.
Chorioretinitis – congenital infection.
Umbilicus – check for omphalitis.
Signs of hypothyroidism – organomegaly, protruding tongue with umbilical hernia, large fontanelle.

## INITIAL INVESTIGATIONS

### *1 Serum bilirubin*

If bilirubin is >300 µmol/litre, or if the child has early or prolonged jaundice, determine the 'split' bilirubin, i.e. conjugated and unconjugated levels. If it is unconjugated, proceed as follows:

### *2 Mother's and baby's blood group*

The commonest combination giving rise to incompatibility is mother O and baby A, but others are possible. Rhesus disease is now rare and is usually known about prior to delivery. Incompatibility of minor blood groups may also give rise to jaundice.

### *3 Hb, WCC, reticulocyte count*

### *4 Blood film*

Nucleated RBCs, erythroblasts – Rh incompatibility.
Microspherocytes – ABO incompatibility.
Fragmented RBC – sepsis, G-6-PD deficiency.

### *5 Direct Coombs' test*

Positive in Rh disease, but seldom positive in ABO or minor blood group haemolysis.

### *6 Urine*

**6.1 Clinitest** For reducing substances (galactosaemia).

**6.2 Microscopy and culture**

### *7 Thyroid function tests*

Verify that screening was done at birth. If not, for persisting or serious jaundice check $T_4$ and TSH levels.

## TREATMENT

Exposure of a jaundiced infant to light of a wavelength near the maximum absorption peak of bilirubin (450–460 nm) results in the photo-isomerization of unconjugated bilirubin to non-toxic isomers. It should be used when the unconjugated bilirubin level approaches that which may be hazardous. In a well, term baby, if the level is kept below 350 μmol/litre (20 mg/dl) the risk of kernicterus is negligible, hence most would commence phototherapy at a level somewhere between 300 and 350 μmol/l. Small, sick, septic, acidotic, asphyxiated neonates are more prone to kernicterus at any given level of bilirubin, hence phototherapy is commenced at lower levels than those above.

## *Jaundice in the first 24 h*

It is due to haemolytic disease until proven otherwise.
Investigate as above, but also send serum for antibodies to toxoplasma, rubella and CMV, and consider a full septic screen for bacterial infection.

## *Prolonged jaundice*

$>$1 week.

### *1 Aetiology*

The most common cause by far is breast milk jaundice. This is possibly due to a steroid present in breast milk, 3α, 20β-pregnanediol, or to high levels of β-glucuronidase in breast milk, which increase unconjugated bilirubin in the GI tract, thus increasing the enterohepatic circulation.

Also consider the following:

Hypothyroidism (may not have the typical clinical features).
Galactosaemia.
Crigler–Najjar, Gilbert's disease.
Conjugated hyperbilirubinaemia/obstructive jaundice hepatitis; biliary atresia, choledochal cyst, inspissated bile syndrome; alpha-1-antitrypsin deficiency.

### *2 Management*

Measure level of conjugated and unconjugated bilirubin.
Check urine for infection and reducing sugars.

**2.1 Unconjugated hyperbilirubinaemia (breast fed)** When found in a well, breast-fed baby, who had routine thyroid function screening at birth, whose urine is uninfected and without reducing sugars, and whose physical examination is normal, it is highly likely to be due to breast milk jaundice and probably needs no further tests. Parents should be reassured and told that mild jaundice may continue for many weeks. Temporary cessation of breast feeding may improve jaundice within 48 h, but is not recommended because of the (frequently terminal) interruption to milk supply. If breast feeding is temporarily halted, continue to express breast milk until feeding is resumed.

**2.2 Unconjugated hyperbilirubinaemia (bottle fed)** When in a bottle-fed baby, this needs thorough investigation as above. Also check:

G-6-PD levels.
Blood 'galactose screen' for galactose-1-phosphate uridyl transferase.
$T_4$ and TSH.
Should be seen by a paediatrician.

**2.3 Conjugated hyperbilirubinaemia** Immediate referral to a paediatrician. The fear is that of missing biliary atresia until it is too late to operate (about 7–8 weeks). A mixed conjugated/unconjugated picture can be due to hepatitis reaction from infection. The following tests should be considered:

Full septic work-up.
Abdominal (liver) ultrasound.
Clotting studies.
Hepatitis B surface antigen.
TORCH screen.
Liver scan.
Mini-laparotomy for exclusion of biliary atresia and for liver biopsy.

Galactose screen for galactose-1-phosphate uridyl transferase.
Alpha-1-antitrypsin level.
Urine and serum amino acids.

### IF THE BABY IS ILL

Admit and perform a full septic work-up.

## 17.7 Measuring infant growth

It is a basic mandatory requirement in following up both sick and healthy children that weight, height and head circumference be measured and plotted against age on percentile charts (see Chapter 3). Until age 2 years, supine length is measured instead of standing height (which is slightly less); hence at the changeover there may be a sudden drop in the child's measured longitudinal growth. Parents often worry or are made to worry about sudden weight loss. In many cases this will only be a reflection of the inconsistency between different weighing scales, or else it may represent the difference between a full and empty bladder, bowel or stomach. In monitoring weight gain, the trend over a period of time is much more important than a single measurement.

In the absence of growth charts, some of the following very crude figures may be of use.

### 1 Weight

Weight loss of up to 10% of birth weight in the first days of life is acceptable. Newborn babies should regain their birth weights by 1 week of age (10 days for prems).

Weight gain is 150 g/wk (25 g/day) until 6 months of age. An infant can be expected to double his birth weight by 4 months of age.

### 2 Length

Length increases by 0.75 cm/wk from term to 3 months of age, and then 0.5 cm/wk until 6 months. In premature babies, length increases by 1 cm/wk until term.

### 3 Head circumference

Head circumference increases by about 0.5 cm/wk until 3 months, and 0.25 cm/wk until 6 months.

### 4 Chronological vs corrected age

Growth measurements are usually plotted on percentile charts that assume birth at term. In the case of a child born prematurely, plotting growth against chronological age is clearly inappropriate. This problem can be circumvented by plotting growth against corrected age.

Corrected age = post-natal age minus the number of weeks that the child was premature.

The difference between corrected and chronological age loses significance after 1.5 years for head circumference, 2 years for weight and 3.5 years for height.

Chapter 18

# Ear, nose and throat

## 18.1 Blocked nose

Most young infants are virtual obligatory nose-breathers. A blocked nose necessitates mouth-breathing which is a struggle, in turn made worse by feeding. Hence these children are miserable and feed poorly. If there is a history of blocked nose since birth, pass a soft catheter down each nostril to exclude choanal atresia or stenosis. If it passes easily, then one can assume that the blockage is due to secretions.

### TREATMENT

1. Often none is necessary if the child can still feed well.
2. Normal saline drops – often effective and are free of side effects.
3. Topical vasoconstrictors – ephidrine 0.5% nose drops. Use only for 48 h. Prolonged use will result in 'rhinitis medicamentosa', i.e. rebound nasal congestion (Toohill, R. J. *et al.* (1981) Rhinitis medicamentosa. *Laryngoscope,* **91**, 1614–1621).
4. Sucking out the nose with a nasal cannula, passed until it reaches the nasopharynx, will exclude choanal atresia and relieve symptoms.

## 18.2 Herpes gingivostomatitis

Primary severe oral/labial herpes simplex infection occurs in children from infancy to 3 years. Thereafter it may present or recur as 'cold sores'. The initial presentation is that of an ill child with fever, halitosis and refusal to feed. On examination, the gums are swollen, bleed readily and are associated with shallow very painful ulcers on gums, buccal mucosa, palate, tongue and lips, with regional lymphadenopathy.

## NATURAL HISTORY

Spontaneous recovery occurs usually within 10 days.

## TREATMENT

### *1 Admit*

Admission to hospital is only indicated if the child is not able to maintain adequate hydration, or for parental relief. The child should be kept in a single room, isolated if possible from neonates and other young children.

### *2 Maintain hydration*

Small amounts of fluids by mouth, given frequently. A soft bland diet with extra fluids should be offered but not forced. Occasionally 2–3 days of IV fluids are required. Attention to hydration is far more important than ensuring an adequate caloric intake during the illness.

### *3 Mouth care*

Thymol or chlorhexidine 0.2% mouth wash. Difflam spray or almost any topical local anaesthetic provides some relief, but if children resist their application, then simply await spontaneous resolution.

### *4 Antiviral drugs*

Topical idoxuridine, acyclovir and interferon (*Lancet* (1988) **i**, 150–152) have all been advocated. Their routine use in this disabling but self-limited condition is controversial but most do not advocate it.

### *5 Much parental support*

The natural history needs to be explained and expectations of a quick cure or recovery lowered. Nevertheless, constant reassurance that in a matter of a few days the ordeal will be over and that no harm will come to the child is helpful.

## DIFFERENTIAL DIAGNOSIS

Herpangina due to group A Coxsackie tends mainly to affect the throat. It causes a milder illness, although treatment is the same. Stevens–Johnston syndrome affects other mucous membranes and is associated with a rash.

# 18.3 Epistaxis

Nose bleeds are most commonly idiopathic, or due to trauma (nose-picking). In the hospital setting it is most commonly seen in children on chemotherapy who are thrombocytopenic. Frequently, bleeding is from Little's area and, in most cases, pressure on the soft part of the nose provides adequate haemostasis.

## AETIOLOGY

1. Idiopathic.
2. Trauma – nose-picking, others.
3. Infections – local, EBV.
4. Severe cough – pertussis, cystic fibrosis.
5. Thrombocytopenia – usually due to malignancy or its treatment.
5. Other bleeding diathesis.

## TREATMENT

### *1 Digital pressure*

Applied to the soft part of the nose for 15 min with the child upright.

### *2 Topical adrenaline*

Spray with xylocaine. Soak a small piece of cotton wool in adrenaline 1:2000 ± cocaine 5–10% and apply to bleeding point for 10 min (longer pressure may cause necrosis).

### *3 Anterior nasal pack*

Xylocaine spray followed by packing with ribbon gauze impregnated with adrenaline (1:5000) and/or cocaine (5%). Some use BIPP gauze (bismuth iodoform and liquid paraffin paste).

### *4 Morphine*

IV bolus 0.1 mg/kg, repeat × 2. Anecdotally (in the author's experience) very helpful, especially if used in conjunction with any of the above.

### *5 Post-choanal packing*

Sometimes required for severe bleeds. Pass a Foley's catheter down either or both nostrils. Inflate when it reaches the hypopharynx. Then gently withdraw catheters until they wedge in the posterior nares. To maintain traction, the catheters may be tied together or taped to the forehead.

### *6 Correct bleeding diathesis*

Administer platelet transfusion in oncology patients with platelet count $<20\,000/mm^3$ (see Section 9.12). Consider steroids or IVGG for ITP (see Section 9.8.1).

### *7 Blood transfusion*

As necessary.

### *8 Cautery*

Best done by ENT surgeons. Can use chemical cautery (e.g. silver nitrate) or electrocautery.

# 18.4 Ingested foreign body (FB)

Usually coins or buttons.

## CLINICAL FEATURES

If the article is lodged in the oesophagus, gagging, coughing, retching or drooling may be observed. Occasionally, presentation will be that of mediastinitis, i.e. dysphagia, dyspnoea, fever, pain, swelling in neck. Most ingested objects will pass asymptomatically into the stomach and will, after several days, appear in the stool.

## INVESTIGATIONS

X-ray – neck, chest and abdomen. Place of lodgement views are best, i.e. maximum dimension of the oesophagus is in the coronal plane and that of the trachea is in the sagittal plane. Radiolucent FB may require fluoroscopic screening of barium swallow or diagnostic oesophagoscopy.

## MANAGEMENT

### *1 Any object lodged in the oesophagus must be removed endoscopically that day*

### *2 FB in stomach*

Natural passage can be confidently expected (although parents are advised to check all faeces until the object is passed). This applies to coins and buttons as well as to open safety pins, needles and sharp objects.

### *3 Kirby grips ('Bobby pins') – an exception*

They pass easily as far as the duodenojenunal flexure, but in children <7 years of age they are often too long and rigid to proceed further, hence laparotomy is frequently necessary.

**Axiom** If a sharp object remains at the same point for >10–14 days *or if symptoms arise, it should be removed at laparotomy*

## PREVENTION

Coins and buttons are unsuitable play objects for children under 5 years of age – see also 'Button (disc) battery ingestion', Section 5.3.

# 18.5 Foreign bodies in ear and nose

### *1 Ear*

Sedation is often necessary.
Have the following equipment available:

Large speculum.
Suitable light source – preferably head mirror or head lamp.
Fine forceps, small crocodile forceps, skin hook.
Soft suction catheter.

Suction is often useful for smooth round objects. Irrigation is tried if suction fails and if the tympanic membrane is intact. Useful for friable material but not for objects that may swell such as foam.

Seek ENT specialist assistance rather than trying and failing repeatedly.

### *2 Nose*

Presents with irritated blocked nose, or haemopurulent unilateral offensive discharge.
Sedation is usually required.
Use local anaesthetic spray or pack soaked with cocaine and adrenaline.
Auriscope or head mirror with good light source are useful for nasal examination.
Remove as per 'Ear' (above).
Consult ENT specialist if there is difficulty after first attempt.

Chapter 19

# Other problems

## 19.1 Sudden infant death syndrome (SIDS)

Unexpected death in an infant, for which a thorough post-mortem examination fails to find an adequate cause, is called SIDS. It is the most common cause of death in infancy excluding the neonatal period, with an incidence of 2 per 1000 live births and a peak age incidence of 6 weeks to 4 months. Recognized risk factors include people of lower socioeconomic groups, high parity, short birth intervals, low birth weight, prematurity, infants who have had a near miss SIDS, subsequent siblings of SIDS victims, infants of drug-dependent mothers.

### AETIOLOGY

SIDS has been related by numerous theories to environmental temperature, vagal response to fear, cardiac conduction abnormalities, poor central respiratory control or obstructive apnoea, metabolic disorders, surfactant deficiency, and others. All have some basis. None appears as a single obvious cause.

### POST-MORTEM INVESTIGATIONS IN CASUALTY

Often none is carried out. Some tests to consider are:

*1 Examination*
Look for signs of illness and non-accidental injury.

*2 Bacteriology*
CSF (microscopy, protein, sugar, culture), blood culture, suprapubic urine aspirate, throat and nose swab.

*3 Virology*
CSF, faeces (a rectal swab is inadequate) sent directly to the laboratory, nasopharyngeal mucus trap for respiratory viruses, clotted blood for serology.

#### *4 Biochemistry*
Urea and electrolytes. N.B. Blood specimens may be taken by intracardiac puncture.

## MANAGEMENT IN THE ACCIDENT DEPARTMENT

1. Provide a room or privacy for the parents.
2. If only one parent is present and agrees, contact the other parent or relatives. Ensure that a suitable person is looking after the siblings.
3. Take a detailed but sympathetic history from parents. Record this and examination findings in the child's notes.
4. Explain to the parents the nature of cot death and address the fact that they will inevitably feel some culpability for a death which they could not avoid.
5. Explain that the coroner will require a post-mortem examination which will be conducted with dignity, and that a statement to the police will be required.
6. Clothe the infant and make him/her presentable, then encourage the parents to see and hold the baby for as long as they desire.
7. Advice regarding lactation – anything from no treatment, simple analgesia, tight brassieres, thiazide diuretics, bromocryptine if severe.
8. Irrespective of the time of day or night, contact the family GP.
9. In most areas there will be a cot death parent support group. Many of these groups provide a round-the-clock service and should be contacted that day or the following morning.

### People to contact the next day
1. Coroner's office.
2. GP and/or cot death parent support group.

### Follow-up
Either a paediatrician, the family GP or a member of the admitting firm associated with the attempted resuscitation of the child should meet with the parents several weeks after the death, to discuss the autopsy findings, more about SIDS, and most importantly to allay the strong feelings of guilt that prevail in parents of children with SIDS.

### ***Parents having a subsequent baby***

#### *1 Contacts*
It is imperative that there be increased input from health visitor and GP, who should provide counselling and facilitate rapid access to medical advice should it be needed.

#### *2 Home apnoea monitor*
It is unlikely that home monitoring prevents SIDS in subsequent children. It may, however, be a source of considerable reassurance or severe

anxiety to parents. It is a socially highly invasive intervention and given that the benefits are questionable it should not be recommended lightly. If it is offered, it should be provided only after full training has been given in its use, basic stimulation techniques, and mouth-to-mouth and mouth-to-nose resuscitation.

### *3 Health visitor to make extra home visits*

### *4 Direct access*

There should be direct access to GP, paediatrician or health visitor when needed.

### *5 Vaccination of subsequent child*

Unrestricted (Griffin *et al.*, 1988).

## Further reading

Griffin, M. R., Ray, W. A., Livengood, J. R. and Schaffner, W. (1988) Risk of sudden infant death syndrome after immunization with the diphtheria-tetanus-pertussis vaccine. *New Engl. J. Med.*, **319**, 618–623

Hunt, C. E. *et al.* (1987) Sudden infant death syndrome – 1987 perspective. *J. Pediatr.*, **110**, 669–678

Milner, A. D. (1987) Recent theories on the cause of cot death. *Br. Med. J.*, **295**, 1366–1368

Milner, A. D. and Ruggins, N. (1989) Sudden infant death syndrome. *Br. Med. J.*, **298**, 689–690

# 19.2 Child abuse

Injuries or conditions that violate community standards and the law concerning the treatment of children form the basis of child abuse.

Child neglect and emotional deprivation also form part of the syndrome. Sexual abuse is considered separately.

## PRESENTATION

One should have a moderate index of suspicion with all childhood trauma. Suspect child abuse if:

1. Injury is reported some time after the incident.
2. One cannot match the injury with the likely results of the proffered explanation for the injury.

3. The finding of additional injuries while examining the injuries under discussion.
4. Finding signs of physical trauma when child presents for another reason, e.g. a cough.
5. Burns and scalds, occasionally in unusual sites (e.g. genitalia) – these are frequently due to cigarettes.
6. Fabrication of illness in children by the parents, i.e. Munchausen syndrome by proxy (*Arch. Dis. Child.* (1982) **57**, 92–98).
7. Characteristic injury patterns such as digital bruises, cuts on upper lip, rib fractures, spiral fractures, subdural haematomata.

## MANAGEMENT

Admit all suspected cases to hospital.
Scrupulous recording of the parents' (and child's) history and the physical findings. Clinical photographs are very helpful.
Examine the eyes for retinal and subconjunctival haemorrhages which suggest vigorous shaking.
Assess physical, intellectual and emotional well-being of the child and the interaction of the child with the parents and others.
Notify the paediatric registrar and duty social worker.
A 'Place of Safety Order' may be required to empower hospital staff to keep the child in hospital until the nature of the child's domestic environment is clarified.
Skeletal x-ray survey (or bone scan), platelet count, prothrombin time and partial thromboplastin time.

Thereafter the management rests with a multidisciplinary team which may consist of social worker, health visitor, GP, police, nursing staff, paediatrician and occasionally psychologist and psychiatrist.

## PREVENTION

We are better at prediction than prevention, but increased visits by health visitors, lower threshold for hospital admission, early enrolment in play group or nursery and other community maternal supports might be beneficial.

In order to offer such services, one must identify families with recognized risk factors such as:

1. Unwanted pregnancy.
2. Prematurity and prolonged course in neonatal intensive care.
3. Social isolation.
4. Youthful parents.
5. Financial, housing and health difficulties.
6. Physically or intellectually handicapped child.
7. Parents who have been abused as children.
8. Depressed mother.
9. Previous non-accidental injury.

## Further reading

Addy, D. P. (1985) Talking points on child abuse. *Br. Med. J.*, **290**, 259–260
Carty, H. (1988) Brittle or battered? *Arch. Dis. Child.*, **63**, 350–352

See the good series entitled 'ABC of child abuse' commencing in *Br. Med. J.* (1989) **298**, 727, and appearing in alternate issues for the ensuing 4 months.

# 19.3 Childhood sexual abuse (CSA)

This is an emotionally charged area and one that is still poorly understood. It may involve oral, anal and vaginal sexual interference, and child pornography and prostitution. Its sequelae include physical and psychological trauma and sexually transmitted disease. CSA may occur without evidence of anogenital contact and conversely physical abnormalities may have an innocent explanation. Principal indicators of sexual abuse are listed in Table 19.1.

Most cases of CSA involve someone well known to the child and in half of all cases a relative is the perpetrator. The natural father is involved in between 25% and 33% of all cases.

Once there is a suspicion of sexual abuse, further history-taking and examination should be done by someone experienced in the field. Increasingly, women police surgeons are being appointed, but it is important that men remain involved. It is crucial to inform the police surgeon and if possible have her present when examining the child. A medical examination must be sensitively performed by a skilled doctor. Repeated examination should be avoided (therefore clinical photography and facilities for genital swabs should be available at the time of examination, to avoid medical 'assaults' on the child).

## MANAGEMENT OF PROBABLE CHILD SEXUAL ABUSE

### *1 Protect the child*

After disclosure, the child and perhaps other members of the family are at heightened risk from the perpetrator, who may also put additional pressure on the child to ensure her (or his) silence. It is preferable to persuade the abuser (if identified) to leave home or ensure that he stays away from the child; however, if this is not possible or there is doubt about the ongoing safety of the child, protective care of the child in hospital or a foster home may be prudent.

**Table 19.1 Principal indicators of sexual abuse* (From Hobbs, C.J. and Wynne, J.M. (1987) *Arch. Dis. Child.*, 62, 1182–1187, with permission of Dr Hobbs and the publishers)**

*1. Presumptive indicators*
Direct report from the child
Sexually transmitted disease
Pregnancy
Genital or anal trauma

*2. Possible indicators*
Preschool:
- Inappropriate or excessive sexual interest, masturbatory activity
- Genital or anal inflammation, discharge, bleeding or pain (also apparent pain on sitting or walking)

School age:
- Decrease in performance
- Truancy
- Enthusiasm for attendance even when ill
- Conversion hysteria
- Anxiety, depression, obsession
- Change in appetite
- Sleep disturbance

Adolescence:
- Antisocial behaviour
- Truancy, running away
- Depression, poor self-esteem
- Drug abuse
- Self-injury or overdose
- Promiscuity or prostitution
- Anorexia or obesity
- Overt concern about pregnancy
- Adoption of mother role

* This list is not exhaustive, and some seriously abused children will show none of these indicators, effectively concealing the abuse.

### 2 Siblings
They should be seen and examined in every case.

### 3 Work with other agencies
Social workers, child psychologist or psychiatrist, police and paediatrician must work together. Refer all cases to the regional child abuse coordinator or the duty social worker.

### 4 General assessment
Paediatricians should make a general assessment of the health, growth, development and emotional/behavioural aspects of the child.

General examination should include a search for bruises, bites, burns, grip or slap marks and careful documentation of the site including photographs if possible.

### *5 Examination of the anogenital region.*

It is important but not pre-eminent.

**5.1 Anus** May show reddening, 'tyre swelling', bruising, loss of normal fold pattern, single posterior or multiple tears, scars and skin tags, dilated veins. Dilatation of the anus and reflex anal dilatation (RAD) on minimal skin traction to the buttocks are important signs that must not, however, be judged in isolation. RAD has been noted as a finding in children not sexually abused (*Br. Med. J.* (1989) **298**, 802–803).

**5.2 Female genitalia** Labial bruising, tears of the posterior fourchette and hymen, dilatation of the hymen (more than 0.5 cm in prepubertal girls), swelling, scars and distorted shape around hymen.

N.B. Infection should be sought in the oropharynx, vagina and anus.

## FORENSIC SAMPLES

These are relevant in cases of acute sexual assault/rape (within 48–72 h). Explanation to and consent from the child where possible is most important.

Have the police surgeon or a member of the police child abuse team present at the time of collecting the samples.

Collect samples of the child's clothing that have stains that might be semen or blood.

Comb out samples of pubic and head hair.

Cotton wool swabs should be taken of internal vulva and vagina. Swabs moistened with normal saline should be collected from anus and external vulva. Give all samples to the police, who will arrange with the regional forensic science laboratory to test for spermatozoa and acid phosphatase.

### Other samples

Collect a swab in gonoccocal transport medium to be sent to the hospital bacteriology laboratory.

## Further reading

Anon. (1988) Child abuse after Cleveland. *Lancet*, ii, 132–140

DHSS (1988) *Diagnosis of Child Sexual Abuse: Guidance for Doctors*, HMSO, London

Herman Giddens, M. E. and Frothingham, T. E. (1987) Prepubertal female genitalia – examination for evidence of sexual abuse. *Pediatr.*, **80**, 203–208

Hobbs, C. J. and Wynne, J. M. (1987) Management of sexual abuse. *Arch. Dis. Child.*, **62**, 1182–1187

James, D. V. and Collings, S. (1989) False allegations of child abuse. *Lancet*, **i**, 48

## 19.4 Failure to thrive (FTT)

FTT implies a failure to gain weight such that the weight progressively drops off from the expected weight centile. Centiles of length and head circumference are initially well preserved, although in long-standing FTT linear growth will also be affected. Children who are disproportionately short for their weight have short stature (see Chapter 14) which is a separate entity, although there is some overlap with FTT. Some children reportedly will not eat and yet demonstrate normal growth (see Section 12.1).

Normal growth can only occur if each of the following is adequate:

1. Environmental and social situation.
2. Nutrition.
3. Organ and tissue homeostasis.
4. Genetic, chromosomal, constitutional factors.

There may be some overlap between these factors.

Berwick and co-workers (*Arch. Dis. Child.* (1982) **57**, 347–351) found that in approximately one-third of hospital admissions for failure to thrive, no cause was found; in one-third, the cause was inadequate nutrition or environmental/social factors, and in the remainder, an organic cause was found.

### CLINICAL FEATURES

A complete history, observation of the interaction between parents and child, thorough examination and occasionally simple focused laboratory investigations will usually reveal the cause of FTT. Establishing and plotting the pattern of the child's growth from birth is an integral part of the assessment.

#### *1 History*

**1.1 Intake** What foods are consumed; how much is taken; how often; how is it made up; who makes it up; is it well taken; how long does the child take to eat each meal; age at which solids were introduced?

**1.2 Output**
Vomit: frequency, projectile, volume, colour (bile is green not yellow), relationship to meals.
Stools: frequency, colour, watery, mucus, bulky offensive (steatorrhoea).
Urine: frequency, infection.

**1.3 Birth** Weight, gestation, mode of delivery, perinatal complications.

**1.4 Past history** Chronic illness, recurrent chest or urine infections.

**1.5 Family history** Consanguinity, other family members affected.

**1.6 Developmental history** Milestones.

### *2 Examination*

Plot weight, height and head circumference.
Inspect – general impression of nutritional status – ? wasted, thin.
  Sparsity of hair. Interaction of child with parents, peers, staff.
  Abdominal protuberance (coeliac disease).
  Muscle wasting – seen best in gluteals.
  Painful walk – scurvy.
  Bow legs, costochondral 'rosary' – rickets.
  Bruising – neglect, decreased clotting factors.
Feel – muscle bulk, subcutaneous fat deposits.
  Ankle/sacral oedema – hypoproteinaemia.
Hands – clubbing, koilonychia, palmar erythema.
Head and neck – anaemia, icterus, central cyanosis.
  Glossitis, number of teeth (normal = age in months – 6), gingivitis (scurvy), fundi – papilloedema (subdural effusion) fontanelle, spider naevi.
Abdomen – protuberant in coeliac disease.
  Hepatosplenomegaly, masses, ascites.
Anus – excoriated, fissured (Crohn's disease).
  Digital examination (Hirschsprung's typically has an empty rectum).
Test feed – pyloric mass.
Chest – hyperinflation, tachypnoea, Harrison's sulcus.
CVS – heaves, thrills, murmurs.

## INVESTIGATIONS

There are no routine tests. Some of the following may be appropriate. See also Section 12.12. Many of the following tests are described in greater detail in Section 12.9:
Test feed – weight before and after each breast feed for 24 h.
FBC – microcytic or macrocytic anaemia suggests iron or $B_{12}$/folate deficiency. Acanthocytosis in abetalipoproteinaemia.
Urea, creatinine – chronic renal disease.
Bicarbonate – low in metabolic acidosis.
Urine – microscopy and culture;
  metabolic screen;
  SG/osmolarity – diabetes insipidus;
  pH – renal tubular acidosis has high urine pH with metabolic acidosis.

Electrolytes.
Xylose absorption test.
Serum alpha-tocopherol (vitamin E) – fat malabsorption.
$B_{12}$, red cell folate – malabsorption.
Clotting profile – vitamin K deficiency in steatorrhoea.
Alkaline phosphatase – high in rickets.
Liver function tests – including total protein and albumin.
Stools – ova, cysts, parasites;
fatty acids, fat globules;
tryptic activity;
3-day faecal fat collection;
pH – low in CHO malabsorption.
Sweat test – cystic fibrosis.
Small bowel biopsy – villus atrophy in coeliac disease;
*Giardia* (may use the 'String test' instead).

## Comments on causes of FTT

N.B. In one-third of cases no cause is found.

### 1 Inadequate physical and social environment

When history and examination provide no obvious cause for FTT, the child (and mother) is often admitted to hospital where possible organic causes are investigated. While in hospital the infants may feed well and gain weight. The mother may have misjudged the adequacy of her breast milk supply or else made up the feeds incorrectly (see below). Alternatively, there are a number of social difficulties recognized in families which may provide the child with a suboptimal domestic environment in which to grow. These include:

(a) infant born within 18 months of a sibling;
(b) mother is young, single, depressed;
(c) obstetric complications and a premature child which among other things mitigate against satisfactory bonding between mother and child;
(d) families in lower socioeconomic groups.

Poor physical care of the child may be apparent. The physical examination must be rigorous and inquiry must be made into the psychosocial background of the family. The involvement of GP, health visitor, social worker, and psychologist or psychiatrist may be necessary. When a child is failing to thrive because of sheer physical neglect, he may need to be removed from the parents' custody. The chances of rehabilitation of the family in these circumstances are poor.

### 2 Inadequate nutrition, i.e. poor intake or increased losses

#### 2.1 Poor intake

*2.1.1 Maternal causes* One should always suspect underfeeding irrespective of what the mother says about the quantity given. It is difficult for a mother breast feeding a child to know how much milk her child takes.

Leaking of breast milk signifies a draught reflex, not adequacy of milk supply. A contented baby is not necessarily receiving sufficient breast milk. Several test feeds (weigh baby before and after feeding) may occasionally resolve the issue, although the anxiety that this generates may diminish lactation. Therefore, a low test feed is of dubious significance.

Artificially-fed babies may be underfed because of errors in making up the feed, insufficient volumes, defective teat, maternal anxiety, inadequate mothering, parental food fads.

*2.1.2 Infant causes* Some babies are restless, difficult and do not suck steadily. Congenital abnormalities such as cleft palate and Pierre Robin syndrome (small jaw, cleft palate, glossoptysis) cause feeding difficulties. Children with severe CNS defects (cerebral palsy) and floppy infants (e.g. Down's syndrome, chronic spinal muscular atrophy) may feed poorly. Congenital heart disease with heart failure causes dyspnoea which is made worse by feeding.

### 2.2 Excessive nutritional losses

*2.2.1 Vomit* Gastro-oesophageal reflux is the most common cause. Others are pyloric stenosis, Hirschsprung's disease, recurrent volvulus. Renal causes of vomit include UTI, chronic renal failure and renal tubular disorders. Many inborn errors of metabolism can cause FTT with or without vomiting. Foetal alcohol syndrome and lead poisoning can present with FTT.

*2.2.2 Diarrhoea/steatorrhoea* FTT with chronic diarrhoea is likely to be due to malabsorption (see Sections 12.9 and 12.12). The commonest causes are coeliac disease and cystic fibrosis (CF). CF typically causes growth failure soon after birth and the child is often very hungry. Coeliac disease causes growth failure when gluten is introduced into the diet and the child is often irritable, anorectic and has a protuberant abdomen.

Other causes include allergic enteropathy (cows' milk protein or soya milk intolerance) and chronic inflammatory bowel disease. Ulcerative colitis will typically have chronic diarrhoea with stools containing mucus and blood. Crohn's disease has a very variable mode of presentation. Weight loss and anorexia can occur with no bowel symptoms at all.

## 3 Chronic illness

Chronic illness of any body system may result in FTT. The mechanism is often unclear.

**3.1 Infection** Increases metabolic requirements while decreasing input of energy through anorexia or vomiting, e.g. UTI, TB, CF, inflammatory bowel disease, immune deficiency.

**3.2 Organ failure** Chronic failure of kidneys, liver, heart or lungs. Heart failure usually is accompanied by poor feeding, sweating and a large liver. Congenital heart disease with or without heart failure or cyanosis may cause FTT. Cyanosis will be self-evident. Renal tubular acidosis may be asymptomatic apart from FTT.

**3.3 Neurological** Babies with cerebral palsy and other CNS lesions may have trouble feeding, vomit frequently often due to gastro-oesophageal reflux, and possibly have poor tissue utilization of energy. A history of perinatal difficulties and physical signs of micro- or hydrocephalus, hypertonicity and developmental delay are important clues. Lesions such as subdural haematoma or hydrocephalus can be remedied.

**3.4 Constitutional, genetic, chromosomal** Children with intra-uterine growth retardation (IUGR) may have incomplete postnatal catch-up growth and hence remain small. Intra-uterine infection (rubella, CMV, *Toxoplasma*) may alter the potential for growth. Turner's (XO) and Down's syndromes usually cause short stature in addition to poor weight gain.

**3.5 Metabolic disorders** Inborn errors of metabolism – most can be diagnosed by urine chromatography for organic acids and urine high-voltage electrophoresis for amino acids.

**3.6 Endocrinopathy** Salt-losing congenital adrenal hyperplasia or other hypoadrenocorticism. Occasionally, diabetes mellitus or insipidus will present in this way. Hypothyroidism and growth hormone deficiency tend to cause short stature rather than FTT.

## 19.5 Parenteral nutrition for children

There are occasions when a hospital pharmacy or (total) parenteral nutrition (TPN) unit are unable to assist in preparing parenteral nutrition (e.g. weekends, bank holiday, small hospitals). It is relatively easy to prepare a very serviceable solution. Children requiring long-term TPN will need more support than that detailed here.

There are three stages in providing TPN, either as sole diet or as a supplement to enteral nutrition.

1. Identification of cases.
2. Use of appropriate solutions.
3. Monitoring and back-up services.

## PRINCIPAL INDICATIONS

### *1 Pre-/postoperatively*

### *2 GI problems*

(a) Short bowel syndrome.
(b) Inflammatory bowel disease ± fistulae.
(c) Ileus.
(d) Severe vomiting, e.g. with cytotoxic therapy.
(e) Cystic fibrosis.

### *3 Trauma and burns*

### *4 Unconsciousness, with tube feeding contraindicated*

## WHICH TPN SOLUTION ? (See Table 19.2)

**Table 19.2 Parenteral nutrition solution**

| | *Volume* (ml) | *CHO/N/fat* (g) | *Calories* (kcal) |
|---|---|---|---|
| 20% dextrose | 350 | 70 | 280 |
| 50% dextrose | 200 | 100 | 400 |
| Vamin 14 (electrolyte free) | 200 | 2.8 | 70 |
| Pred-el (trace element soln) | 40 | – | – |
| | 790 | | |
| Intralipid 20% | 200 | 40 | 360 |
| Vitlipid/Solivito | 10 | – | – |
| | 210 | | |

Non-protein:protein calorie ratio 15:1 (should be >7:1).
Grams carbohydrate:grams fat 4.25:1 (should be approx. 4:1)

*Notes*

*1. Infusion mix*
Infuse the Vamin/dextrose mixture, with added trace elements, through a separate line from the intralipid solution; if infusing through a single cannula, join the infusions with a 'Y' connector as close as possible to the infusion site. Calcium and heparin in combination rapidly 'crack' intralipid solutions, giving a theoretical risk of fat embolism.

*2. Vitamins*
The addition of vitamins is not important in the short term. Fat-soluble vitamins are provided in Vitlipid. Most other vitamins are found in adequate quantities in Solivito which comes as a powder and should be reconstituted using a 10 ml ampoule of Vitlipid, the whole of this being diluted in the 200 ml of 20% intralipid.

*3. Electrolytes*
Sodium and potassium should be added as indicated by the day's electrolyte values. Typical intakes are 2–3 mmol/kg/day for sodium and 1–2 mmol/kg/day for potassium. Solutions commonly available are:

'Strong NaCl' = 30% = 5 mmol Na/ml.
'Strong KCl' = 15% = 2 mmol K/ml.

## FLUID REQUIREMENTS

Infusion rates which provide adequate fluid volume and calories – see Table 19.3.

Typical fluid requirements are:

1. For children of 1 year old and above:
   (a) for the 1st 10 kg: 100 ml/kg/day;
   (b) for the 2nd 10 kg: 50 ml/kg/day;
   (c) for the 3rd and each subsequent 10 kg: 25 ml/kg/day.

e.g. 16 kg child: 1000 ml + 6 × 50 = 1300 ml/day
= 54 ml/h

**Table 19.3 Guideline infusion rates for TPN**

| *Weight* (kg) | *Vamin dextrose* (ml/h) | *Intralipid* (ml/h) |
|---|---|---|
| 10 | 33 | 9 |
| 12 | 37 | 10 |
| 14 | 40 | 11 |
| 16 | 43 | 11 |
| 18 | 46 | 12 |
| 20 | 49 | 13 |
| 24 | 53 | 14 |
| 28 | 56 | 15 |
| 32 | 59 | 16 |
| 36 | 63 | 17 |
| 40 | 66 | 18 |

TPN, total parenteral nutrition.

**Table 19.4 Monitoring children receiving TPN**

| | *Daily* | *Weekly* | *p.r.n.* |
|---|---|---|---|
| Serum | Na | LFT | Trace elements: Mg, Zn |
| | K | Creatinine | Immunoglobulins |
| | Ca | FBC | Blood culture |
| | Urea | Triglycerides | |
| | Glucose | | |
| Urine | Glucose | Na | |
| | | K | |
| | | Urea | |
| | | ? Creatinine clearance | |

TPN, total parenteral nutrition; LFT, liver function tests; FBC, full blood count.

2. For children of less than 1 year use the following figures:

| | | |
|---|---|---|
| up to 1 mo | 180 ml/kg/day | = 7.5 ml/kg/h |
| 1–2 mo | 150 ml/kg/day | = 6.25 ml/kg/h |
| 2–4 mo | 120 ml/kg/day | = 5 ml/kg/h |
| 4–6 mo | 110 ml/kg/day | = 4.6 ml/kg/h |
| 6–12 mo | 100 ml/kg/day | = 4.2 ml/kg/h |

## NURSING CARE

Routine nursing care of a child on TPN consists of 4-hourly observation of temperature, pulse, respiratory rate and urine output.

## INVESTIGATIONS (see Table 19.4)

## COMPLICATIONS (see Table 19.5)

**Table 19.5 Complications of TPN**

*1. Cannulae and catheters*
Migration
Embolization
Extravasation
Thrombosis

*2. Infection*
Especially with central lines
Avoid by using central line for TPN only, and careful sterile preparation of fluids

*3. Metabolic*
Glucose disturbances
Azotemia
Hyperammonaemia – seems principally related to glycine intake
  Arginine exerts protective effect
Fat overload after prolonged IV intralipid ± fat emboli
  ? Related to lipid cracking by Ca/heparin
Acidosis – effect of high $Cl^-$ content, and ratio of anionic to cationic amino acids

*4. Liver*
Fatty infiltration – essential fatty acid deficiency if intralipid not used
Cholestatic jaundice – multifactorial

*5. Solution incompatibilities*
Heparin and calcium together can 'crack' intralipid, leading to flocculation.
Vitamins A, C and riboflavin best given by mixing Solivito in Vitlipid, and infusing it in with intralipid

*6. Trace elements deficiency*
Adequate amounts of all except chromium and selenium provided by 40 ml/litre of Ped-el

TPN, total parenteral nutrition.

Appendix I

# Abbreviations

The following are the abbreviations used throughout the text, most of which are defined at their first mention therein:

**ACTH** adrenocorticotrophic hormone
**ADH** antidiuretic hormone
**AE** atopic eczema
**ANA+** antinuclear antibodies positive
**ANC** absolute neutrophil count
**AP** anteroposterior
**APSGN** acute post-streptococcal glomerulonephritis
**APTT** activated partial thromboplastin time
**ARF** acute renal failure
**5-ASA** 5-aminosalicylic acid
**ASD** atrial septal defect
**ASOT** antistreptolysin-O titre
**AST** aspartate aminotransferase
**ATN** acute tubular necrosis
**AV** atrioventricular
**AXR** abdominal x-ray

**BCG** bacille Calmette-Guérin (vaccine)
**BM** basement membrane
**BMA** bone marrow aspiration
**BP** blood pressure

**CCF** congestive cardiac failure
**CD** Crohn's disease
**CDH** congenital dislocation of the hips
**CF** cystic fibrosis
**CFU** colony-forming units
**CHO** carbon, hydrogen, oxygen (carbohydrate)
**CIBD** chronic inflammatory bowel disease
**CIE** countercurrent immune electrophoresis
**CM** cows' milk
**CMA** cows' milk allergy
**CMV** cytomegalovirus
**CNS** central nervous system

| | |
|---|---|
| **CP** | cerebral palsy |
| **CPAP** | continuous positive airway pressure |
| **CPR** | cardiopulmonary resuscitation |
| **CRP** | C-reactive protein |
| **CSA** | childhood sexual abuse |
| **CSF** | cerebrospinal fluid |
| **CT** | computed tomography |
| **CVC** | central venous catheter |
| **CVH** | combined ventricular hypertrophy |
| **CVP** | central venous pressure |
| **CVS** | cardiovascular system |
| **CXR** | chest x-ray |
| **DC** | direct current |
| **DDS** | diaminodiphenylsulphone |
| **DIC** | disseminated intravascular coagulation |
| **DMSA** | $^{99m}$Tc dimercaptosuccinic acid |
| **DMSO** | dimethyl sulphoxide |
| **DNA** | deoxyribonucleic acid |
| **DT** | (combined) diphtheria and tetanus (vaccine) |
| **DTP** | diphtheria, tetanus, pertussis (vaccine) |
| **DTPA** | $^{99m}$Tc diethylenetriamine penta-acetic acid |
| **DXRT** | deep x-ray therapy |
| **EAR** | expired air resuscitation |
| **EBV** | Epstein–Barr virus |
| **ECF** | extracellular fluid |
| **ECG** | electrocardiogram |
| **ECM** | external cardiac massage |
| **EEG** | electroencephalogram |
| **ELISA** | enzyme linked immunosorbent assay |
| **EM** | electron microscopy |
| **EMH** | estimated mature height |
| **ENT** | ear, nose and throat |
| **ESR** | erythrocyte sedimentation rate |
| **ETT** | endotracheal tube |
| **F VIII** | factor VIII (coagulation factor) |
| **F IX** | factor IX (coagulation factor) |
| **FB** | foreign body |
| **FBC** | full blood count |
| **FDP** | fibrin degradation products |
| **FEF** | forced expiratory flow |
| **FEV$_1$** | forced expired volume in 1 second |
| **FFA** | free fatty acids |
| **F/H** | family history |
| **FIBA** | factor (VIII) inhibitor bypassing activity |
| **FRC** | functional residual capacity |

**FSH** follicle-stimulating hormone
**FTT** failure to thrive

**GA** general anaesthesia
**GABHS** group A beta haemolytic streptococci
**GCS** Glasgow Coma Scale
**GFR** glomerular filtration rate
**GGT** gamma-glutamyl transferase
**GI** gastrointestinal
**GIT** gastrointestinal tract
**GN** glomerulonephritis
**GOR** gastro-oesophageal reflux
**G-6-PD** glucose-6-phosphate dehydrogenase
**GTT** glucose tolerance test

**Hb** haemoglobin
**HBOT** hyperbaric oxygen therapy
**HCG** human chorionic gonadotrophin
**Hct** haematocrit
**HHV-6** human herpesvirus 6
**HIV** human immunodeficiency virus
**HLA** human leucocyte antigen
**HM** human milk
**HNI** human normal immunoglobulin
**HSP** Henoch–Schönlein purpura
**HT** hypertension
**HUS** haemolytic uraemic syndrome

**IA** intra-arterial
**ICP** intracranial pressure
**ICU** intensive care unit
**IF** intrinsic factor
**IFB** intrabronchial foreign body
**IgE** immunoglobulin E
**IgG** immunoglobulin G
**IgM** immunoglobulin M
**IM** intramuscular(ly)
**IO** intraosseous
**IPPV** intermittent positive pressure ventilation
**ITP** idiopathic thrombocytopenic purpura
**IUGR** intra-uterine growth retardation
**IV** intravenous(ly)
**IVGG** intravenous gamma globulin
**IVH** intraventricular haemorrhage
**IVP** intravenous pyelogram

**JCA** juvenile chronic arthritis

**KPTT** kaolin partial thromboplastin time
**KS** Kawasaki syndrome

**LAD** left axis deviation
**LDH** lactate dehydrogenase
**LFT** liver function tests
**LH** luteinizing hormone
**LHRH** luteinizing hormone releasing hormone
**LMB** Laurence–Moon–Biedl syndrome
**LOC** loss of consciousness
**LP** lumbar puncture
**LV** left ventricle
**LVH** left ventricular hypertrophy

**MCH** mean corpuscular haemoglobin
**MCHC** mean corpuscular haemoglobin concentration
**MCN** minimal change nephritis
**MCT** medium-chain triglycerides
**MCU** micturating cystourethrogram
**MCV** mean corpuscular volume
**$MEF_{50}$** maximum mid-expiratory flow rate
**MMR** measles, mumps, rubella (vaccine)
**MRSA** methicillin-resistant *Staphylococcus aureus*
**MSU** mid-stream urine

**NGT** nasogastric tube

**OFC** occipitofrontal circumference
**OM** osteomyelitis

**PAS** para-aminosalicylic acid
**PCV** packed cell volume
**PD** peritoneal dialysis
**PDA** patent ductus arteriosis
**PEEP** positive end expiratory pressure
**PEFR** peak expiratory flow rate
**$PGI_2$** prostacyclin
**PKU** phenylketonuria
**PPD** purified protein derivative
**PR** (a) per rectum; (b) pulse rate
**PS** pulmonary stenosis
**PT** prothrombin time
**PTT** partial thromboplastin time
**PUO** pyrexia of unknown origin
**PW** Prader–Willi syndrome

**RAD** (a) reflux anal dilatation; (b) right axis deviation
**RAST** radioallergosorbent test(s)
**RBC** red blood cell (count)
**RDW** red (blood cell volume) distribution width
**RF+** rheumatoid factor positive
**RhF** rheumatoid fever

**RNA** ribonucleic acid
**RSL** renal solute load
**RSV** respiratory syncytial virus
**RV** residual volume
**RVH** right ventricular hypertrophy

**SA** (a) septic arthritis; (b) surface area
**SC** subcutaneous(ly)
**SD** standard deviation
**S/E** side effects
**SEM** standard error of the mean
**SFC** simple febrile convulsions
**SG** specific gravity
**SGOT** serum glutamic oxaloacetic transaminase
**SIADH** syndrome of inappropriate antidiuretic hormone
**SIDS** sudden infant death syndrome
**SLE** systemic lupus erythematosus
**SPA** suprapubic aspiration
**SR** slow release
**SRT** slow-release theophylline
**SSPE** subacute sclerosing panencephalitis
**SUFE** slipped upper femoral epiphysis
**SVC** superior vena cava
**SVT** supraventricular tachycardia
**SXR** skull x-ray

**$T_3$** triiodothyronine
**TAG** triacyl glycerides
**TAPVD** total anomalous pulmonary venous drainage
**TAR** thrombocytopenia absent radii
**TB** tuberculosis
**TBG** thyroxine-binding globulin
**TCA** tricyclic antidepressants
**TGV** transposition of the great vessels (arteries)
**TIBC** total iron binding capacity
**TLC** total lung capacity
**TMP** trimethoprim
**TOF** tracheo-oesophageal fistula
**TORCH** toxoplasmosis, other, rubella virus, cytomegalovirus and herpes simplex viruses
**TPA** tissue plasminogen activator
**TPN** total parenteral nutrition
**$T_3$RU** triiodothyronine resin uptake
**TSH** thyroid-stimulating hormone

**UC** ulcerative colitis
**UDT** undescended testes
**U + E** urea + electrolytes

**URTI** upper respiratory tract infection
**US** ultrasound
**UTI** urinary tract infection

**VA** ventriculo-atrial
**VF** ventricular fibrillation
**VMA** vanillylmandelic acid
**VP** ventriculoperitoneal
**VSD** ventricular septal defect
**VT** ventricular tachycardia
**VTEC** verocytotoxin-producing *E. coli*
**VU** vesico-ureteric

**WCC** white cell count

**ZIG** zoster immune globulin

# Index